Comprehensive Manual of

Taping, Wrapping, & Protective Devices

5th Edition

Melvin Lewis, PhD, AT-Ret
Ken Wright, DA, AT-Ret
Scott Barker, MS, ATC
Randy Deere, DA, AT-Ret

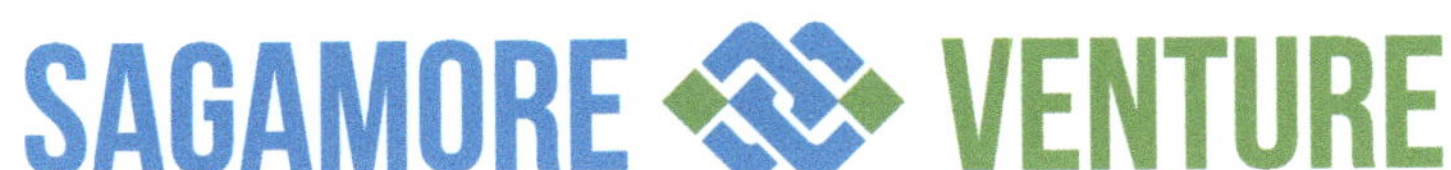

Publishers: Joseph J. Bannon/Peter Bannon
Sales and Marketing Manager: Misti Gilles
Marketing Assistant: Kimberly Vecchio
Director of Development and Production: Susan M. Davis
Graphic Designer: Marissa Willison
Technology Manager: Mark Atkinson

Library of Congress Control Number: 2017941956
ISBN print edition: 978-1-57167-851-5
ISBN ebook: 978-1-57167-852-2
Printed in the United States.

SAGAMORE VENTURE
1807 N. Federal Dr.
Urbana, IL 61801
www.sagamorepublishing.com

The authors, along with all contributors to this text, would like to dedicate this text to all athletic trainers, physical therapists, physiotherapists, prospective allied health students, related health care professionals, athletic coaches, and sports consumers.

DISCLAIMER

The procedures in this text are based on current research and recommendations from professionals in sports medicine and related health care professions. The information is intended to supplement, not substitute, recommendations from a qualified physician, qualified health care professional, or medical equipment specialist. Sagamore-Venture, LLC and the authors disclaim responsibility for any adverse effects or consequences resulting from the misapplication or injudicious use of the material contained in the text. It is also accepted as judicious that the health care professionals, sport industry professionals, and students must work under the guidance of a licensed physician, qualified health care provider, and medical equipment specialist.

Contents

Sponsors

Medco Sports Medicine, 25 Northpointe Parkway, Suite 25, Amherst, NY 14228

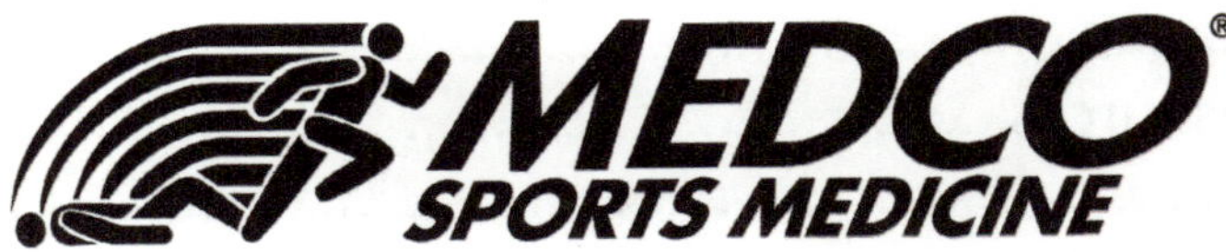

Cramer Products, 153 W Warren Street, Gardner, KS 66030

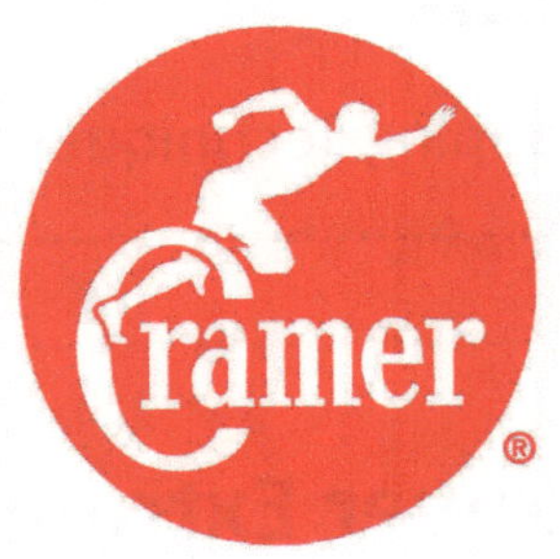

PRO Orthopedic Devices, Inc., 2884 East Ganley Road, Tucson, AZ 85706

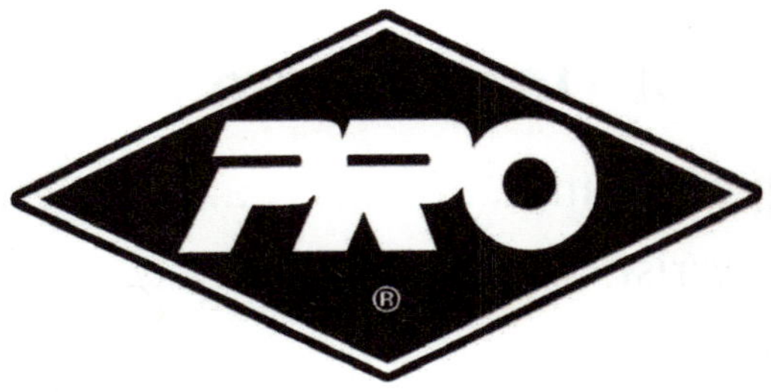

BSN Medical, Inc., 5825 Carnegie Boulevard, Charlotte, NC 28209

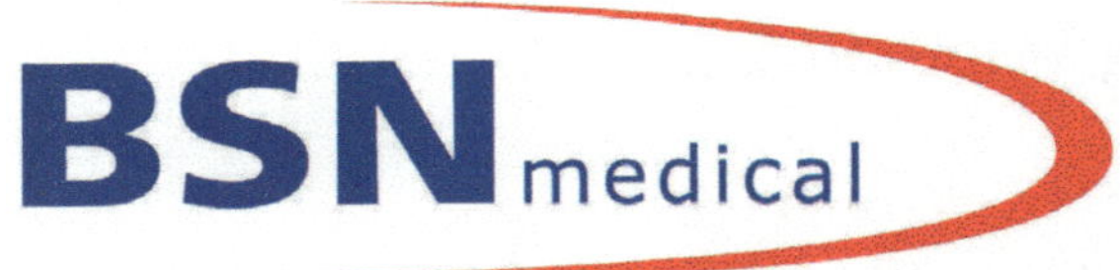

an SCA company

Johnson & Johnson Products, 75 Nassau Terminal Road, New Hyde Park, NY 11040

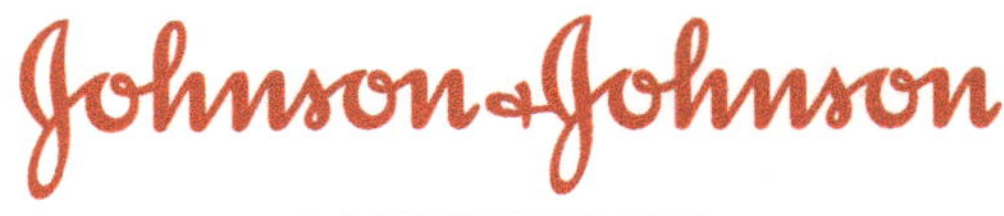

CONSUMER INC.

Preface

Recognized as the most comprehensive text in taping, wrapping, and protective devices for health care professionals, the fifth edition (2017) has been enhanced by the addition of selected audio and video segments, kinesiology taping techniques, and an in-depth visual display of protective devices. Obtaining knowledge from renowned experts in sports medicine health care, this text displays and describes a step-by-step process in the application of taping and wrapping products along with a listing of protective devices that could be utilized in preventing the severity of injuries. The *Comprehensive Manual of Taping, Wrapping & Protective Devices* features online supplements along with instructional resources.

Online Companion Resources

Online companion resources include video, images, and other resources the authors have provided as supplemental information for the text. A list of videos available include the following:

- Knee Compression - Elastic Wrap
- Elbow Compression - Elastic Wrap
- Wrist/Hand Compression - Elastic Wrap
- Great Toe Taping
- Toe Splint Taping
- Plantar Fasciitis Taping
- Ankle - Closed Basket Weave Taping
- Ankle - Open Basket Weave Taping
- Shin Splint Taping
- Achilles Tendon Taping
- Knee Joint Wrap
- Hamstring Wrap
- Quadriceps Wrap
- Hip Flexor Wrap
- Hip Adductor Wrap
- Acromioclavicular (AC) Joint Taping
- Glenohumeral Joint Taping
- Glenohumeral Joint Wrap
- Elbow Hyperextension Taping
- Elbow Epicondylitis Wrap
- Forearm Splint Taping
- Wrist Taping
- Thumb Spica Taping
- Finger Splint Taping
- Hyperextension of Phalanges Taping
- Contusion to Hand Taping

These resources are found online and accessible only by creating an account using the one-time passcode provided in the back of the text (pg 232). For more information about the use of or policies regarding the code for online companion resources, please visit www.sagamorepub.com

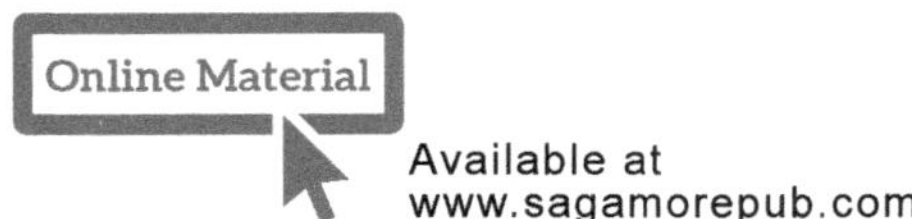

The icon indicates that an instructional video is available for the technique using the Online Companion Resources.

Special Thanks

The authors would like to thank Sagamore-Venture Publishing, LLC, Medco Sports Medicine, Cramer Products, PRO Orthopedic Devices, BSN Medical, and Johnson & Johnson Products for providing the financial support for this educational project. Without their support, we would not have been able to complete the 5th edition of *Comprehensive Manual of Taping, Wrapping, & Protective Devices*. The authors would also like to thank the following individuals for their assistance in the development of this manual: Ms. Reata Strickland as cover designer of text, Mr. Kyle Fondren as graphic designer and photographer, Mr. Keith Davis as photographer, and Ms. Kendra Wright for serving as guest reviewer, and past editors/ reviewer (Mr. William Whitehill, Mr. Bud Carperter, Mrs. Katy Curren Casey, Mr. James Dodson, Dr. A. Louise Fincher, Mr. Tim Garl, Ms. Ginger Gilmore, Dr. Ronnie Harper, Ms. Sherry Kimbro, Mr. Donald Lowe, Mr. Henry Lyda, Mr. William McDonald, Dr. Alice McLaine, Mr. Lindsy McLean, Ms. Lorraine Michel, Mr. Russell Miller, Mr. Ken Murray, Mr. Chris Patrick, Mr. Ralph Reiff, Mr. Ed Ryan, Dr. Patrick Sexton, Dr. Vincent Stilger, Mr. Hunter Smith, Mr. Buddy Taylor, and Mr. Charles Vosler) of the *Comprehensive Manual of Taping and Wrapping Techniques* and *Preventive Techniques: Taping/ Wrapping Techniques and Protective Devices* for their input and expertise.

Acknowledgments

Jeff Allen, MEd, LAT, ATC, The University of Alabama, Tuscaloosa, AL

George Borden, MSc, AT-Ret, The Society of Sports Therapists, Glasgow, Scotland (United Kingdom)

Rodney Brown, MA, LAT, ATC, The University of Alabama, Tuscaloosa, AL

Samuel Brown, MS, OTC, Medical Affairs Manager, BSN Medical, Asia Pacific Region, Tokyo, Japan

E. Lyle Cain, MD, Andrews Sports Medicine & Orthopaedic Center, Birmingham, AL

R. T. Floyd, EdD, ATC, The University of West Alabama, Livingston, AL

Fred Hina, MA, ATC, University of Louisville, Louisville, KY

Ron Medlin, MS, ATC, Baltimore Ravens, Owings Mills, MD

Tim Neal, MS, ATC, Concordia University, Ann Arbor, MI

Dexter Nelson, MSc. CAT(C) Emeritus, Mount Royal University, Calgary, Alberta

Álvaro García-Romero, MSc, PT, Camilo José Cela University, Madrid, Spain

Keith Waldon, Member of the Society of Sports Therapists (MSST) & Chartered & State Registered Physiotherapist (MCSP)(HCPC)

Ron Walker, EdD, ATC, CSCS, University of Tulsa, Tulsa, OK

Katherine Reinecke, PT, DPT, M.S., Memorial Hermann Sports Medicine & Rehabilitation, Houston, TX

Norman Waldrop, MD, Andrews Sports Medicine & Orthopaedic Center, Birmingham, AL

About the Authors

Melvin Lewis, PhD, AT-Ret

Dr. Melvin Lewis is an assistant professor in the Sports Business Management Graduate Program and fellow of the Alabama Program in Sports Communication at The University of Alabama. He is a member of the North American Society for Sport Management. Dr. Lewis earned all three of his higher education degrees from The University of Alabama. He received a doctor of philosophy degree in 2003, master of arts degree in 1996, and a bachelor of science degree in 1994. Additionally, Dr. Lewis was presented the "Penny Allen" service award for faculty in 2016 at The University of Alabama. He has more than 15 years of experience delivering industry essential sports medicine supplies and capital equipment to the sport industry. Dr. Lewis was the National Sales Director for Medco Sports Medicine before departing to academia. Dr. Lewis received certificates of training for Carew International Essentials of Branch Management Leadership in 2011, Carew International Dimensions of Professional Selling Facilitator Training in 2010, and The Counselor Salesperson in 2005. He was an assistant athletic trainer for the Buffalo Bills Professional Football Organization for four years. Prior to joining the Buffalo Bills full time in 1996, Dr. Lewis was an intern for the Buffalo Bills in 1995 and the Los Angeles Raiders Professional Football Organization in 1994. Dr. Lewis earned the Southern Region Fellowship for Doctoral Scholars in 2000 and the Professional Football Athletic Trainer's Ethnic Minority Scholarship in 1994. Dr. Lewis has published several scholarly articles, book chapters, and presentations. His current research focuses on sport-consumer behavior and technology in sports.

Ken Wright, DA, AT-Ret

Dr. Ken Wright is a Professor of Sports Business Management Program at The University of Alabama. Dr. Wright received his doctor of arts from Middle Tennessee State University (1984), master of science from Syracuse University (1976), and a bachelor of science degree from Eastern Kentucky University (1974). He has served as head athletic trainer at the University of North Carolina at Charlotte and Morehead State University and as assistant athletic trainer at Ohio University. Inducted into the National Athletic Trainers Association Hall of Fame (NATA) in 2014, Dr. Wright has also received the Sayers "Bud" Miller Distinguished Educator of the Year Award (2000), Most Distinguished Athletic Trainer Award (2006), and Athletic Trainer Service Award (1996) from the NATA. Dr. Wright has numerous publications to his credit, including a series of 13 videos (*Sports Medicine Evaluation and Sports Medicine Taping*), a computer-assisted instructional program (*Sports Injuries*) and textbooks (*Basic Athletic Training, 6th edition*, 2013, *The Comprehensive Manual of Taping & Wrapping Techniques, 5th edition*, 2017), and *Orthopaedic Immobilization Techniques, 1st edition* (2014). Ken has been involved with the United States Olympic Committee as an athletic trainer, educator and invited presenter at national and international sports medicine and sport management conferences. Additionally, he has served on the editorial board of the *Journal of Athletic Training, Physical Therapy in Sport, and Sports Medicine Update*, and as chair and/or member on various NATA, USOC, and USADA committees. In 2012, Dr. Wright was appointed as a member of the board of directors of the United States Anti-Doping Agency.

Scott Barker, MS, ATC

Scott Barker is the head athletic trainer and adjunct faculty for the graduate athletic training education program at California State University, Chico. He received his master of science degree in exercise and sport sciences with a specialization in athletic training from the University of Arizona (1985) and his bachelor of science degree in physical education from the University of Arizona (1984). Barker served for eight years on the National Athletic Trainers Association Education Council Continuing Education Committee and for nine years on the National Athletic Trainers Association Education Multimedia Committee. During this time, Mr. Barker helped with the inception and development of the National Athletic Trainers' Association Virtual Library (online continuing education courses). Barker has received numerous awards in the area of educational multimedia in athletic training including the 2000, 2001, 2002, 2004, 2005, and 2008 National Athletic Trainers' Association, Educational Multimedia Committee, Educational Software Production Contest ATC Commercial Winner; the 2006 National Athletic Trainers' Association, Educational Multimedia Committee, Educational DVD/Video Production Contest ATC Commercial Winner; the 2006 National Athletic Trainers' Association Continuing Education Excellence Award; and the 2007 MERLOT Classic Award for Exemplary Online Learning Resource. Barker has been an invited presenter at 15 National Athletic Trainers' Association Annual Meeting and Clinical Symposium conferences.

Randy Deere, DA, AT-Ret

Dr. Randy Deere is a retired professor and program coordinator for the Graduate Sport Administration Program Athletic Administration Concentration at Western Kentucky University. Dr. Deere received his doctor of arts degree from Middle Tennessee State University in 1992, master of arts degree from Austin Peay State University in 1979, and a bachelor of science degree from Middle Tennessee State University in 1978. Dr. Deere spent 14 years as a collegiate athletic trainer before moving into university teaching. Dr. Deere's research interest focuses on online instructional pedagogy. Dr. Deere received the W. H. Mustaine Distinguished Service Award from the Kentucky Association of Health Physical Education Recreation and Dance (KAHPERD) in 2007, the University PE Teacher of the year award from KAHERD in 1998, and the WKU Faculty Service Award for the College of Health and Human Service in 2004. Dr. Deere has numerous national publications and presentations and served as *KAHPERD Journal* editor from 1993 until 2008. Additionally, Deere has served as a reviewer for Wolters Kluwer/Lippincott Williams and Wilkins and created the PowerPoint supplements for *Applied Sports Medicine for Coaches* in 2009. He served as a Doping Control Officer for the United States Anti-Doping Agency from 2002 until 2008.

PART I
Basic Fundamentals

Chapter 1
Taping Techniques, Wrapping Techniques for Support, and Protective Devices

EDUCATIONAL OBJECTIVES

Upon completing this chapter, the reader will be able to do the following:

- Identify anatomical structures and landmarks critical for correct taping procedures
- Explain philosophies and principles surrounding the proper use of adhesive and elastic tape and elastic wrap applications
- Select the proper supplies and specialty items used for taping, wrapping, or protective devices
- Describe the body preparation issues (for taping and wrapping) as they relate to hair removal, skin preparation, spray adherent, skin lubricants, and underwrap or cohesive tape
- Demonstrate correct application of taping wrapping and protective devices
- Explain the purposes for supportive wrapping techniques for anatomical joints and related structures

Introduction

The fundamentals of taping techniques, wrapping techniques for support, and protective devices are important to understand due to the increased population of active individuals. Scholars, health care professionals, and medical equipment specialists collaborated on this chapter to highlight the philosophies, identifications, applications, and other key components that revolve around taping techniques, wrapping techniques for support, and protective devices.

Proper Assessment of Injury

Before applying a preventive technique (tape, wrap, and/or device), a qualified physician or qualified health care professional should complete a proper injury evaluation. Following the injury evaluation, a qualified health care professional can then recommend proper taping techniques. This ensures that proper taping and wrapping techniques and protective devices are applied for support and stabilization. Also, developing a thorough knowledge of taping application fundamentals is imperative for the qualified health care professional.

Principles of Physical Rehabilitation

Supportive techniques, in conjunction with a rehabilitation program, enhance an individual's return to activity. Please note that taping and wrapping procedures are NOT a substitute for proper injury rehabilitation. You should follow specific instructions regarding injury rehabilitation and supportive taping and wrapping techniques and protective devices, as outlined by a qualified physician or qualified health care professional. You, as the qualified health care professional, need to develop a thorough knowledge of taping application fundamentals.

Fundamentals of Taping Procedures

Philosophies of Adhesive and Elastic Tape Application

With tape application, you must consider proper angle, direction, and tension. Adhesive tape is traditionally marketed as nonelastic, white tape. Currently, adhesive tape comes in multiple colors. Elastic tape has the ability to contract and expand and is commonly used in areas that require greater freedom of movement. Elastic tape also has the characteristics of conformability and strength. Additionally, it can be placed on the body part with fewer wrinkles and at unique angles. When you apply elastic tape, you must apply proper tension. The choice of adhesive or elastic tape in the application of a preventive technique is at your discretion.

Purpose of Taping

The primary purpose for tape application is to provide additional support, stability, and compression for the affected body part. Through proper application, taping techniques can be applied to shorten the muscle's angle of pull; to decrease joint range of motion; to secure pads, bandages, and protective devices; and to ap-

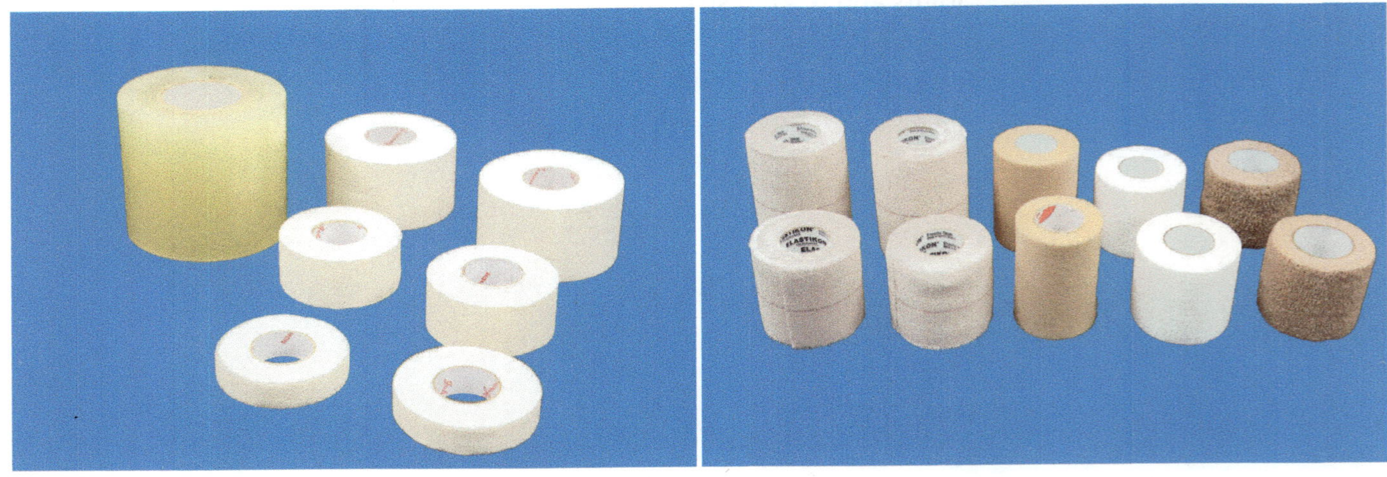

ply compression to control swelling. With the availability of commercial durable medical goods (braces and sleeves), you must have a comprehensive understanding of anatomy, physiology, and biomechanics, along with indications and contraindications of taping/wrapping versus bracing.

Medical Supplies: Adhesive, Elastic, and Cohesive Tape

The terms of choice for this text will be *adhesive tape*, *elastic tape*, and *cohesive tape*. Adhesive tape is traditionally marketed as nonelastic white tape. Elastic tape provides greater freedom of mobility to the affected body part and is marketed as elastic tape. Both adhesive and elastic tapes are produced in a variety of widths. Cohesive (self-adherent) tape is a dressing material that will adhere to itself but not to other surfaces. This product comes in a variety of widths, lengths, and colors. Additionally, adhesive and elastic tapes are used to secure a wrap. In the preparation of some body parts, skin protection must be considered, such as a Band-Aid with a lubricant. The metric table is displayed for international conversion use.

Selection of Proper Supplies and Specialty Items

One of the most critical aspects of taping techniques is the selection of proper supplies. Your selection depends on the number and types of sports or physical activities your organization offers and the frequency of injury in those activities. Purchasing supplies depends on budget, philosophy of medical staff regarding taping techniques, and occurrence of injury. Give special consideration to these additional supplies: benzoin (spray adherent), adhesive versus elastic tape, width of adhesive and elastic tape, cohesive tape, and length and width of elastic wraps.

METRIC TABLE

The metric table is displayed for international conversion use.

Inches	Centimeters
1	2.5
1.5	3.8
2	5.1
3	7.6
4	10.2
6	15.2
8	20.3
12	30.5

Inches	Centimeters
24	61
36	91.4
48	121.9
60	152.4
72	182.9
96	243.8
120	304.8

inch x 2.54 = centimeter
centimeter x .39 = inch

Preparation of Body Part to Be Taped

In preparing the body for taping application, consider these items:

- **Removal of Hair (optional):** The individual should shave the affected body part. This will ensure a solid foundation for the tape, will allow for easy tape removal, and will reduce skin irritation.
- **Clean the Area:** After hair removal, make sure the skin is clean and moisture free.
- **Special Considerations:** Skin protection is important. Provide special care if the skin has allergies, tape or tape adherent, infections, or open and closed wounds.

- **Spray Adherent (optional):** Spray the affected area with an adherent to aid in the adhesive quality.
- **Skin Lubricants:** In areas of high friction or sensitivity, a skin lubricant such as a heel and lace pad will reduce the possibility of irritation.
- **Underwrap or Cohesive Tape:** *Underwrap* is a foam wrap that is used when the individual is allergic to tape, whereas *cohesive tape* is a self-adherent tape that sticks to itself. Both of these products are used to hold heel and lace pads in place at high friction areas. The use of either underwrap or elastic tape over the entire taping area can compromise the stability of the taping technique. When applying an elastic wrap, do not use underwrap material.
- **Proper Body Position:** Ask the individual to assume an anatomically correct and comfortable body position

Application and Removal of Taping Procedures

To tear tape, hold the adhesive or elastic tape firmly on each side of the proposed tear line. With proper tension applied on the tape, pull away the free end at an angle so that the force crosses the lines of the fabric and backcloth at a sharp angle. The tear then occurs sequentially through the backcloth. The more quickly you perform this maneuver, the more evenly tape edges will be torn. Some brands of elastic tape are extremely hard to tear by hand. Cut these elastic tape brands with scissors to ensure proper tape application and neatness.

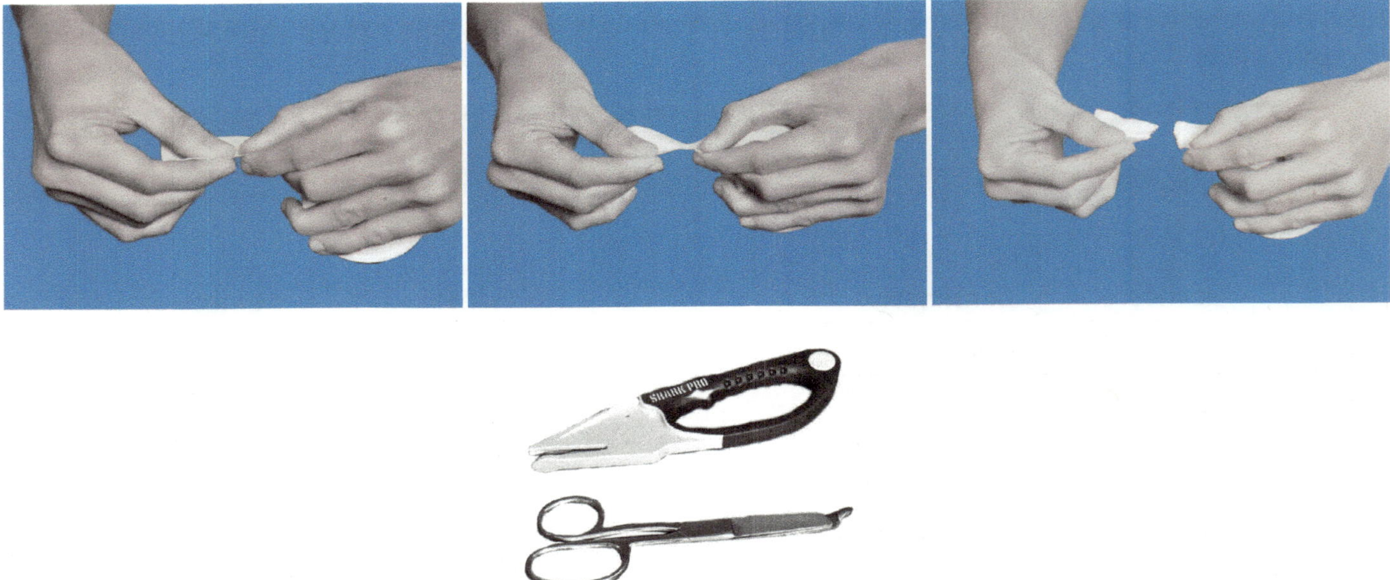

Remove adhesive and elastic tape easily by using bandage scissors or a specially constructed tape cutter. Apply a small amount of lubricant on the tip of the cutting device to allow the instrument to slip under the tape more readily, thus allowing you to remove the tape with ease. Avoid bony prominences by moving the scissor/cutter along the natural channels or in areas of greatest soft tissue cushion. Once you complete this, remove the tape from the skin in a constant and gradual manner. It is preferred that the tape be removed in the opposite direction from which it was applied. When pulling the tape from the skin at an angle of 180 degrees, exercise care to minimize removal of skin tissue and skin irritation. It is recommended that you apply pressure to the skin (pull the skin away from the tape), which will reduce the possibility of skin irritation. The daily use of a tape remover is recommended to help keep the skin clean and to prevent skin irritations and/or infections. Tape remover and/or alcohol will aid in the removal of tape mass and adherent from the skin.

TIPS FROM THE FIELD

Taping Procedures

- Know what body part and injury to which you are providing support and/or compression.
- Cover sensitive body parts (nail/nipple) and wounds with a protective covering.
- When applying a technique, learn to stand at a comfortable and stationary position and place the body part to be taped at your elbow height.
- When practicing, start with small length and width elastic wraps so you can learn common techniques such as figure of eight and joint spica. Once you have become proficient with wraps, then use adhesive and elastic tape.
- Apply proper tension to the tape so that circulation and neurological function will not be compromised.
- When applying a taping technique, follow the tape with your hand to smooth out all wrinkles.
- Overlap tape one half of its width to avoid spaces that could cause cuts and friction burns.
- Always angle the tape in order for the tape ends to meet at the anchor strips. If you do not succeed, retry the angle at a sharper degree.
- When applying closure strips, always apply proximal to distal.
- Upon completing the taping procedure, make sure you check for neatness and gaps, adequate support, and proper function of the affected area. In certain situations, the individual might be asked to perform function tests to establish appropriate technique application.
- Anchor the wrap with tape, but do not put on too tightly as it may cut off circulation.
- **PRACTICE!**

Sport-Specific Rules on Taping

If you apply supportive techniques to an individual, you should be aware of specific rules governing tape application in that particular sport. Your application must fall within the guidelines established for each sport by appropriate governing bodies.

Precautions

Before you apply any techniques, the individual's skin temperature should be normal. To reduce the chance of skin irritation, after any therapeutic treatment, allow adequate time for the skin to return to its normal temperature. When applying support techniques, consider the safety of the individual your priority. Improper tape application can cause further injury. With all injured individuals, consult with a qualified physician. Do not use tape application with any disabling conditions.

Fundamental Procedures of Wrapping Techniques for Support

Philosophies of Elastic Wrap Application

Elastic wraps are primarily used to apply either compression or support to injured anatomical structures. Elastic wrap has the ability to contract and expand and is commonly used in areas that need greater freedom of movement. Elastic tape also has the characteristic of conformability and strength. As stated above, the selection of elastic wraps in the application of any preventive technique is at your discretion. You must develop a thorough knowledge regarding the fundamentals of the application of taping and wrapping procedures. During physical activity, supportive wraps are used to aid in muscle function and support and to reduce excessive range of motion. These applications are typically used in competition or practice. Spica wraps are traditionally employed at the hip and shoulder joints. Figure of eight wraps are placed over ankle, knee, elbow, and wrist and hand joints.

Purpose and Application of Elastic Wraps for Support

The primary purpose for the application of an elastic wrap is to provide support and/or compression for the affected body part. Through the proper application, wrapping techniques can be applied to shorten the muscle's angle of pull; to decrease joint range of motion; to secure pads, bandages, and protective devices; and to apply compression to reduce swelling. During physical activity, supportive wraps are used to aid in muscle function and support, reduce excessive range of motion, and aid in securing pads after the proper placement of felt, foam rubber, and protective devices. These applications are usually used for short periods, typically for competition or practice. Common terms for these wraps are *spica*, *figure of eight*, and *pad support*. Spica wraps are traditionally employed at the hip and shoulder joints. Figure of eight wraps are placed over ankle, knee, elbow, and wrist and hand joints.

Medical Supplies—Elastic Wrap

Elastic wrap is defined as a woven fabric that also allows for expansion and contraction and is used for compression or supportive techniques. This product is typically produced in 2-in., 3-in., 4-in., and 6-in. widths.

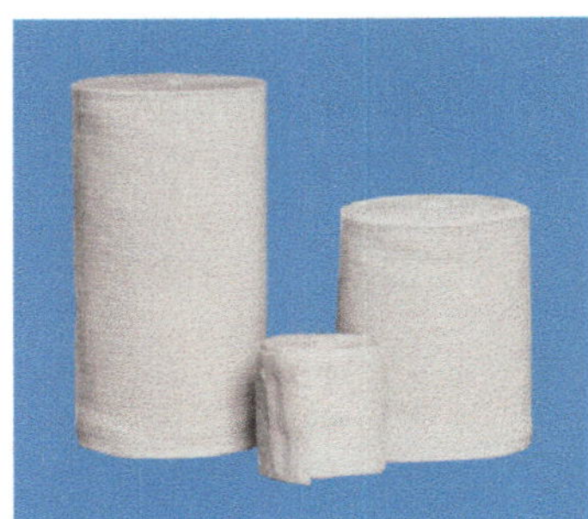

In certain situations, an extra-long length is more desirable. The ankle cloth wrap is a nonelastic cloth that is 2 in. wide and between 72 in. and 96 in. in length. Additionally, adhesive and elastic tape is used to stabilize the wrap. In the preparation of some body parts, consider skin protection, such as a Band-Aid with a lubricant. Depending on the number and types of sports or physical activities an organization offers and frequency of injury in those activities, a variety of supplies should be available. Purchasing supplies depends on budget, philosophy of medical staff regarding taping techniques, and occurrence of injury. Also, give special consideration to benzoin (spray adherent) and the length and width of elastic wraps.

TIPS FROM THE FIELD

Wrapping Procedures

- Know what body part and injury to which you are providing support and/or compression.
- When applying a technique, learn to tape from a comfortable and stationary position and place the body part to be wrapped at your elbow height.
- When practicing, start with small length and width elastic wraps so you can learn common techniques such as figure of eight and joint spica.
- Apply proper tension to the wrap so that circulation and neurological function will not be compromised.
- When applying a wrapping technique, follow the wrap with your hand to smooth out all wrinkles.
- Overlap wrap one half of its width to avoid spaces that could cause cuts and friction burns.
- Upon completing the wrapping procedure, make sure you check for neatness and gaps, adequate support, and proper function of the affected area. In certain situations, the individual might be asked to perform function tests to establish appropriate technique application.
- When applying a compression wrap, always start distally and wrap proximally (toward the heart).
- **PRACTICE!**

Sport-Specific Rules on Wrapping

If you apply supportive techniques to an individual, you should be aware of specific rules governing supportive wrap application in that particular sport or physical activity. Your application must fall within the guidelines established for each sport by appropriate governing bodies.

Preparation of Body Part to Be Wrapped

In preparing the body for taping application, consider these three items:

1. **Clean the Area:** Make sure the skin is clean and moisture free.
2. **Special Considerations:** Skin protection is important. Provide special care if the skin has allergies, tape or tape adherent, infections, or open and closed wounds.
3. **Spray Adherent:** If needed, spray the affected area with an adherent to aid in the adhesive quality.

Proper Body Positioning

Before beginning a wrapping procedure, ask the individual to assume an anatomically correct and comfortable position. When applying a technique, stand at a comfortable and stationary position and place the body part to be taped and/or wrapped at your elbow height. The wrapping techniques presented in this text are the fundamental procedures. Variations can be achieved by adapting these techniques to a particular injury situation. Always give special consideration to the following:

- purpose of the wrapping procedure
- clinical application
- correct anatomical position
- appropriate supply selection

Note: A strong knowledge of anatomy, physiology, and biomechanics is essential.

NOTES:

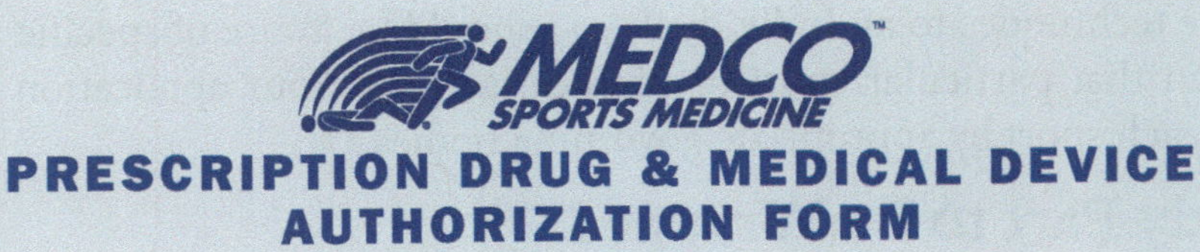

PRESCRIPTION DRUG & MEDICAL DEVICE AUTHORIZATION FORM

If purchasing prescription pharmaceuticals, please complete sections A & B
If purchasing an Automated External Defibrillator (AED) unit or other medical device, please complete sections A & C

Dear Valued Customer,

In order to ship you prescription pharmaceuticals and/or medical devices, we must have authorization from a licensed physician or other authorized prescriber. This individual needs to fill out the form below and fax a copy of this page and a photocopy of their license to 800-222-1934.

If your School/Facility does not have a licensed physician or other authorized prescriber, but is licensed to purchase prescription pharmaceuticals and/or medical devices, please fax a copy of the license and this form for identification to 800-222-1934.

A) Name of School/Facility: ______________________________

Attention: ______________________ Customer #: ______________________

Address: ______________________________

City & State: ______________________ Zip: ______________________

Phone: ______________________ Fax: ______________________

E-Mail: ______________________

B) I hereby authorize the internally designated representatives named below to order prescription products for this School/Facility. (please print)

1. ______________________ 2. ______________________

Type of authorization: ❑ Unlimited ❑ Limited (please attach list of products)

Physician/Authorized Prescriber Signature: ______________________

Physician/Authorized Prescriber Name (please print): ______________________

State License Number: ______________________
(please include photocopy of license)

C) I hereby acknowledge that I am aware that medical devices are intended for use by a physician or a person certified or trained to use such device.

Name (please print): ______________________

Title: ______________________

State License/Certification Number: ______________________

Signature: ______________________ Date: ______________________

Call 1-800-55MEDCO www.medco-athletics.com Fax 1-800-222-1934 MEDCO SPORTS MEDICINE 137

Rx Pharmaceuticals

Figure 1.1 Prescription Medical Device Form Sample

Fundamentals of Protective Devices: Off-the-Shelf and Custom Braces

Philosophies of Protective Device

The use of a protective device can be highly beneficial to the particular body part if properly selected, applied, and worn. To avoid violating the manufacturer's specifications, follow the suggested guidelines for proper selection, application, and maintenance.

Definition of Protective Device

A protective device is a commercial product that is well designed and provides manufacturing liability and proper application instructions. The protective device is worn for protection, support, stability, or compression of an anatomical body part. Off-the-shelf braces are made in standard sizes and are available from merchandise in stock. In certain situations, these braces are called prefabricated braces. Custom braces are made to individual specification and fitted by qualified health care professionals and medical equipment specialists. Because these braces come in contact with the skin, it is highly recommended that daily maintenance should occur. As recommended by the manufacturer and Centers for Disease Control and Prevention (www.cdc.gov/mrsa/environment/athleticfacilities.html), proper steps in cleaning and disinfecting protective equipment should occur on a daily basis. The pads are not to be altered in any way. If they are cut or altered in any manner from the manufacturer, the person who altered the pad assumes all liability.

Purpose of Protective Device

The primary purpose for a protective device is to prevent an injury and to protect injured anatomical structures from further aggravation. Through proper application, a protective device can be applied to add additional protection, support, stability, and compression.

Protective Device: Sport-Specific Equipment, Liability, and Instruction

To ensure safety and product effectiveness, the protective device should have product liability coverage from the manufacturer and instructions for proper application. Sport-specific regulations, rules, and warnings exist concerning proper athletic equipment. Sport-specific equipment is worn as a standard uniform for participation in order to address individuals' safety. Standards of protection have improved through combined efforts of athletic governing bodies, the American Society for Testing and Materials (ASTM), the National Operating Committee on Standards for Athletic Equipment (NOCSAE), and the Hockey Equipment Certification Council (HECC).

Medical Device Authorization

As required, a qualified physician or qualified health care professional must prescribe a custom brace. Prior to this occurring, a qualified physician should complete a proper injury evaluation. Upon the physician's recommendation, a qualified health care professional and a medical equipment specialist can then recommend a custom or off-the-shelf protective device. This ensures that the proper device is applied for protection, support, stability, and/or compression. Also, the qualified health care professional and medical equipment specialist must develop a thorough knowledge of protective devices. See Figure 1.1 for an example of a Medco Sports Medicine Prescription Drug and Medical Device Authorization Form.

Description of Protective Device

A variety of materials is used in the fabrication process of a protective device. The materials consist of different density and resilience. Low-density material absorbs force and high-density material disperses force. Resilience provides the ability to bounce or spring back into the position or shape after being stretched, impacted, or bent.

Selection of Proper Protective Device

The selection of a protective device is based on the optimal level of impacted intensity in regard to density, resilience, thickness, comfort, and specificity. In terms of appropriateness, consider age, size, skill level, and physical activity. Selecting a device that will absorb impact and disperse it before injury or stress occurs to the underlying body part is important. Because a variety of protective devices is available, a qualified physician or qualified health care professional and medical equipment specialist can determine whether the individual is best suited for an off-the-shelf or custom brace.

Application of Protective Device

The qualified health care professional, medical equipment specialist, and individual must be aware of the suggested guidelines, rules, and warnings when applying a protective device. Following the manufacturer's instructions is imperative, as is not modifying a device without a physician's approval. Once a device has been modified, the protection component is compromised, as the safety and liability to the manufacturer are no longer valid.

Precautions

Before applying any protective device, be aware of congenital deformities and scars that may alter the fit of the device. A protective device is an important product to prevent and protect injuries if used within the manufacturer's rules and guidelines. When you apply the support, safety should be your priority. Therefore, do not modify protective devices that are standardized and regulated. With all injured individuals, consult a qualified physician.

When a specialty pad is needed, consider the following criteria:

1. Does the pad meet specific rules and guidelines of the sport? If NO, then do not use the pad.
2. Does the pad perform the function for which it was designed? If NO, then do not use the pad.
3. Will the pad contribute to further injury to the area or to an adjacent area? If YES, then do not use the pad.
4. Will the pad alter the function or void the warranty of a manufactured piece of equipment (e.g., helmet, shoulder pads)? If YES, then do not use the pad.
5. Will the device cause damage and/or harm to others participating? If YES, then do not use the device.

Ask and answer these and other common questions routinely before having a specialty pad constructed.

Sport-Specific Rules on Braces and Special Devices

The use of braces and special devices is beneficial if they are intelligently selected, used in the appropriate setting, correctly fitted, properly applied, and used within the rules and guidelines of the specific sport. Qualified physician approval must be obtained prior to application and use. Three common specialty supplies used in braces and special devices techniques are listed below.

Foam. Whether adhesive or nonadhesive, foam can be used in conjunction with various taping/wrapping procedures to increase efficacy of the technique. Keep these items in mind prior to applying tape or wrap to foam: proper size, thickness, shape, and foam composition.

Felt. Apply this product with many of the same considerations as with foam rubber products. Factors that you should consider in the construction and application of a felt pad are size, varying thickness, and use of either adhesive or nonadhesive felt.

Thermoplastic. This rigid material could allow the injured individual to return to practice and/or competition with an increased awareness that the injury can be protected from further harm. Because of the hard composition of this product, thermoplastic material may be restricted from some sports, be limited to a certain body part, or require padding according to the guidelines of each sport.

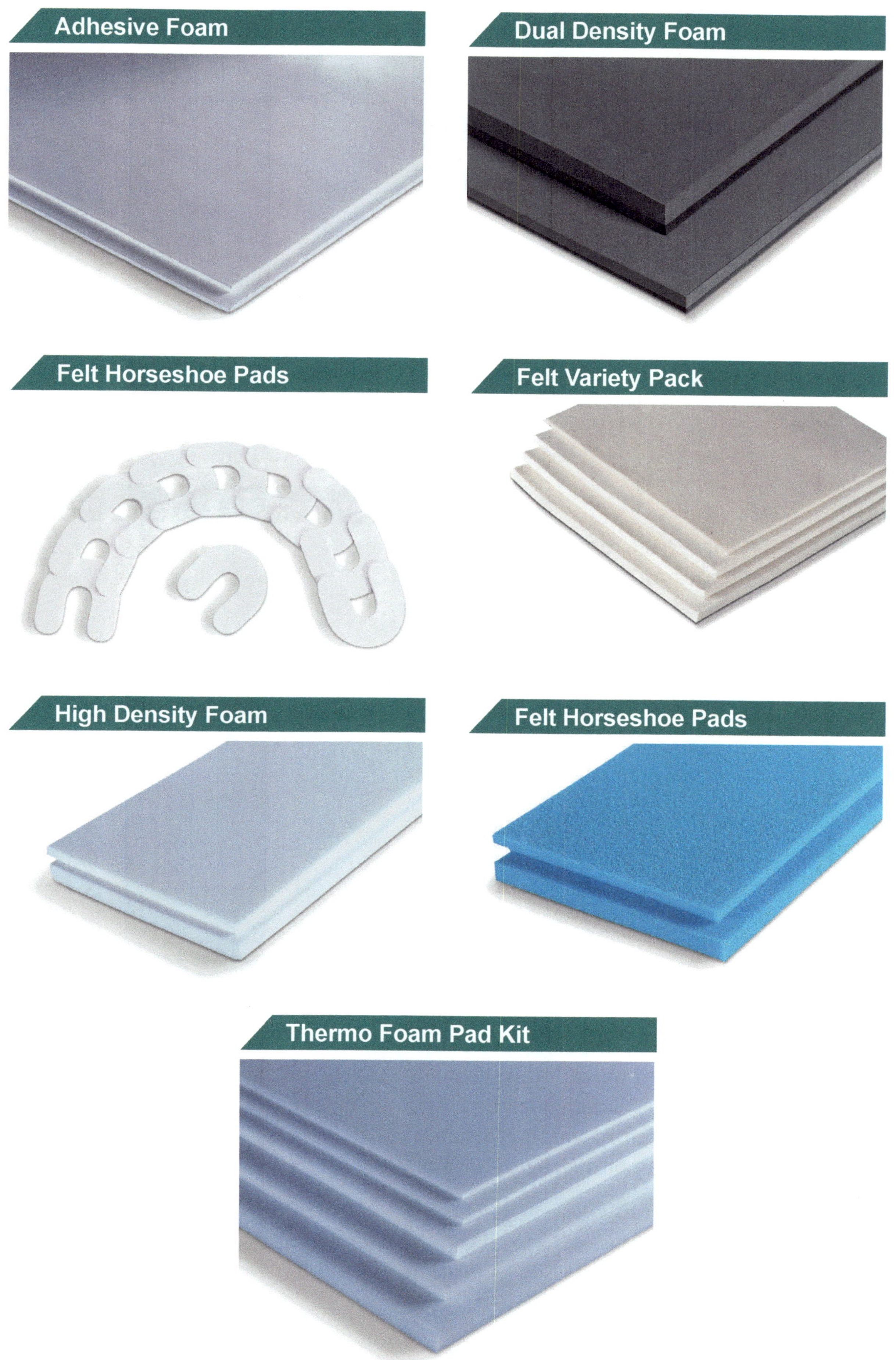
Adhesive Foam
Dual Density Foam
Felt Horseshoe Pads
Felt Variety Pack
High Density Foam
Felt Horseshoe Pads
Thermo Foam Pad Kit

Anatomical Planes

Transverse Plane. A horizontal plane at right angles to the vertical axis of the body. A plane that divides the body into a top and bottom portion.

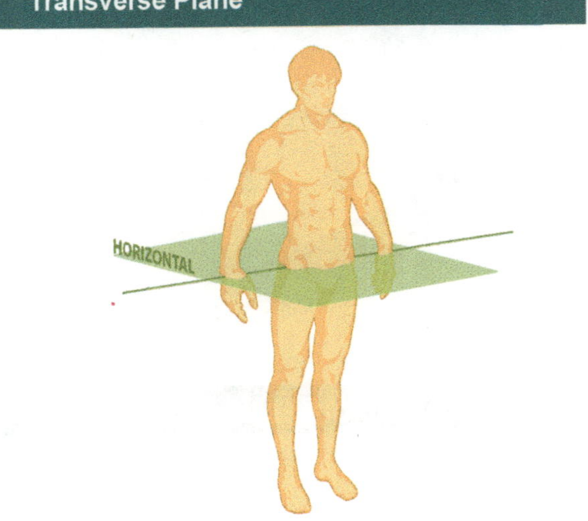

Frontal Plane. A flat surface formed by making a cut, imaginary or real, through the body or a part of it. Planes are used as points of reference by which positions of parts of the body are indicated. In the human subject, all planes are based on the body being in an upright anatomical position.

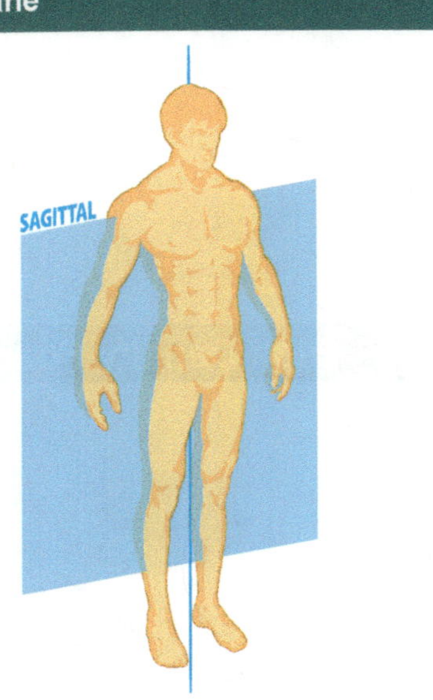

Sagittal Plane. A vertical plane through the longitudinal axis of the body or part of the body, dividing it into right and left parts. If it is through the anteroposterior midaxis and divides the body into right and left halves, it is called a median or midsagittal plane.

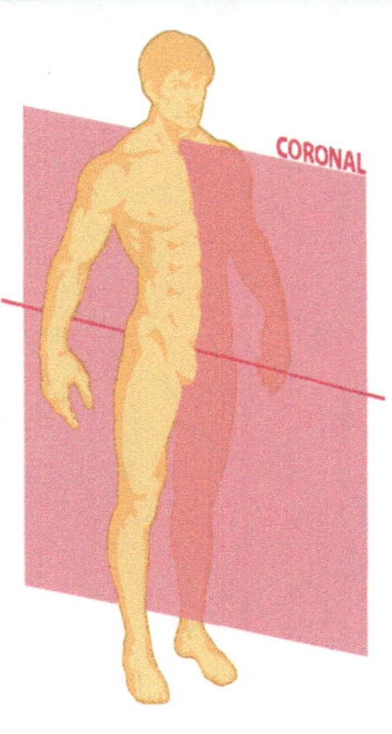

Chapter 2
Basic Fundamentals

EDUCATIONAL OBJECTIVES

Upon completing this chapter, the reader will be able to do the following:

- Identify anatomical structures and landmarks critical for correct taping procedures
- Explain philosophies and principles surrounding the proper use of elastic wrap applications for compression
- Demonstrate correct application of compression wraps and compression sleeves
- Explain the purpose and techniques for the application of compression wraps for the ankle, knee, elbow, wrist, and hand
- Explain philosophies and principles for casting and splinting

Introduction

The fundamentals of compression wrapping are necessary skills needed to properly administer injury care. An injury that occurs from a sprain, strain, or contusion will need immediate first aid attention to assist with the healing process. Compression to the injured area is a key part of the initial injury protocol and will help reduce swelling. A common acronym, PRICES (protection, rest, ice, compression, elevation, and support), lists the essential injury care measures. This chapter will discuss principles for injury care, fundamentals of compression wrapping, compression wraps, compression sleeves, casts, and splints.

Proper Assessment of Injury

Before applying a preventive technique (tape, wrap, and/or device), a qualified physician or qualified health care professional should complete an initial injury evaluation. Following initial injury evaluation, the professional can then recommend proper compression wrapping techniques. This ensures that proper wrapping techniques are applied for compression, support, and stabilization. Also, having a thorough knowledge of wrapping application fundamentals is imperative for the qualified health care professional. With specific written instruction (standing orders) provided by a qualified physician, the qualified health care provider's response to an acute injury should include the basic treatment protocol of protection, rest, ice, compression, elevation, and support (PRICES).

P (Protection). Once an injury has occurred, protect the injury from further damage by removing the individual from participation.

R (Rest). After the evaluation is completed, rest the injury. The length of rest is dependent on the severity of the injury; therefore, rest could easily be longer than 24 hours.

I (Ice). Apply cold to the injured area. This will aid in controlling bleeding and the associated swelling. The most common way to perform this activity is with an ice pack or plastic bags filled with ice covered with a towel. This treatment should be done for 10 minutes, with 3 hours in between treatment, four times per day. *Note:* Persons with known circulation problems must avoid ice. If problems arise, consult a qualified physician.

C (Compression). Using a compression wrap to control swelling, begin the elastic wrap distally (farthest from the heart) to the injury and spiral the wrap toward the heart on the involved extremity. Remove the wrap every 3 hours. *Note:* Compression wraps applied too tightly could interfere with circulation or nerve function. Signs and symptoms include extremities turning blue or pink, numbness and tingling of extremities, and increased pain. If the individual experiences this, remove the elastic wrap and reevaluate the injury!

E (Elevation). Keep the injured body part elevated higher than the heart. This will allow gravity to keep excessive blood and associated swelling out of the injured area.

S (Support). Various techniques can be used to support an injury (i.e., elastic wrap, cohesive tape, first-aid equipment, or compression sleeve). If necessary, place the injured extremity in a first-aid splint. Examples of other supports include the use of crutches for a lower extremity injury or use of a sling for an upper extremity injury.

Fundamentals of Compression Wrapping Procedures

Philosophies of Compression Application

Compression wraps are bandages that cover securely around the body structures. These are made to fit snugly to reduce swelling, increase circulation and provide support. The product selection and application of compression to the effected anatomical structure is at your discretion.

Medical Supplies: Compression Wrap, Cohesive Tape, and Compression Sleeve

Compression application uses snug-fitting stockings and wraps to maintain pressure on anatomical structures. Additionally, adhesive and elastic tapes are used to secure a wrap. Cohesive (self-adherent) tape is a dressing material that will adhere to itself but not to other surfaces. This product comes in a variety of widths, lengths, and colors. A compression sleeve is a commercial product that provides specific compression to anatomical structures (joints and muscles) and is usually sized from small to 4X-large.

METRIC TABLE

The metric table is displayed for international conversion use.

Inches	Centimeters
1	2.5
1.5	3.8
2	5.1
3	7.6
4	10.2
6	15.2
8	20.3
12	30.5

Inches	Centimeters
24	61
36	91.4
48	121.9
60	152.4
72	182.9
96	243.8
120	304.8

inch x 2.54 = centimeter
centimeter x .39 = inch

Proper Body Positioning

Before beginning a wrapping procedure, ask the individual to assume an anatomically correct and comfortable position. When applying a technique, learn to stand at a comfortable and stationary position and place the body part to be wrapped at your elbow height. The wrapping techniques presented in this text are the fundamental procedures. Variations can be achieved by adapting these techniques to a particular injury situation. Always give special consideration to the

- purpose of the wrapping procedure
- clinical application
- correct anatomical position
- supply selection
- *A strong knowledge of anatomy, physiology, biomechanics and pathology is essential.*

Precautions

Before applying a technique, make sure the individual's skin temperature is normal. To reduce the chance of skin irritation, after any therapeutic treatment, allow adequate time for the skin to return to its normal temperature. When applying support techniques, consider the safety of the individual your priority. With all injured individuals, consult a qualified physician.

TIPS FROM THE FIELD

Wrapping Procedures for Compression

- Know what body part and injury to which you are providing compression.
- When applying a compression wrap, always start distally and wrap proximally (toward the heart).
- When applying a technique, learn to stand at a comfortable and stationary position and place the body part to be wrapped at your elbow height.
- Apply proper tension to the tape so that circulation and neurological function will not be compromised.
- Follow the wrap with your hand to smooth out all wrinkles.
- Overlap the wrap one half of its width to avoid spaces that could cause cuts and friction burns.
- **PRACTICE!**

NOTES:

Compression Wraps: Elastic Wrap and Cohesive Tape

Developing a thorough knowledge regarding the fundamentals of the application of wrapping procedures is imperative. In applying a compression wrap, use a spiral pattern, and, beginning distal to the injury, wrap toward the heart. *On a frequent basis, remove the compression wrap to ensure that normal circulation and neurological function is present.

ANKLE COMPRESSION–ELASTIC WRAP

Purpose: Compression

Supplies: 4-in. elastic wrap and 1½-in. adhesive tape

Wrapping Procedures

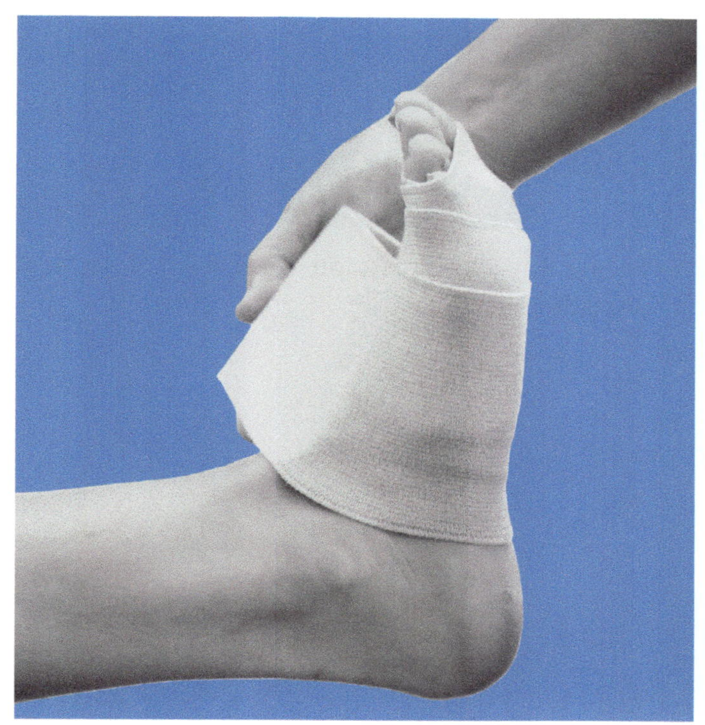

1. Begin the 4-in. elastic wrap at the distal part of the phalanges, spiral the wrap around the foot and ankle and on the distal aspect of the lower leg.

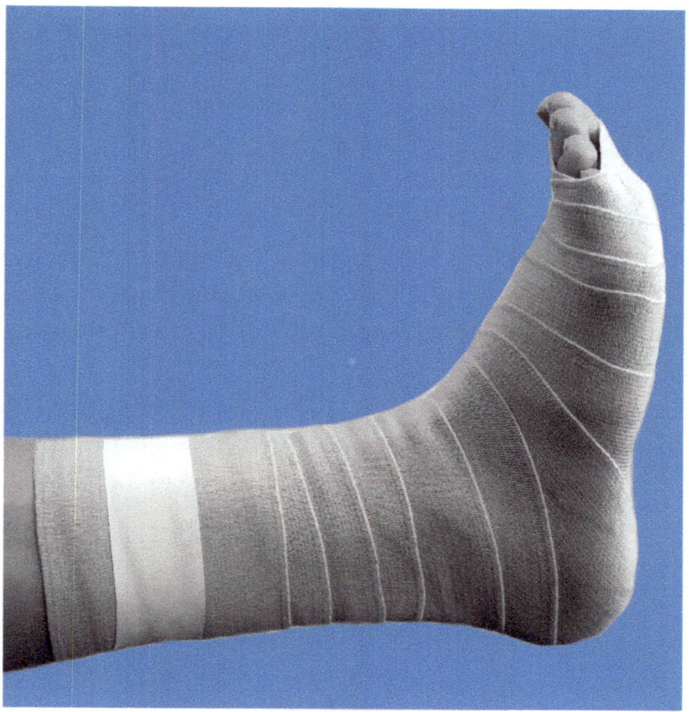

2. Secure the wrap with a small strip of 1½-in. adhesive tape.

**In certain situations, the ankle joint can be at a 90-degree angle or in slightly plantar flexion.*

ANKLE COMPRESSION–COHESIVE WRAP

Purpose: Compression

Supplies: 2-in., 3-in., or 4-in. cohesive tape and 1½-in. adhesive tape

Wrapping Procedures

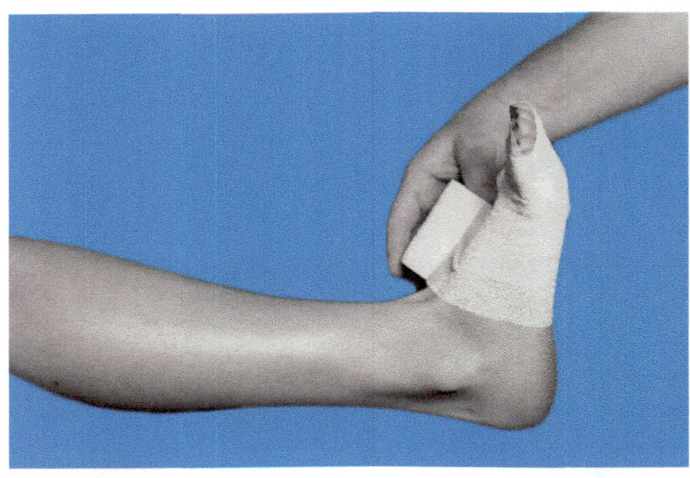

1. Begin the 2-in., 3-in., or 4-in. cohesive tape at the distal part of the phalanges, spiral the wrap around the foot and ankle and on the distal aspect of the lower leg.

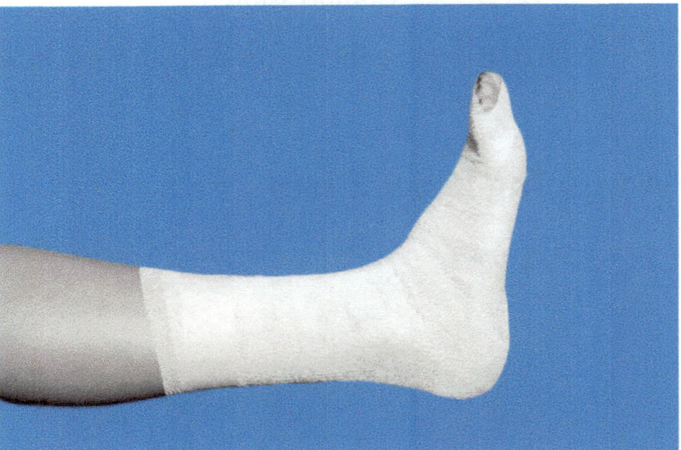

2. Secure the cohesive tape with a small strip of 1½-in. adhesive tape.

**The foot should remain at a 90-degree angle for this procedure.*

KNEE COMPRESSION–ELASTIC WRAP

Purpose: Compression

Supplies: 6-in. extra long elastic wrap and 1½-in. adhesive tape

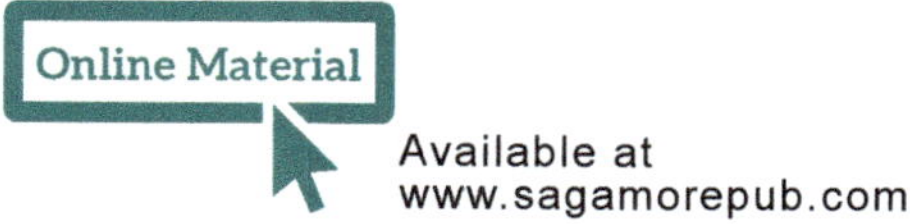

Available at
www.sagamorepub.com

Wrapping Procedures

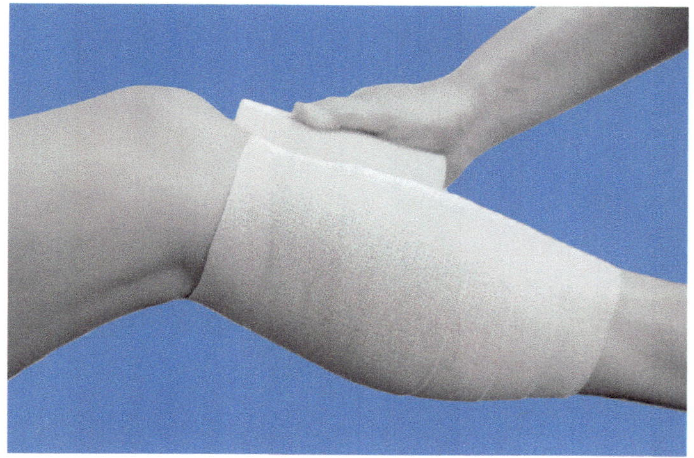

1. Begin the 6-in. elastic wrap around the lower leg, spiral around the leg, knee, and above the knee.

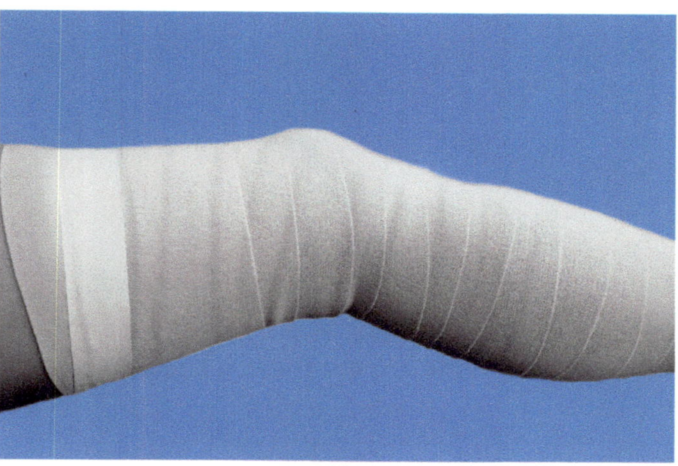

2. Secure the wrap with a small strip of 1½-in. adhesive tape.

KNEE COMPRESSION–COHESIVE TAPE

Purpose: Compression

Supplies: 3-in., 4-in., or 6-in. cohesive tape and 1½-in. adhesive tape

Wrapping Procedures

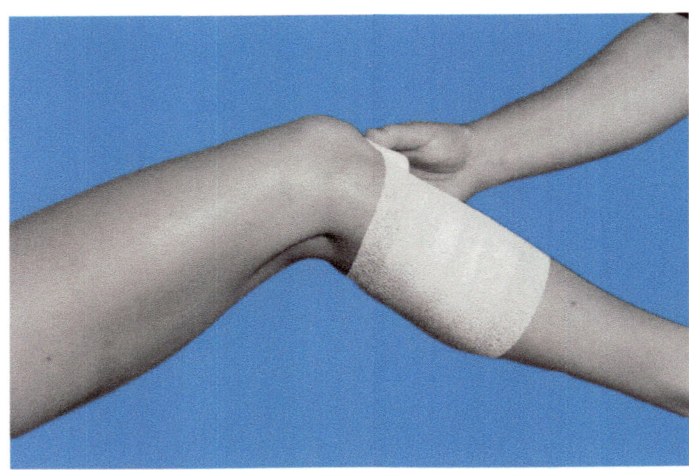

1. Begin the 3-in, 4-in., or 6-in. cohesive tape around the lower leg, spiral around the leg, knee, and above the knee.

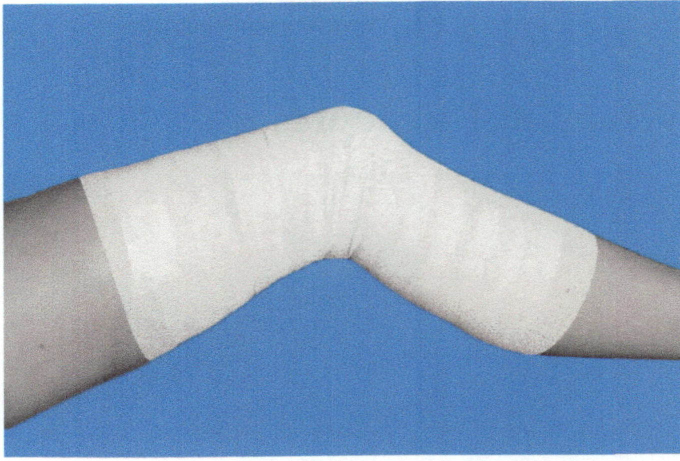

2. Secure the cohesive tape with a small strip of 1½-in. adhesive tape.

ELBOW COMPRESSION–ELASTIC WRAP

Purpose: Compression

Supplies: 6-in. elastic wrap and 1½-in. adhesive tape

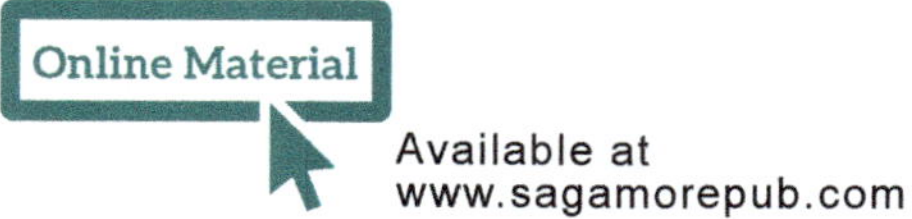

Wrapping Procedures

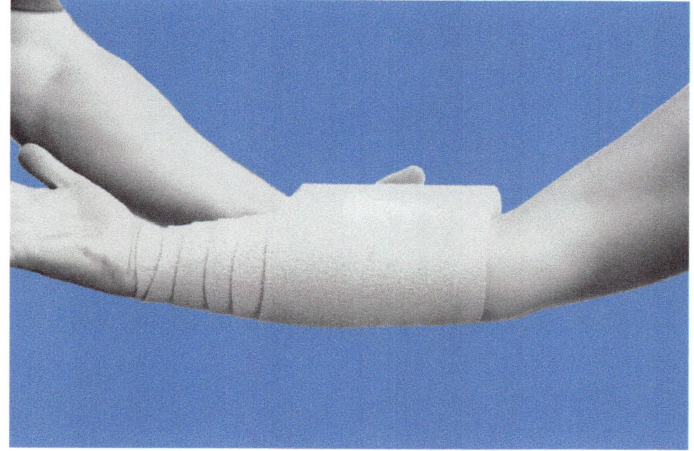

1. Begin the 6-in. elastic wrap at the wrist, spiral the wrap around the forearm and above the elbow joint.

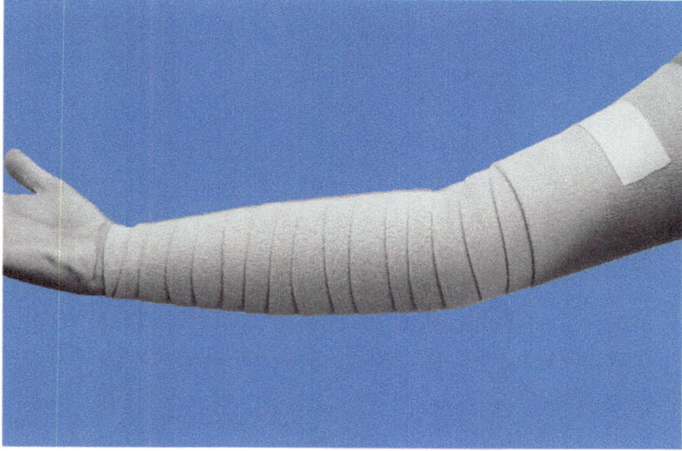

2. Secure the wrap with a small strip of 1½-in. adhesive tape.

ELBOW COMPRESSION–COHESIVE TAPE

Purpose: Compression

Supplies: 3-in. or 4-in. cohesive tape and 1½-in. adhesive tape

Wrapping Procedures

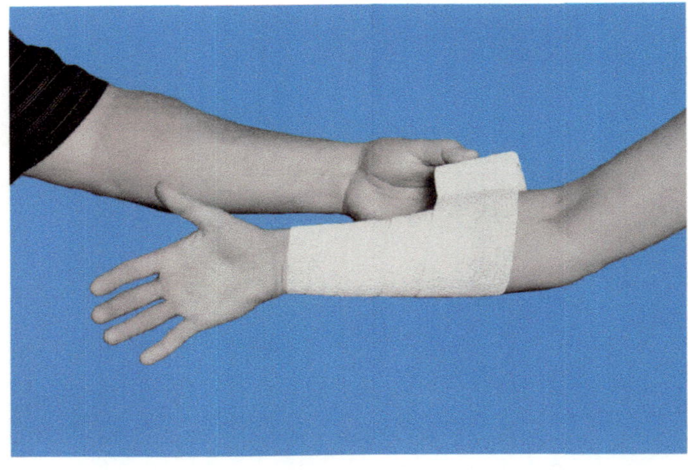

1. Begin the 3-in. or 4-in. cohesive tape at the wrist, spiral the wrap around the forearm and above the elbow joint.

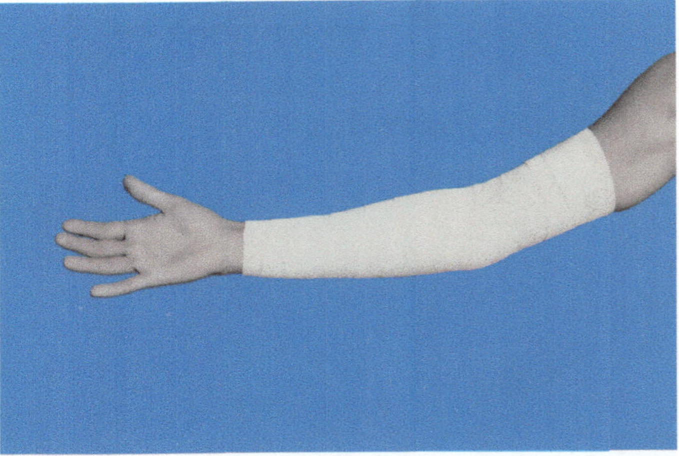

2. Secure the cohesive tape with a small strip of 1½-in. adhesive tape.

WRIST/HAND COMPRESSION–ELASTIC WRAP

Purpose: Compression

Supplies: 4-in. elastic wrap and 1½-in. adhesive tape

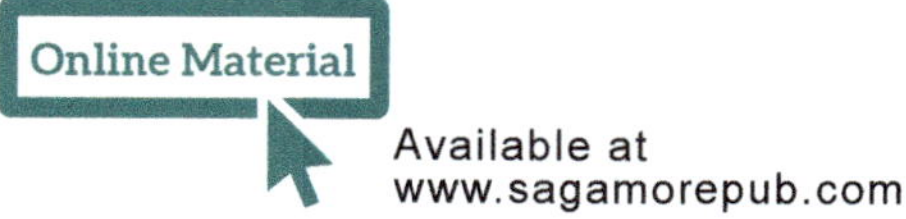

Wrapping Procedures

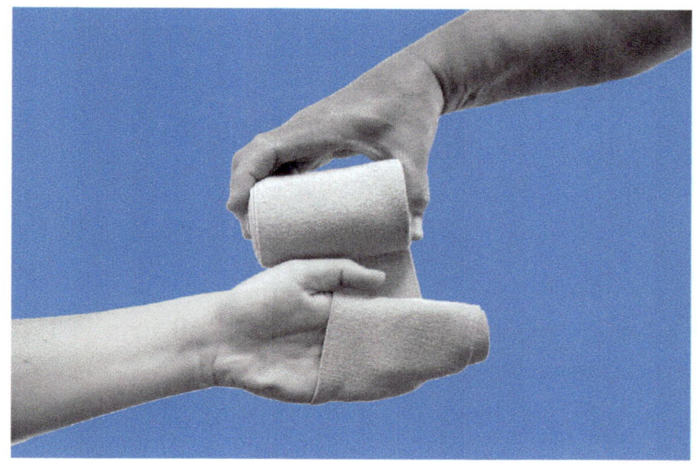

1. Begin the 4-in. elastic wrap at the finger tips, spiral around the hand and above the wrist.

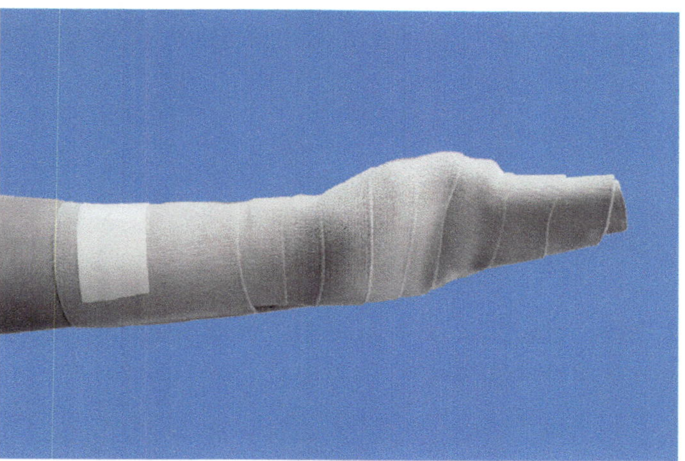

2. Secure the wrap with a small strip of 1½-in. adhesive tape.

WRIST/HAND COMPRESSION–COHESIVE TAPE

Purpose: Compression

Supplies: 2-in. or 3-in. cohesive tape and 1½-in. adhesive tape

Wrapping Procedures

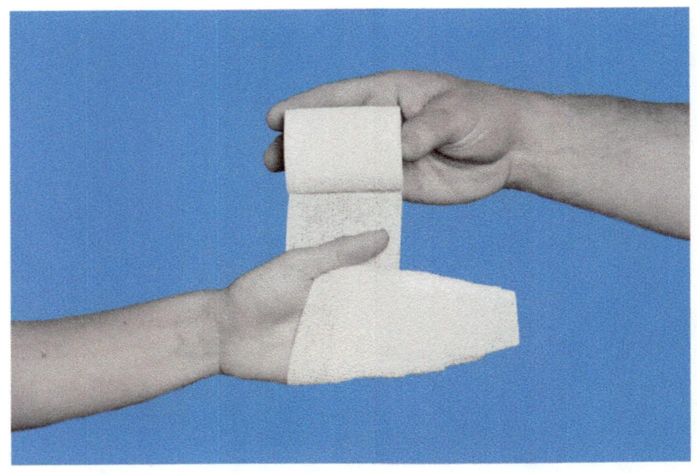

1. Begin the 2-in. or 3-in. cohesive tape at the finger tips, spiral around the hand and above the wrist.

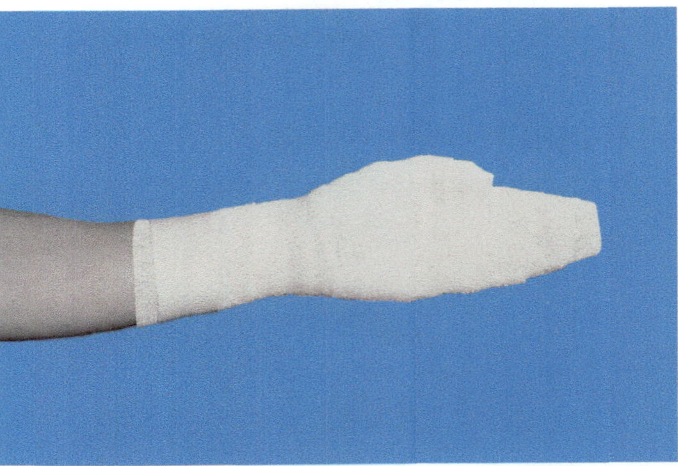

2. Secure the cohesive tape with a small strip of 1½-in. adhesive tape.

Compression Sleeves

Compression sleeves are garments designed to provide pressure to upper and lower body extremities. They may be used for prevention, support, swelling reduction, and to increase circulation. The Nanoflex Supports were manufactured for comfortable support and compression. The silver technology eliminates odor-causing bacteria. Additionally, the polyester filament wicks moisture away from the body.

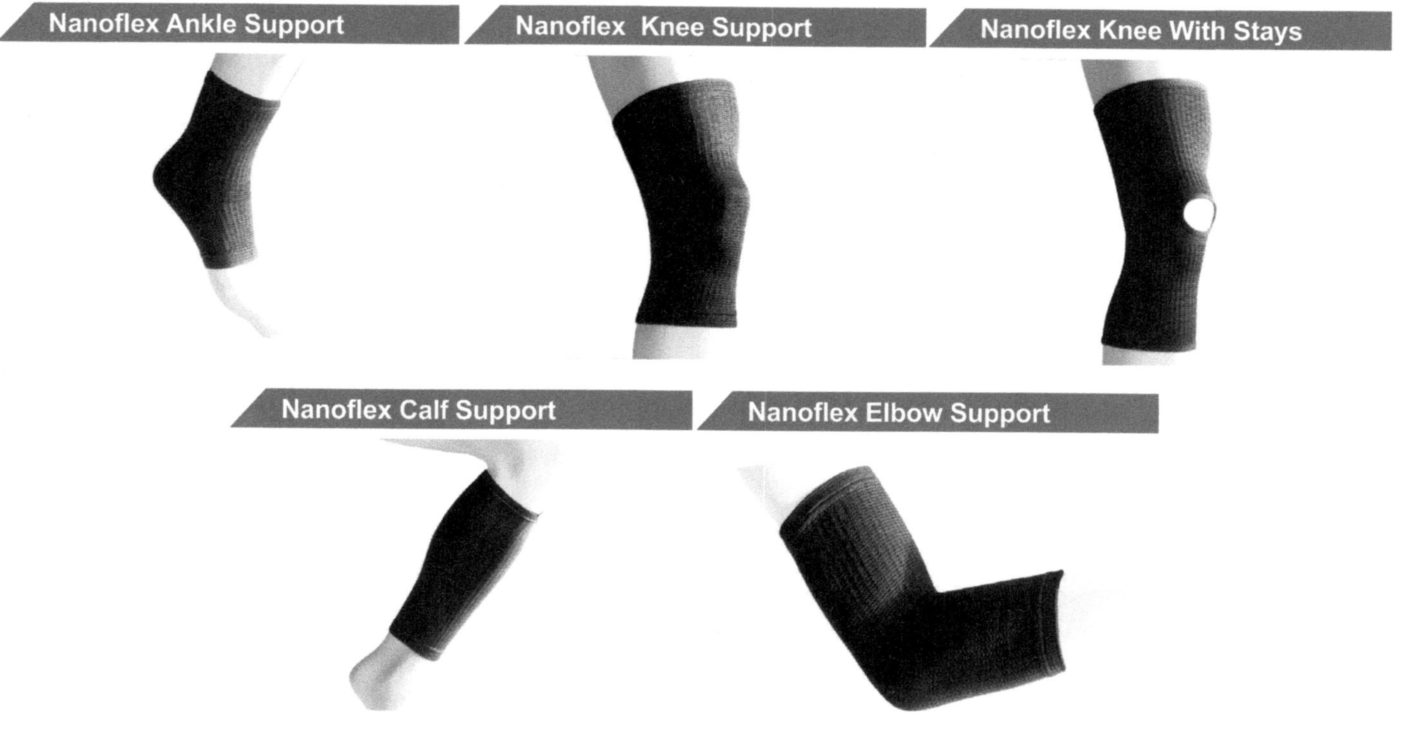

Casts and Splints

An individual who has sustained an injury and requires a cast or splint should be aware of possible complications associated with the use of these immobilization techniques. The most pressing issue is the possibility of developing compartment syndrome. Compartment syndrome is a true orthopedic medical emergency in which delayed treatment could result in permanent functional loss or loss of limb. Compartment syndrome is caused by an increase in pressure within fascial compartments of the forearm and lower leg. This increase in pressure is due to swelling as a result of the body's natural response to injury, lack of elevation of the injured extremity, splint and cast applications that are applied too tightly, or a combination of these factors. Elevated intracompartmental pressure leads to a reduction in venous outflow, which increases interstitial pressure and results in tissue necrosis. Six hours after the development of compartment syndrome, complete functional recovery cannot be guaranteed, and beyond 8 to 12 hours, the damage is irreversible. Qualified health care professionals, coaches, individuals (patient), and parents (if applicable) should be educated about the symptoms of compartment syndrome:

- **Pain:** A steady increase of pain out of proportion to the injury. Pain sensation is greater than that experienced at the time of injury.
- **Pressure:** Cast or splint has the sensation of "being too tight."
- **Paresthesia:** An abnormal or unpleasant sensation that results from injury to one or more nerves. It is often described by patients as numbness and tingling or as a prickly, stinging, or burning feeling; sensation of tingling, burning, or prickling.
- **Pulselessness:** Weak or absence of distal pulse.

If any of these symptoms are present, take the following steps:

1. Contact the provider and advise him or her of the symptoms. If the provider cannot be reached, proceed to the closest emergency room for evaluation.
2. Elevate the extremity above the level of the heart.
3. If the patient is wearing a splint, loosen the compressive dressing that is securing the splint. Loosening can relieve pressure while maintaining immobilization.
4. If the patient is wearing a cast, bi-valve the cast to relieve pressure. Bi-valving is making complete (proximal to distal) longitudinal cuts on the cast to relieve pressure. (For the Qualified Health Care Professional: A short arm cast should be cut on both the dorsal area and the ventral area and the short leg cast should be cut on both the medial area and the lateral area. Be sure to use a cast spreader to "pop" the cast open.)

Generally, these steps may relieve acute symptoms of compartment syndrome; however, the provider must evaluate the individual even if the symptoms subside.

Splint: Splints should be used in the acute setting (injury less than 7 to 10 days postinjury) as opposed to casts because splints can accommodate for swelling commonly associated with injuries. Be sure to evaluate neurovascular status before and after splint application.

Materials:

- cast padding (cotton or synthetic)
- compressive wrap
- bandage tape to secure the compressive wrap
- water to activate the splint resin
- bandage scissors
- splint material: fiberglass cast tape or plaster cast material (prefab = Ortho-glass)

Be sure to use the appropriate size when selecting these materials. The width of the individual's hand is a good indicator of which size should be used. The use of stockinette is contraindicated due to its compressive effect, which may add to the potential of compartment syndrome.

Cast: Individuals should be transitioned into a cast after the acute phase (injury greater than 7 to 10 days postinjury) for proper immobilization. Be sure to evaluate neurovascular status before and after cast application.

Materials:

- stockinette
- cast padding (cotton or synthetic)
- fiberglass or plaster cast tape
- water to activate the cast resin
- bandage scissors

Be sure to use the appropriate size when selecting these materials. The width of the individual's hand is a good indicator of which size should be used.

PART II
Techniques for Lower Extremities

Chapter 3
Foot, Ankle, and Lower Leg

EDUCATIONAL OBJECTIVES

Upon completing this chapter, the reader will be able to do the following:

- Identify anatomical structures and landmarks critical for correct taping procedures
- Describe the purpose for the applications of adhesive and elastic tape
- Select the proper supplies and specialty items used for taping
- Explain the steps in preparing the body for taping, wrapping, or protective device
- Describe and demonstrate the purposes, clinical applications, anatomical structures, supplies needed, pretaping, and taping procedures for anatomical areas
- Identify the proper use and application of protective devices for the foot, ankle, and leg

Introduction

Lower extremity injuries related to the foot, ankle, and lower leg represent a large population. Knowing the basic concepts will prove beneficial for proper injury management. This chapter will improve insight by addressing the terminology, taping techniques, wrapping techniques, protective devices, and musculoskeletal disorders related to the ankle, foot, and lower leg.

Terminology

Dorsal. Upper surface (e.g., top of foot).

Plantar. Ventral aspect of the foot (sole of the foot).

Proximal. Closest to the midline or center of the trunk; nearest to the point of attachment, origin, or other point of reference.

Distal. Away from a center, from the midline, or from the trunk. A point that is greater from point of reference (opposite of proximal).

Plantar flexion. Act of drawing the toe or foot toward the plantar aspect of the proximally conjoined body segment; opposite of dorsiflexion.

Dorsiflexion. Act of drawing the toe or foot toward the dorsal aspect of the proximally conjoined body segment.

Inversion. Act of rotating the pronated foot internally on the ankle; turning the sole of the foot inward.

Eversion. Act of rotating the pronated foot externally on the ankle; turning the sole of the foot outward.

Pronation. Act of rotating the hand or foot internally on its long axis; medial rotation of the forearm, as in turning the palm of the hand downward.

Supination. Act of rotating a hand or foot externally on its long axis; lateral rotation of the forearm, as in turning the palm of the hand upward.

Malleolus. A rounded bony protuberance on each side of the ankle joint.

Pes cavus. High arch; deformities of the foot.

Pes planus. Flat feet.

Stirrup. Any U-shaped loop or piece.

Heel lock. Commonly used in ankle taping, this supportive technique aids in stabilizing the calcaneus; medial and lateral heel locks are usually applied.

Figure of eight. Bandaging of a joint where the initial turn circles the one part of the joint and the second turn circles the adjoining part of the joint to form a figure of eight.

Taping Techniques and Protective Devices

Developing a thorough knowledge regarding the fundamentals of the application of taping/wrapping procedures is imperative. Review Chapter 1 before applying any technique.

Proper Assessment of Injury

Before applying a preventive technique (tape, wrap, and/or device), a qualified physician or qualified health care professional should complete a proper injury evaluation. Following injury evaluation, the professional can then recommend proper taping techniques. This ensures that proper taping techniques are applied for support and stabilization. Also, developing a thorough knowledge of taping application fundamentals is imperative for the professional.

Purpose and Application of Adhesive and Elastic Tape

The primary purpose for tape application is to provide additional support and stability for the affected body part. Through proper application, taping techniques can be applied to shorten the muscle's angle of pull; to decrease joint range of motion; to secure pads, bandages, and protective devices; and to apply compression to reduce swelling.

Medical Supplies and Specialty Items

Purchasing supplies depends on budget, philosophy of medical staff regarding taping techniques, and occurrence of injury. Review Chapter 1 before applying any technique.

Specific Rules on Taping, Wrapping, and/or Protective Device

If you apply supportive techniques to an individual, you should be aware of specific rules governing tape application in that particular sport or physical activity. Your application must fall within the guidelines established for each sport by appropriate governing bodies.

Special Techniques: Adjunct Taping Procedures

The taping techniques presented are the fundamental procedures. Adjunct techniques will be shown to provide additional support; however, you should still follow the fundamental procedures. Variations can be achieved by adapting these techniques to a particular injury situation. Always give special consideration to

- purpose of the taping procedure
- clinical application
- correct anatomical position
- supply selection
- tape/wrap technique or protective device

Preparation of Body Part for Taping

In preparing the body for tape application, consider these items:

- removal of hair (optional)
- clean the area
- special considerations
- spray adherent (optional)
- skin lubricants
- underwrap or cohesive tape
- proper body position

Proper Body Positioning

Before beginning any taping procedure, select a comfortable table height and ask the individual to assume an anatomically correct and comfortable position.

- *Neutral Position of Foot:* When taping the foot, the anatomical position should be slightly plantar flexed (10 to 15 degrees).
- *Neutral Position of Ankle Joint:* With the leg fully extended, the foot should be positioned at a 90-degree angle.

When applying a technique, learn to stand at a comfortable and stationary position and place the body part to be taped at your elbow height.

Anatomical Graphics

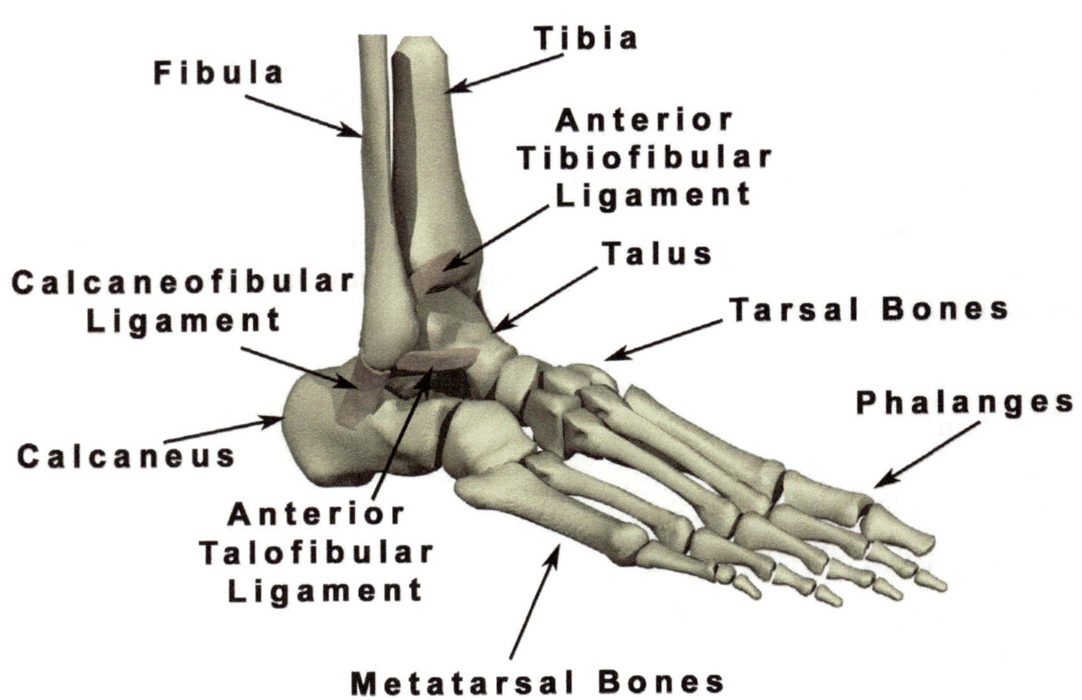

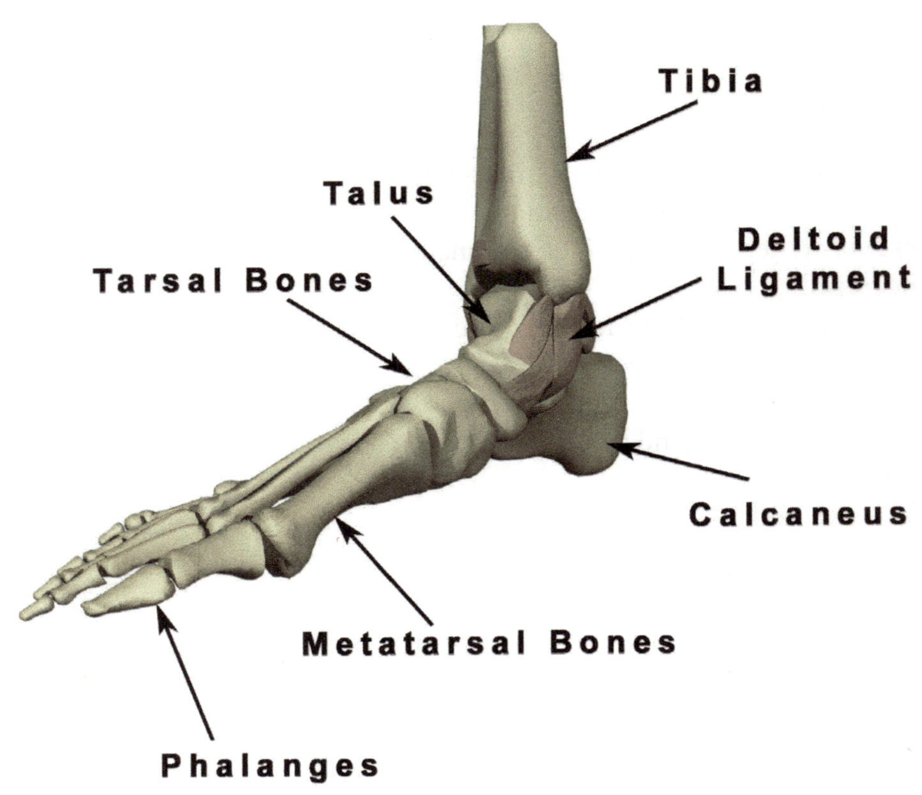

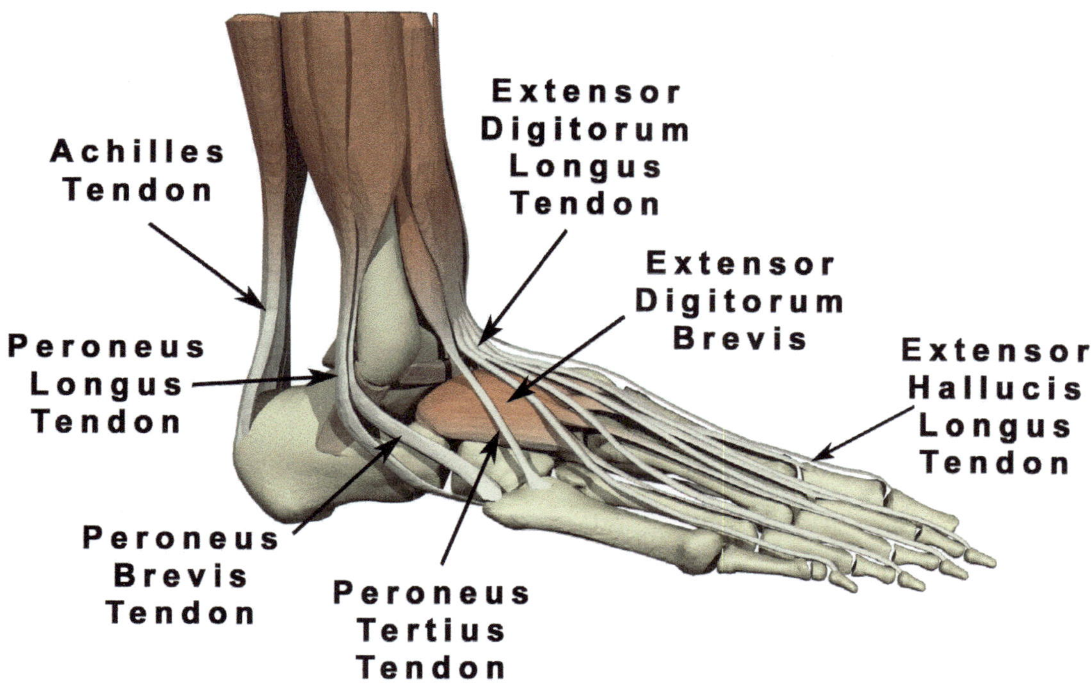
Achilles Tendon
Extensor Digitorum Longus Tendon
Extensor Digitorum Brevis
Peroneus Longus Tendon
Extensor Hallucis Longus Tendon
Peroneus Brevis Tendon
Peroneus Tertius Tendon

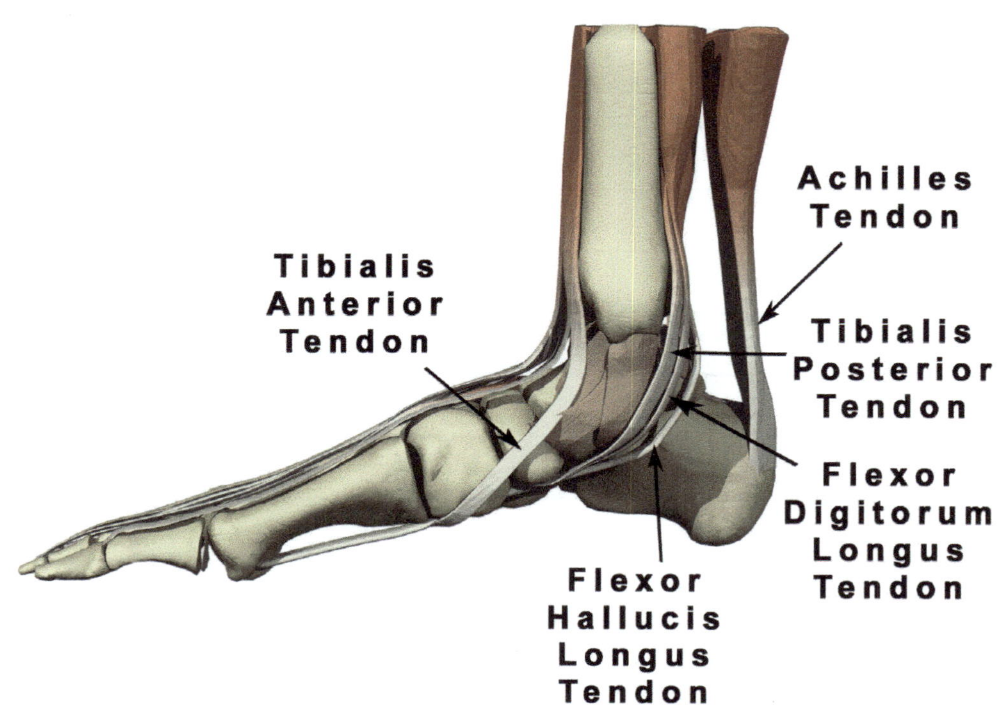
Achilles Tendon
Tibialis Anterior Tendon
Tibialis Posterior Tendon
Flexor Digitorum Longus Tendon
Flexor Hallucis Longus Tendon

Taping Techniques

The taping techniques presented are the *fundamental procedures*. A strong knowledge of anatomy, physiology, biomechanics, and pathology is essential. Developing a thorough knowledge regarding the fundamentals about the application of taping/wrapping procedures is imperative. Review Section A - Chapter 1 before applying any technique. When applying tape to the foot or ankle, pull the tape lateral to avoid excessive tension/compression on the fifth metatarsal.

The Kinesio® Taping Method is a therapeutic taping technique not only offering your patient the support they are looking for, but also rehabilitating the affected condition as well. Please consult Chapter 9 for specific application instructions.

NOTES:

GREAT TOE–DORSAL

Purpose: To limit excessive motion of the first metatarsophalangeal joint (MP Joint), therefore helping to prevent or stabilize a sprain or turf toe

Clinical Application: Sprain to first metatarsophalangeal joint (turf toe)

Anatomical Structure: First metatarsal joint (great toe)

Anatomical Position: Ankle should be placed in neutral position and first MP joint placed in neutral position

Supplies: 1-in. or 1½-in. adhesive tape, and 2-in. elastic tape

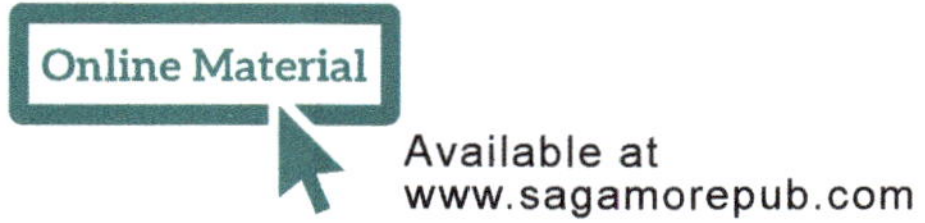

Taping Procedures

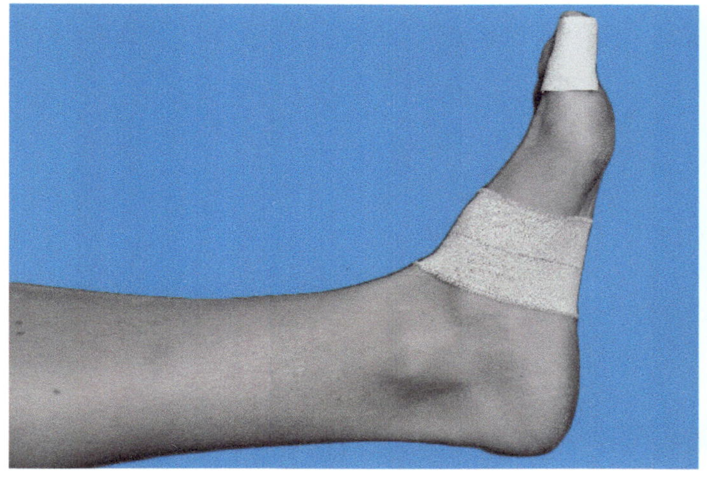

1. Apply two anchor strips.
   a. Apply adhesive anchor strip around distal aspect of the great toe.
   b. Apply elastic anchor strip around the mid-foot. This strip should begin on the dorsal aspect, go lateral, and continue across the plantar aspect to the mid-foot medial portion, crossing the tape ends.

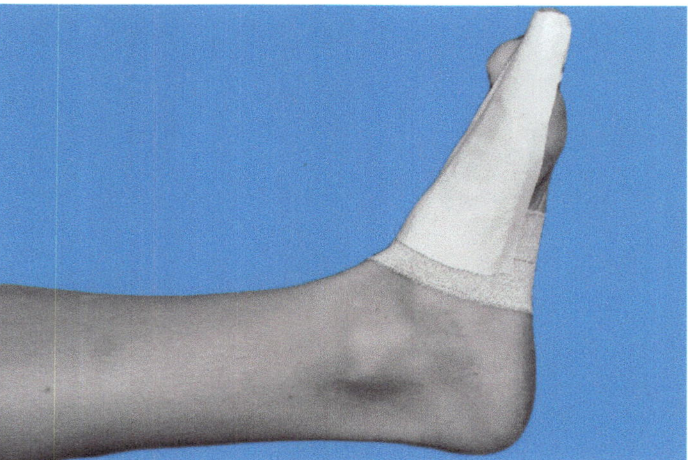

2. Apply four to six strips of adhesive tape to form a fan shape. This will provide adequate support. Place fan-shaped tape from the anchor on the great toe, covering the affected dorsal area and ending on the elastic anchor at the mid-foot.

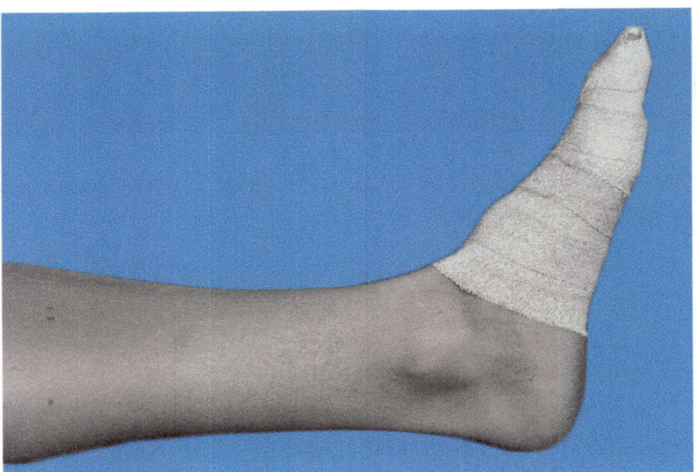

3. Using a continuous strip of elastic tape, apply a figure of eight around the great toe and mid-foot. This will aid in abduction of the first MP joint and should assist in preventing excessive movement, flexion, or extension of the MP joint.

**Upon completion of the procedure, make sure you check for neatness and gaps, adequate support, along with proper function of the affected area. In certain situations, the individual might be asked to perform function tests to establish appropriate technique.*

Adjunct Taping Procedures:

These adjunct taping procedures can be used in conjunction with the basic technique presented.

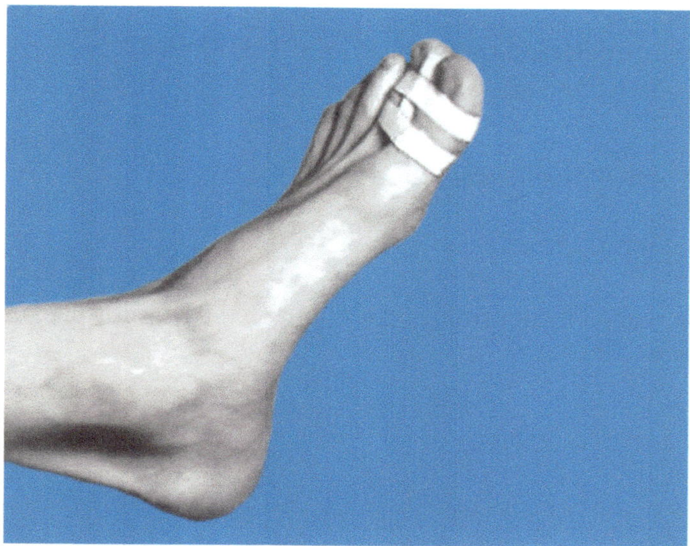

Adjunct Technique A. Apply two circular strips of adhesive tape, around the proximal and distal aspect of first and second phalanges. This is commonly referred to as buddy taping.

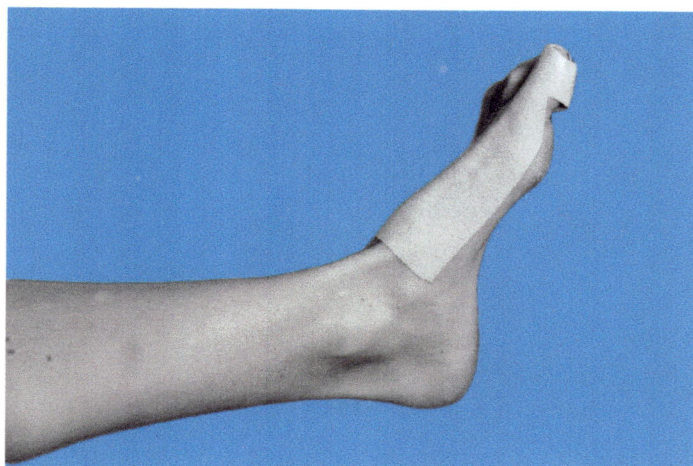

Adjunct Technique B. Apply a strip of moleskin over the Dorsal area.

GREAT TOE–PLANTAR

Purpose: To limit excessive motion of the first metatarsophalangeal joint (MP Joint), therefore helping to prevent or stabilize a sprain or turf toe

Clinical Application: Sprain to first metatarsophalangeal joint (turf toe)

Anatomical Structure: First metatarsal joint (great toe)

Anatomical Position: Ankle should be placed in neutral position and first MP joint placed in neutral position

Supplies: 1-in. or 1½-in. adhesive tape, and 2-in. elastic tape

Taping Procedures

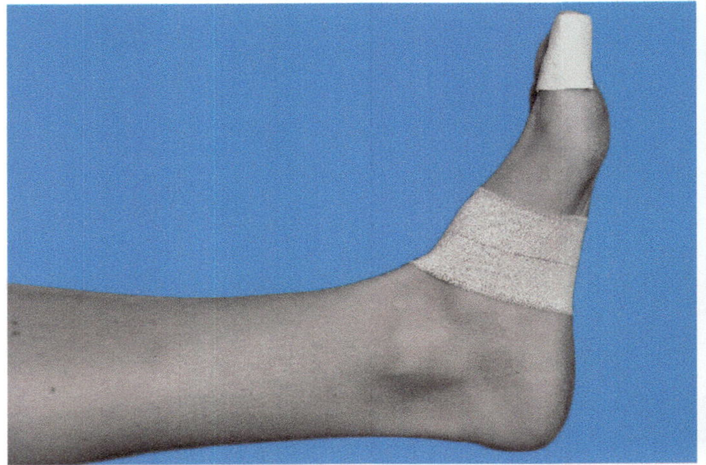

1. Apply two anchor strips.
   a. Apply adhesive anchor strip around distal aspect of the great toe.
   b. Apply elastic anchor strip around the mid-foot. This strip should begin on the dorsal aspect, go lateral, and continue across the plantar aspect to the mid-foot medial portion, crossing the tape ends.

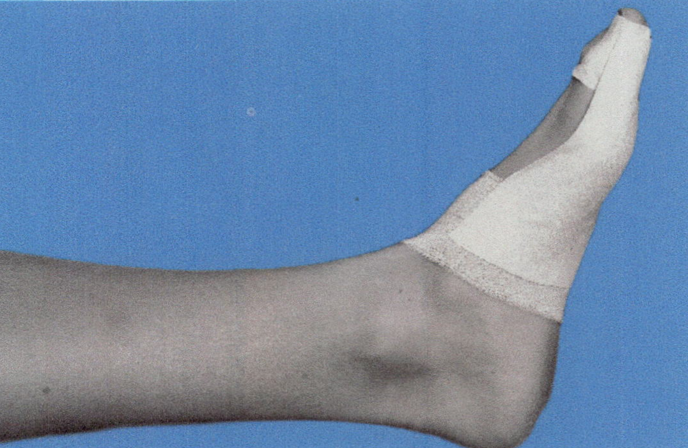

2. Four to six strips of adhesive tape should be applied to form a fan shape. This will provide adequate support. Place fan-shaped tape from the plantar aspect of the anchor on the great toe, covering the affected plantar area and ending on the elastic anchor at the mid-foot.

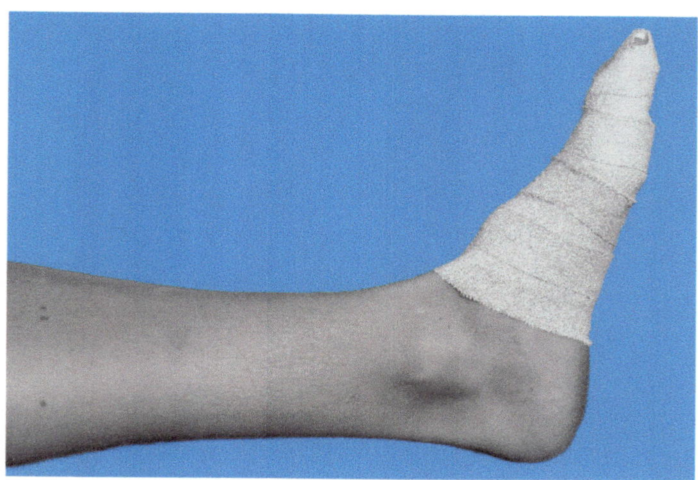

3. Using a continuous strip of elastic tape, apply a figure of eight around the great toe and mid-foot. This will aid in abduction of the first MP joint and should assist in preventing excessive movement, flexion or extension of the MP joint.

**Upon completion of the procedure, make sure you check for neatness and gaps, adequate support, along with proper function of the affected area. In certain situations, the individual might be asked to perform function tests to establish appropriate technique.*

Adjunct Taping Procedures:

These adjunct taping procedures can be used in conjunction with the basic technique presented.

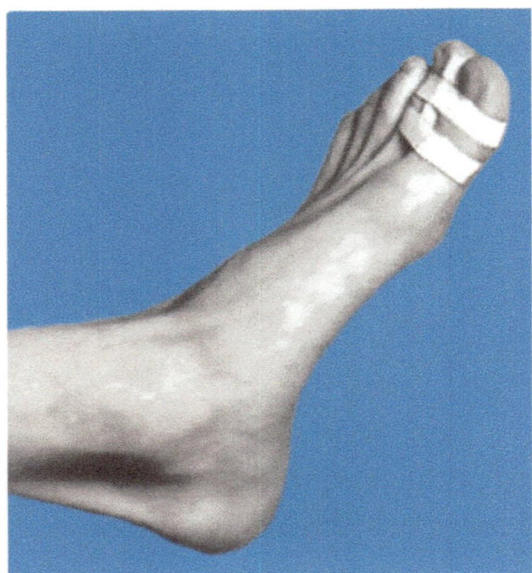

Adjunct Technique A. Apply two circular strips of adhesive tape, around the proximal and distal aspect of first and second phalanges. This is commonly referred to as buddy taping.

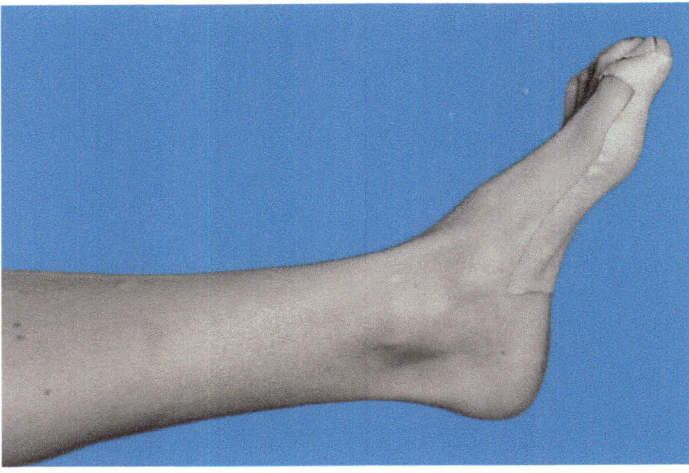

Adjunct Technique B. Apply a strip of Moleskin over the plantar area.

HEEL

Purpose: To provide compression and support to the calcaneus fat pad and underlying tissue

Clinical Application: Contusion to the heel area

Anatomical Structure: Calcaneus (Heel)

Anatomical Position: Place ankle joint in neutral position

Supplies: 1-in. or 1½-in. adhesive tape

Pre-taping Procedure: Apply tape adherent to affected area

Taping Procedures

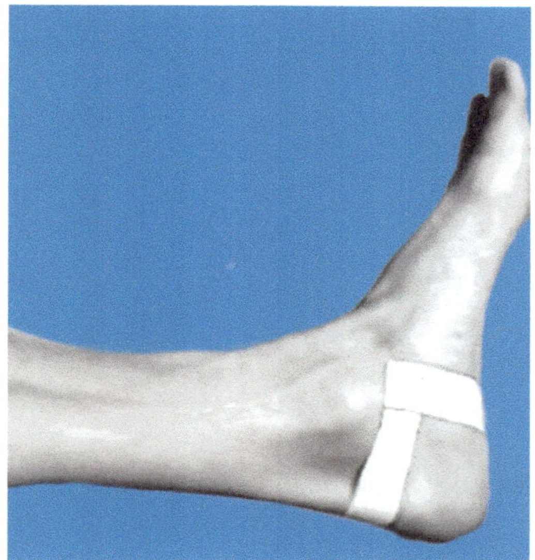

1. Apply anchor strips (medial to lateral) to enclose affected heel area.
   a. Across the heel (plantar surface).
   b. Around the heel (posterior surface).

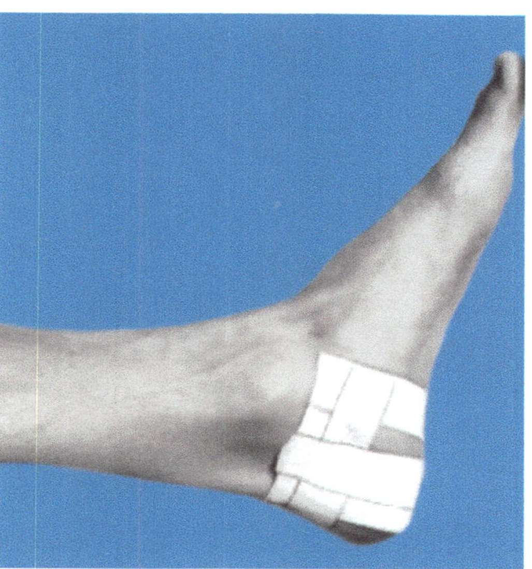

2. Using an alternative method, apply four to six strips of tape that apply direct pressure to the heel. Overlap these support strips one half of the tape width. The tape should be applied proximal to distal on the plantar surface of the foot.

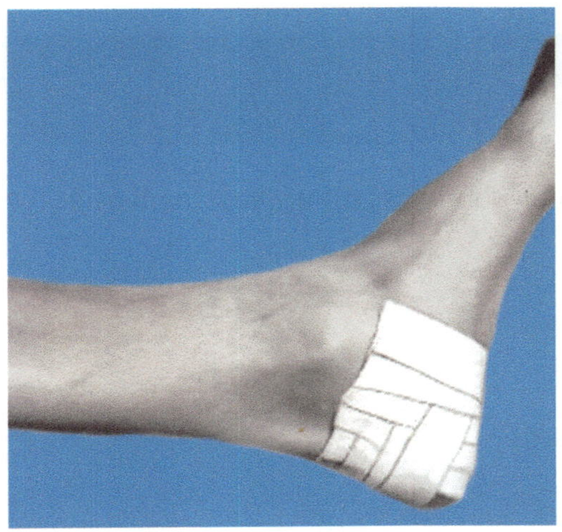

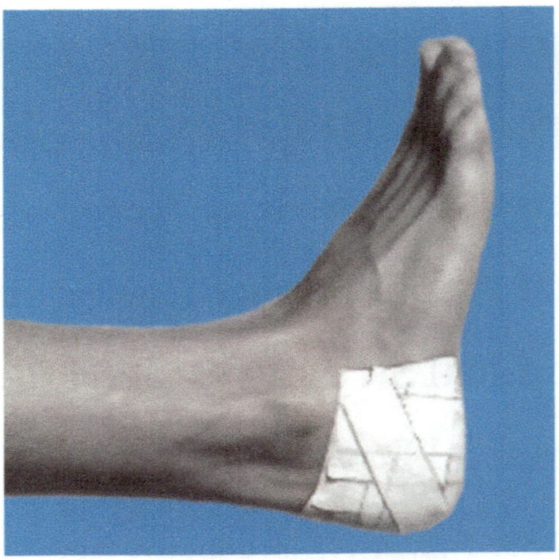

3. To cover the entire heel area, apply a diagonal strip of tape starting on the medial aspect, crossing the heel, and ending on the lateral aspect.

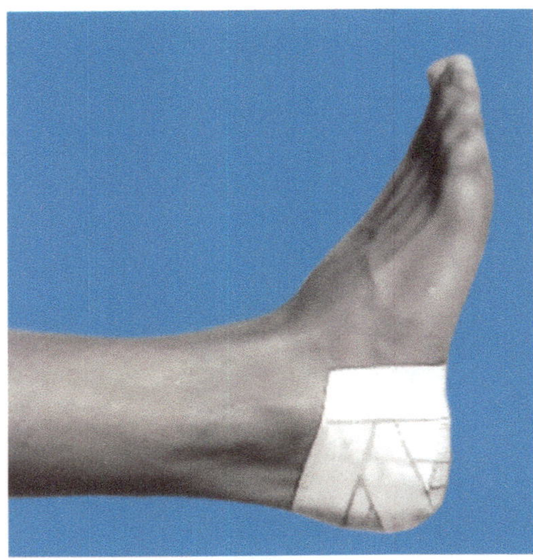

4. To close, place an anchor strip around the heel, from the medial to lateral side of the foot.

**Upon completion of the procedure, make sure you check for neatness and gaps, adequate support, along with proper function of the affected area. In certain situations, the individual might be asked to perform function tests to establish appropriate technique.*

METATARSAL ARCH

Purpose: To elevate the metatarsal heads

Clinical Application: Dropped metatarsals, contusions, strains, and sprains

Anatomical Structure: Metatarsal arch

Anatomical Position: Ankle should be positioned in a slight plantar flexed position

Supplies: ¼-in. or ½-in. felt, 2-in. or 3-in. elastic tape, and 1½-in. adhesive tape

Pre-taping Procedure

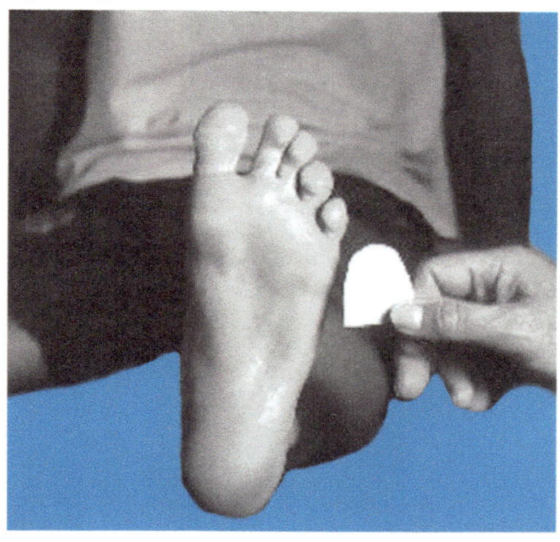

First, cut a ¼-in. or ½-in felt piece in a diamond shape (metatarsal pad) with all sides slightly tapered.

Taping Procedures

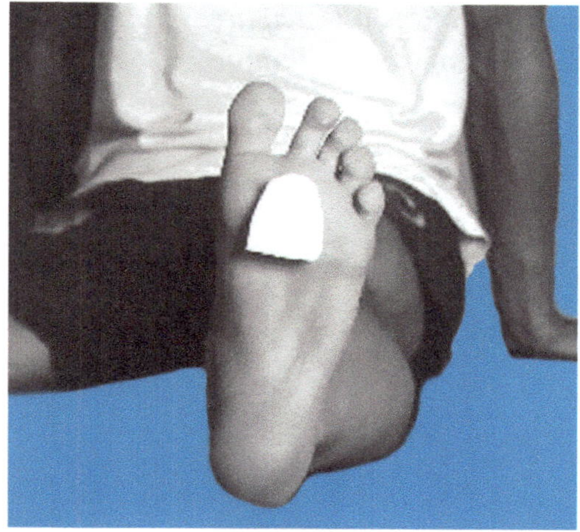

1. Place the metatarsal pad proximal to the heads of the second through fourth metatarsals.

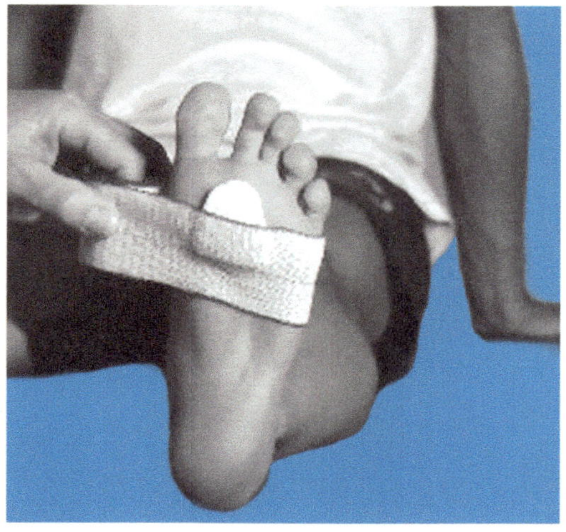

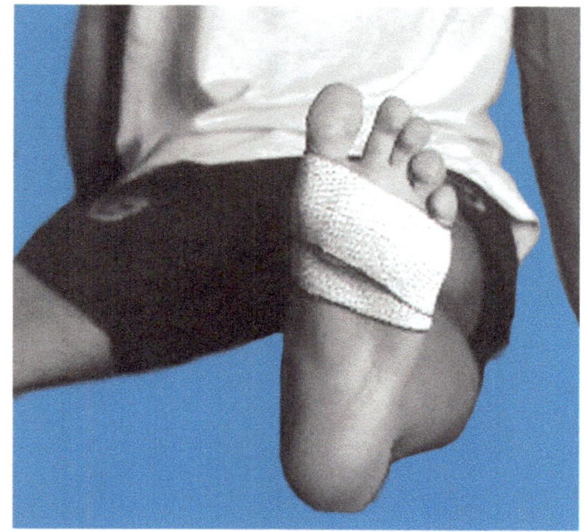

2. Secure this supportive pad to the foot by using elastic tape. It is preferred that this circular strip begin on the dorsal aspect, go lateral, and continue across plantar aspect to medial portion of the foot, crossing the tape ends.

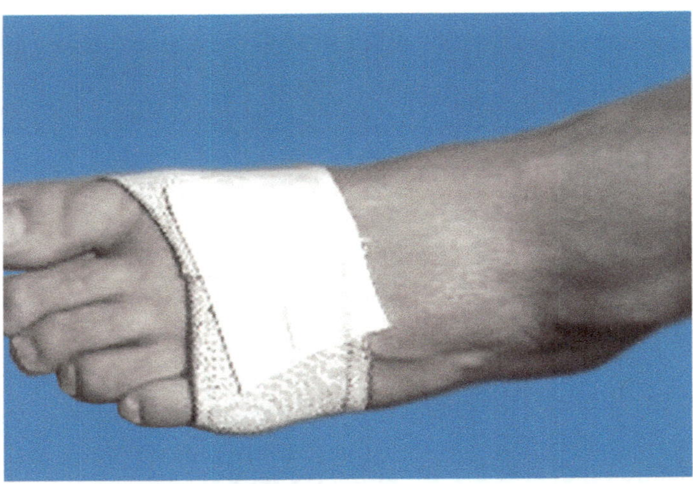

3. Apply a strip of 1½-in. adhesive tape over the tape ends to secure the elastic tape.

**Upon completion of the procedure, make sure you check for neatness and gaps, adequate support, along with proper function of the affected area. In certain situations, the individual might be asked to perform function tests to establish appropriate technique*

MEDIAL LONGITUDINAL ARCH

Purpose: To support the bones, ligaments, muscles, and accessory components on the plantar surface of the foot

Clinical Application: Arch sprains, shin splints, and common overuse injuries

Anatomical Structure: Plantar surface of the foot

Anatomical Position: Ankle should be positioned in a slight plantar flexed position.

Supplies: 1-in. and 1½-in. adhesive tape, 2-in. elastic tape, and heel and lace pad

Pre-taping Procedure: Place the heel and lace pad over the individual's posterior aspect of the heel

Taping Procedures

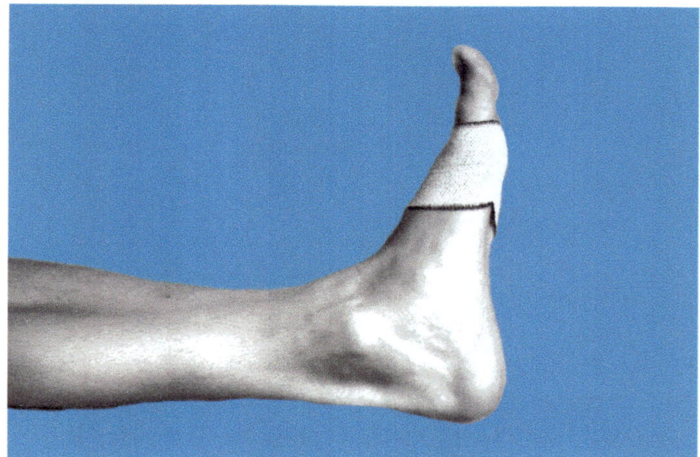

1. Place an anchor strip of 2-in. elastic tape around the metatarsals. This circular strip should begin on the dorsal aspect, go lateral, and continue across the plantar aspect to the medial portion of the foot, crossing the tape ends.

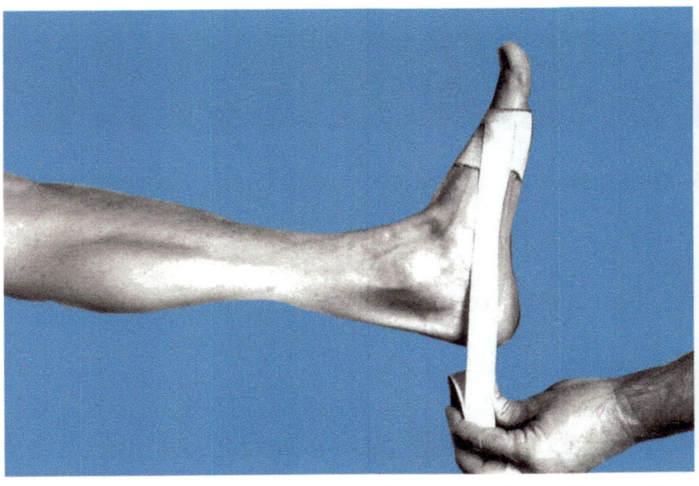

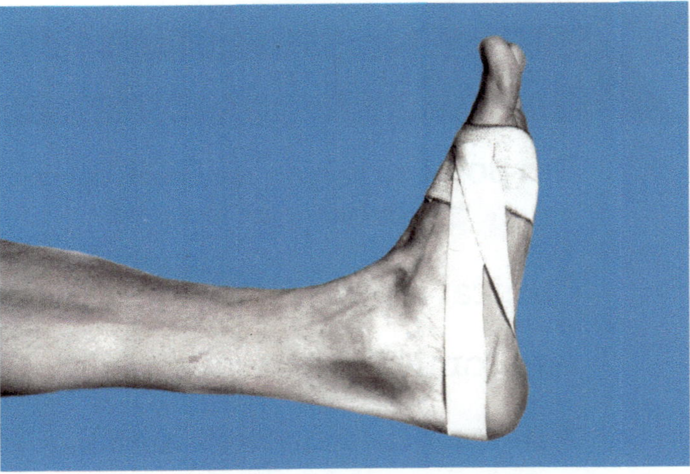

2. Next, starting at the medial aspect of the first MP joint, apply 1-in. adhesive tape along the medial margin of the foot and around the heel, pulling diagonally across the plantar surface and ending on the medial aspect of the first MP joint.

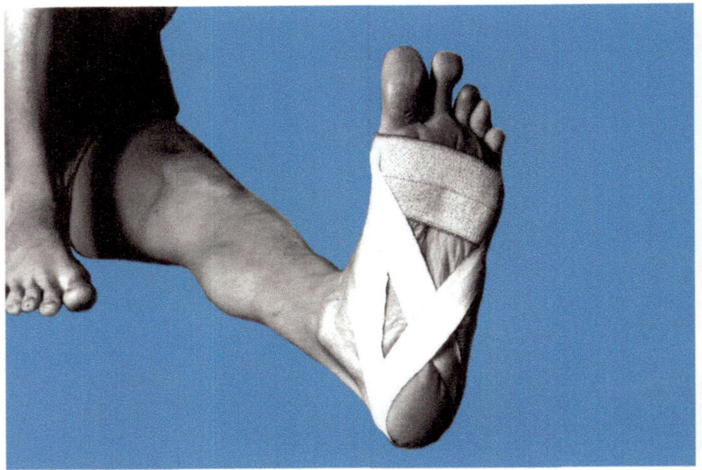

3. Start at the lateral aspect of the fifth MP joint and place a strip of 1-in. adhesive tape on the outside of the foot and around the heel, pulling diagonally across the plantar surface and going back to the lateral aspect of the fifth MP joint. Repeat steps 2 and 3. Remember to overlap the tape one half of its width.

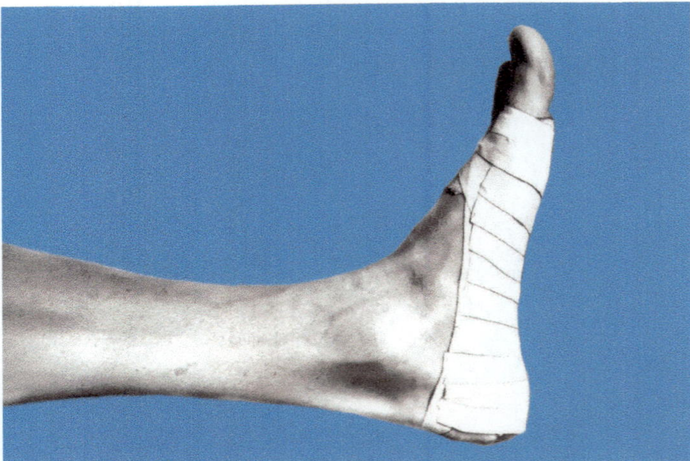

4. Starting at the proximal aspect of the foot, apply strips of tape from the lateral to medial side. The tape strips should cover the entire plantar surface of the foot. This should provide additional support to the inner longitudinal arch.

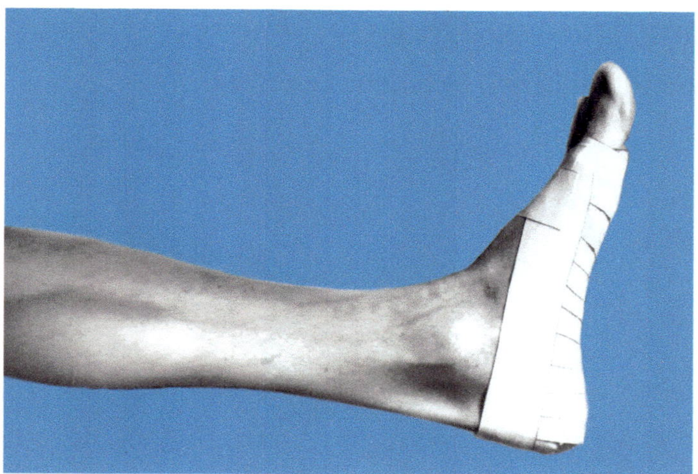

5. To close, apply a 1½-in. adhesive anchor strip from the medial aspect of the first metatarsal, around the heel, and to the lateral aspect of the fifth metatarsal head.

**Upon completion of the procedure, make sure you check for neatness and gaps, adequate support, along with proper function of the affected area. In certain situations, the individual might be asked to perform function tests to establish appropriate technique.*

Adjunct Taping Procedures: Medial Longitudinal Arch

This adjunct taping procedure can be used in conjunction with the basic technique presented.

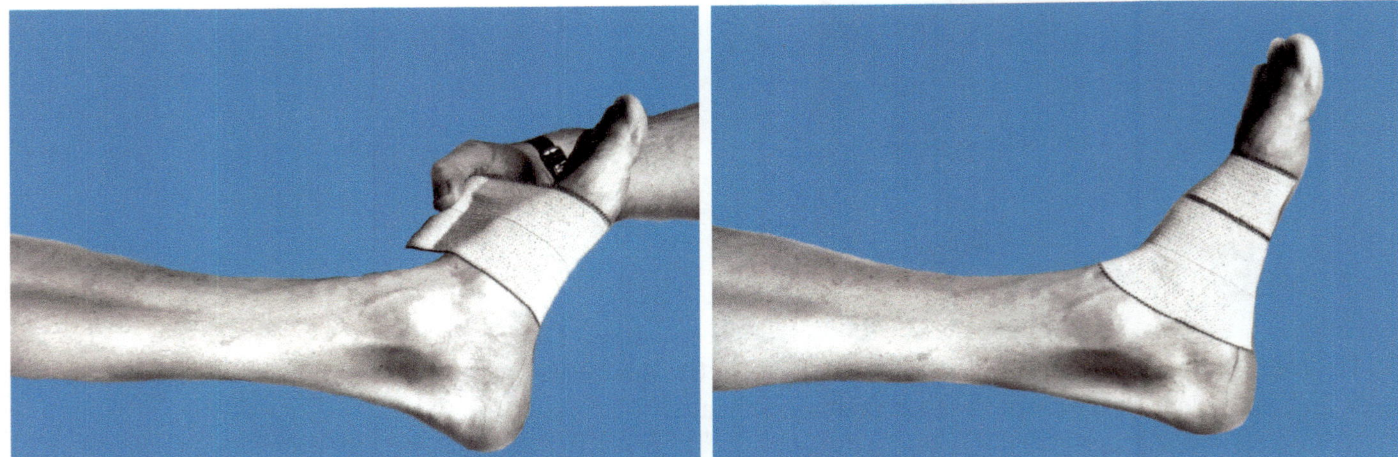

Technique A. Apply 3-in. elastic tape around the mid-foot area. It is preferred that this circular strip begin on the dorsal aspect, go lateral, and continue across the plantar aspect to the medial portion of the foot, crossing the tape ends.

TOE SPLINT

Purpose: To aid and support the injured phalanx

Clinical Application: Contusions, sprains, and strains to the phalanges of the foot

Anatomical Structure: Phalanges

Anatomical Position: Neutral position

Supplies: ½-in. adhesive tape and gauze, felt, and/or foam rubber

Pre-taping Procedure: Cut gauze, felt, or foam rubber to appropriate size

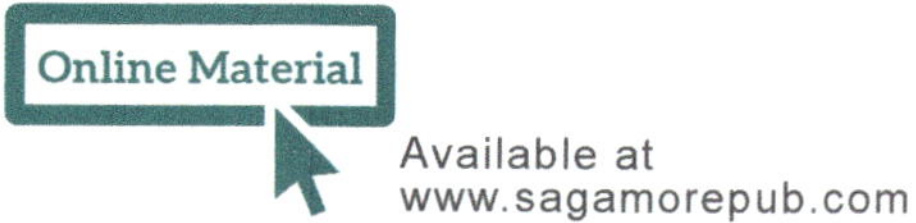

Available at www.sagamorepub.com

Taping Procedures

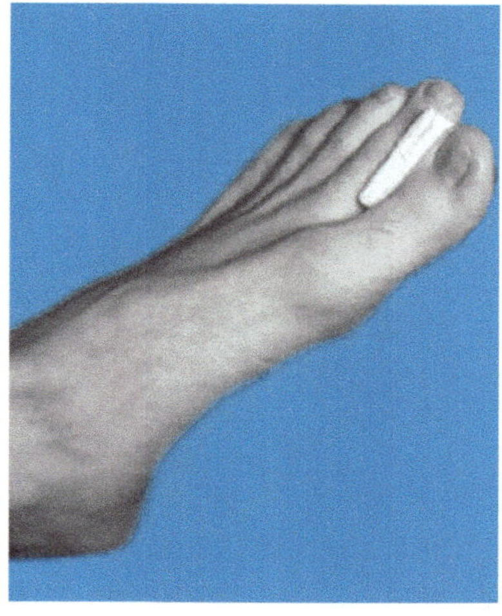

1. Place gauze between the affected and adjacent phalanges.

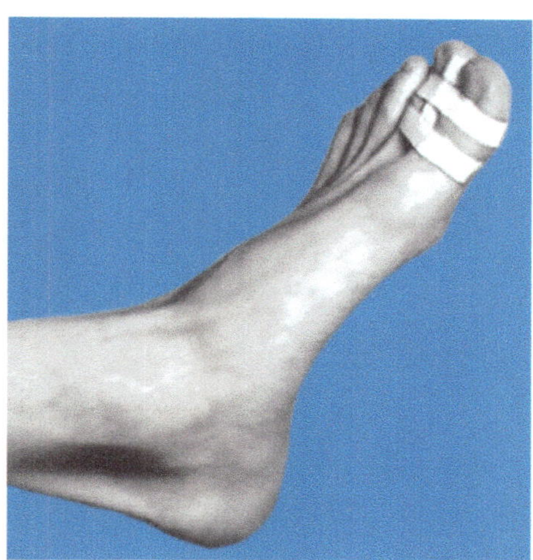

2. Then apply the ½-in. adhesive tape around both phalanges. This technique is known as buddy taping.

**Upon completion of the procedure, make sure you check for neatness and gaps, adequate support, along with proper function of the affected area. In certain situations, the individual might be asked to perform function tests to establish appropriate technique.*

PLANTAR FASCIITIS

Purpose: To aid in the reduction of stress on the plantar fascia and related foot structures

Clinical Application: Plantar fasciitis

Anatomical Structure: Plantar surface of the foot

Anatomical Position: Ankle placed in a slightly plantar flexed position

Supplies: 3-in. adhesive felt (moleskin), 2-in. elastic tape, and 1½-in. adhesive tape

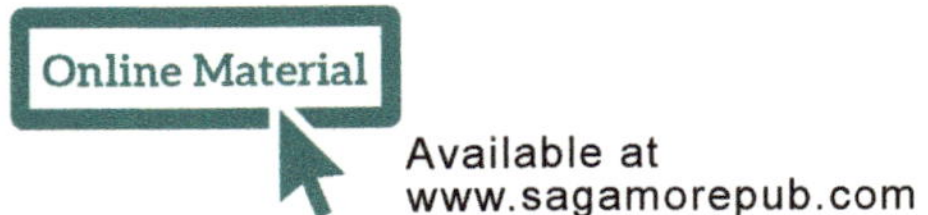

Pre-taping Procedure

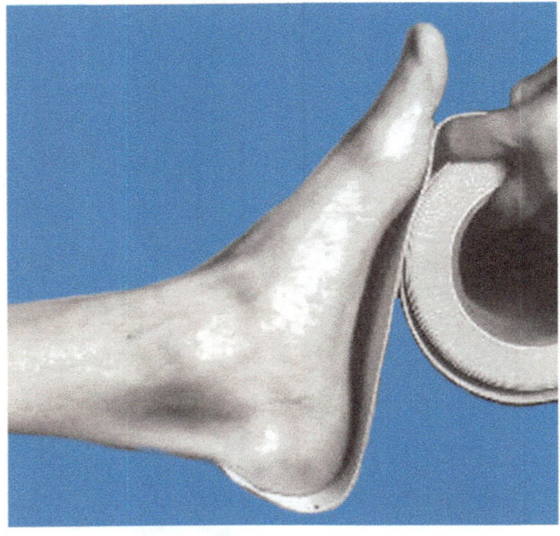

Before you begin, cut the adhesive felt to the length that measures from the metatarsal heads to the posterior aspect of the heel.

Taping Procedures

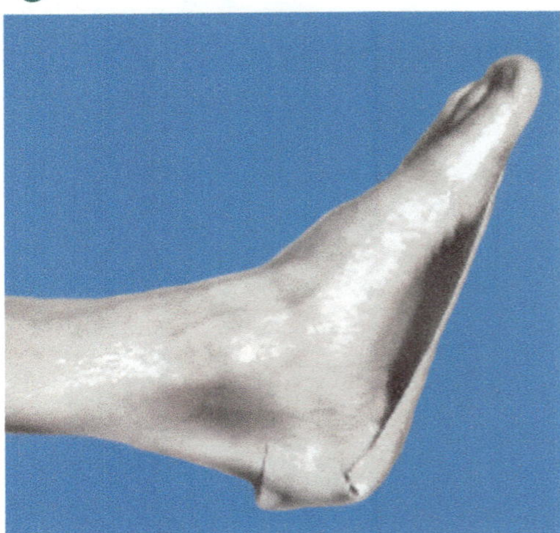

1. With the ankle slightly plantar flexed, apply the adhesive felt strip at the posterior aspect of the heel and firmly pull toward the metatarsal heads. To eliminate binding, cut a V on both edges of the adhesive felt where the felt crosses the heel area. Once adequate tension is applied, press the adhesive felt against the plantar aspect of the foot.

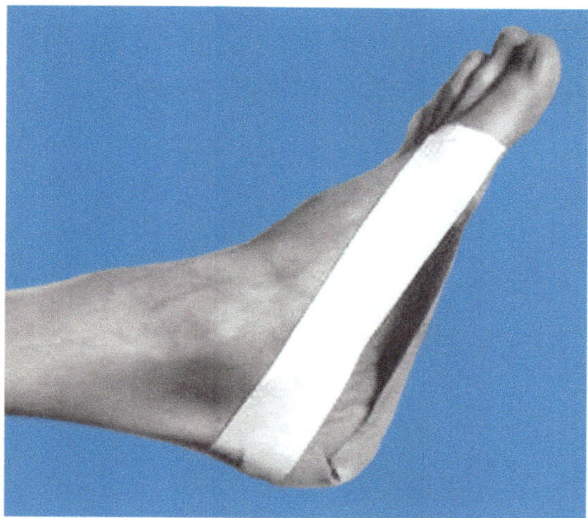

2. Apply a 1½-in. adhesive anchor strip from the medial aspect of the first metatarsal, around the heel, to the lateral aspect of the fifth metatarsal head.

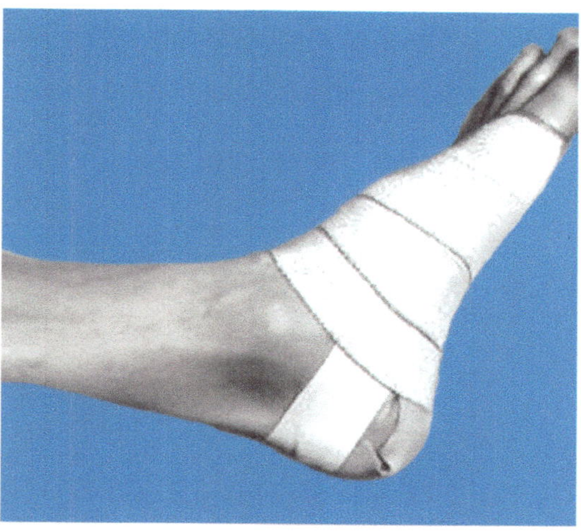

3. Apply 2-in. elastic tape around the mid-foot area. This circular strip should begin on the dorsal aspect, go lateral, and continue across the plantar aspect to the medial portion of the foot, crossing the tape ends.

**Upon completion of the procedure, make sure you check for neatness and gaps, adequate support, along with proper function of the affected area. In certain situations, the individual might be asked to perform function tests to establish appropriate technique.*

Adjunct Taping Procedures: Plantar Fasciitis

These adjunct taping procedures can be used in conjunction with the basic technique presented.

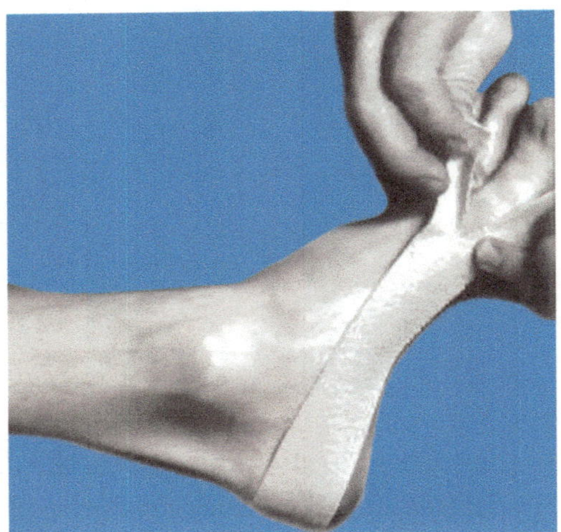

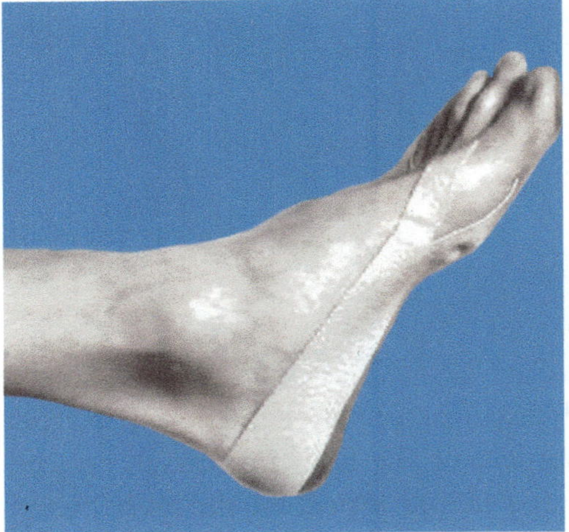

Technique A. The individual should be instructed to slightly plantar flex the ankle and flex the phalanges. Apply a 2-in. adhesive felt anchor strip from the medial aspect of the first metatarsal head, around the heel, to the lateral aspect of the fifth metatarsal head (allow 1 in. additional length on both ends of this strip). Split both ends of this strip of moleskin lengthwise approximately 2 in., and place the ends of the tape on the dorsal and plantar aspect of the first and fifth metatarsals.

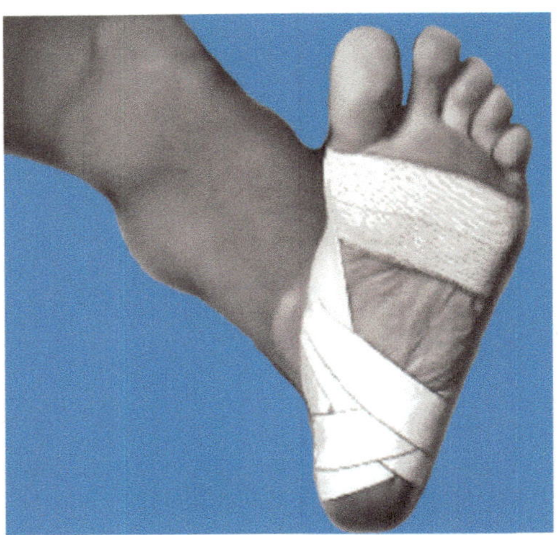

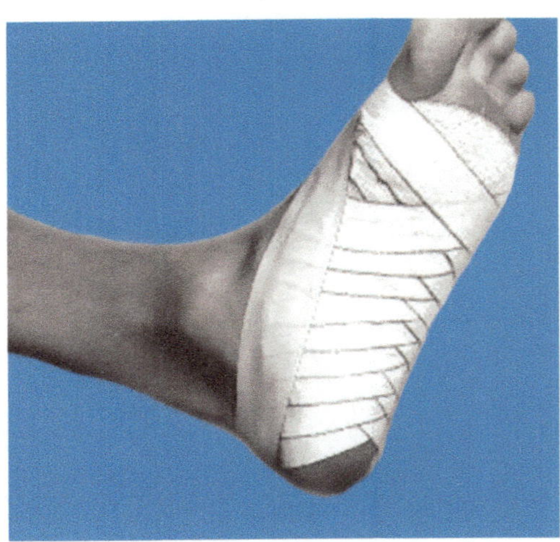

Technique B: X Pattern technique by following these steps:

1. Apply a 1½ in. adhesive tape anchor strip from the medial aspect of the first metatarsal head, around the heel, to the lateral aspect of the fifth metatarsal head.
2. Place an anchor strip of 2-in. elastic tape around the head of the metatarsals (lateral to medial). It is preferred that this circular strip begin on the dorsal aspect, go lateral, and continue across the plantar aspect to medial portion of the foot, crossing the tape ends.
3. Starting at the proximal aspect of the foot (heel), apply strips of 1-in. adhesive tape in a diagonal fashion (45 degrees). Alternate the application of the 1-in. strips from lateral to medial, and vice versa. Cover the entire plantar surface of the foot with the tape strips.
4. Apply a closure strip of 1½-in. adhesive tape from the medial aspect of the first metatarsal head, around the heel, to the lateral aspect of the fifth metatarsal head.

ANKLE–CLOSED BASKET WEAVE

Purpose: To support and stabilize the ankle joint for INVERSION sprains

Clinical Application: Sprains

Anatomical Structure: Ankle joint

Anatomical Position: Ankle joint in neutral position

Supplies: 1½-in. or 2-in. adhesive tape and heel and lace pads

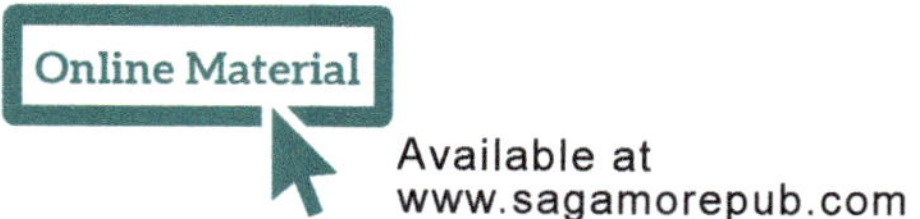

Pre-taping Procedure

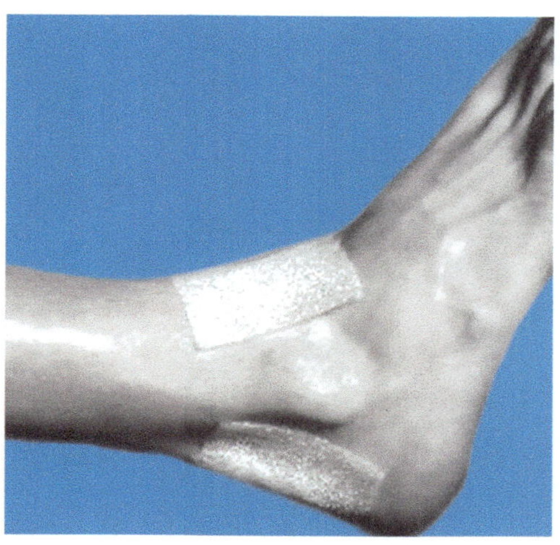

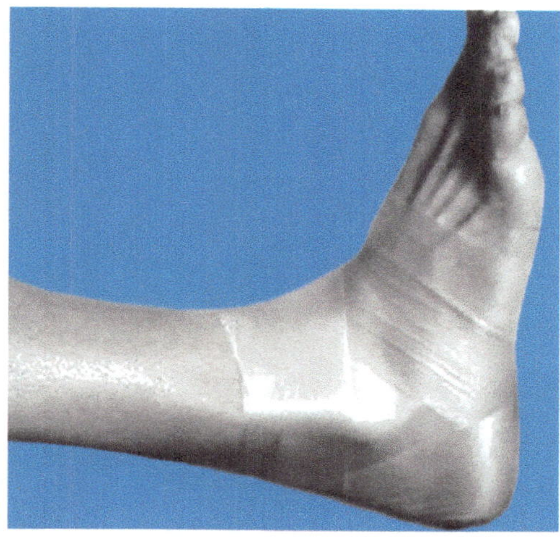

Before you begin taping, apply lubricated heel and lace pads at high friction areas: one at the distal aspect of the Achilles tendon and the other at the dorsal aspect of the ankle joint. Additionally, apply underwrap to secure the two heel and lace pads in place and reduce skin irritation. It is critical that the foot remain at a 90-degree angle for this procedure.

Taping Procedure

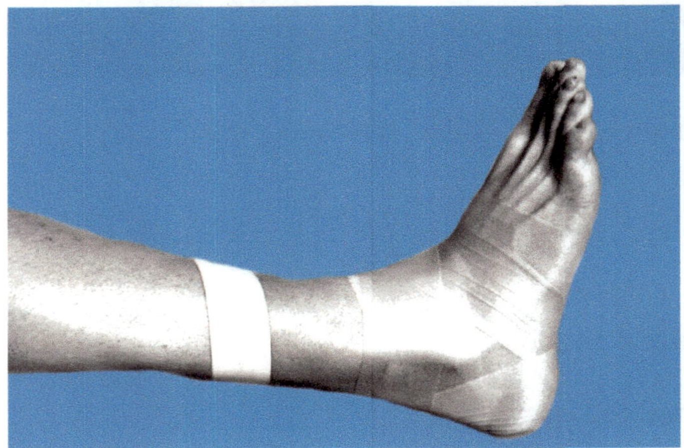

1. Because the leg at this site is slightly conical shaped, apply the tape at a slight angle. Apply an adhesive tape anchor strip around the lower leg at approximately the musculo-tendon junction of the gastrocnemius. Because the leg at this site is not cylindrically shaped, angle the tape slightly to conform to the leg.

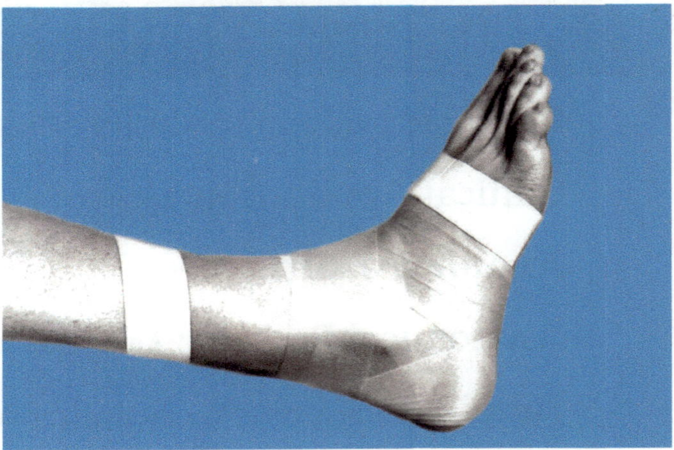

2. Apply an additional anchor at the instep. Remember that excessive tension on the fifth metatarsal could cause pain on weight bearing.

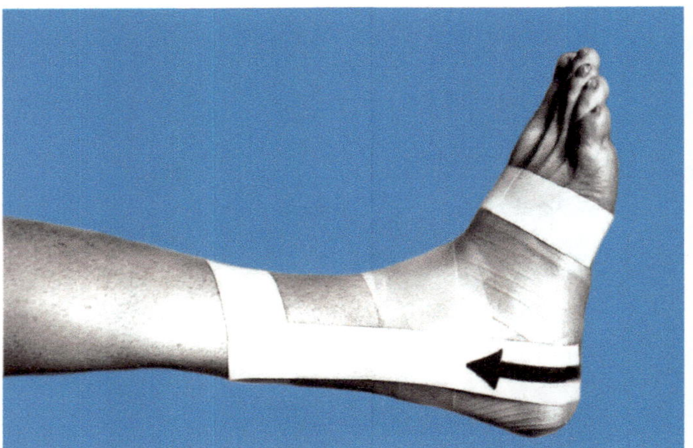

3. Apply the first of three stirrup strips. Beginning on the medial aspect of the upper anchor, continue this stirrup down the inside of the leg, over the medial malleolus, across the plantar aspect of the foot, over the lateral malleolus, and up the lateral aspect of the leg, ending at the lateral aspect of the upper anchor. Apply proper tension to cause some eversion of the foot, thus helping to reduce inversion.

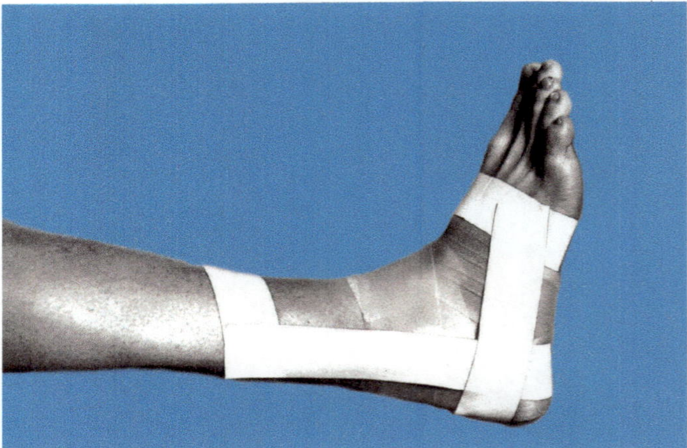

4. Apply the first of three horseshoe strips. The first horizontal strip is started on the medial aspect of the foot, continues toward the heel and below the medial malleolus, crosses the Achilles tendon below the lateral malleolus, and ends on the lateral aspect of the foot.

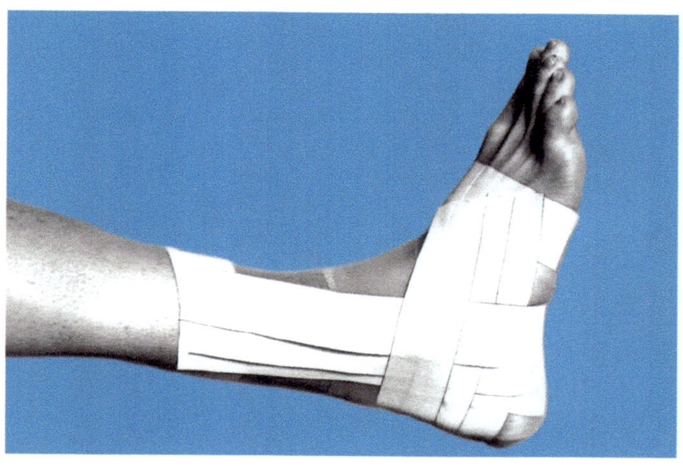

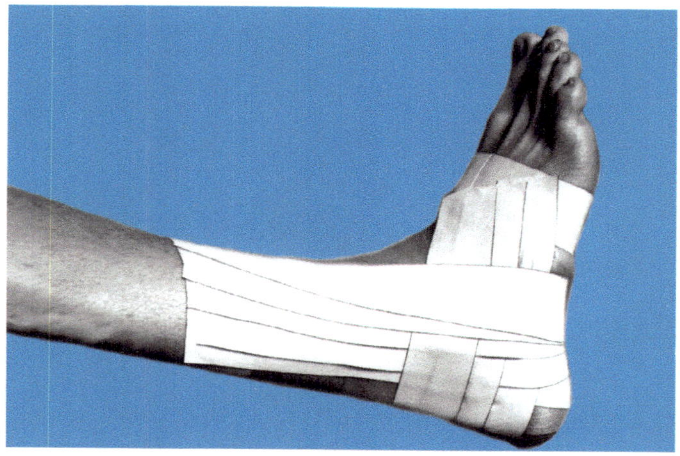

5. Repeat Steps 3 and 4 twice, overlapping the tape one half of its width. These interlocking strips should provide additional support for this technique. The completed portion of this closed basket weave has sets of interlocking stirrups and horseshoe strips. Apply a proximal anchor for support. For proper adherence, apply compression to the tape so that the tape conforms to the body part.

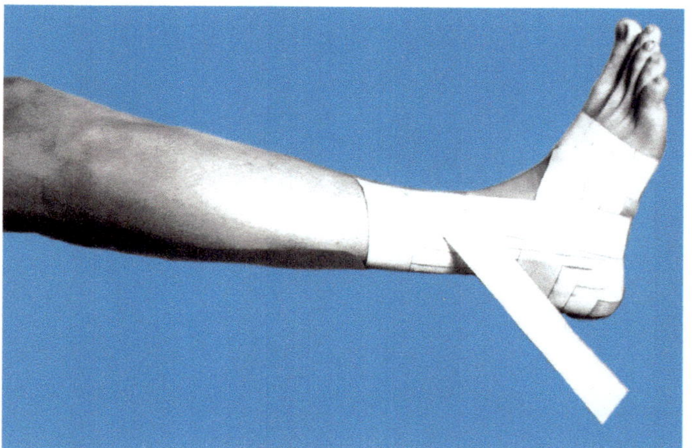

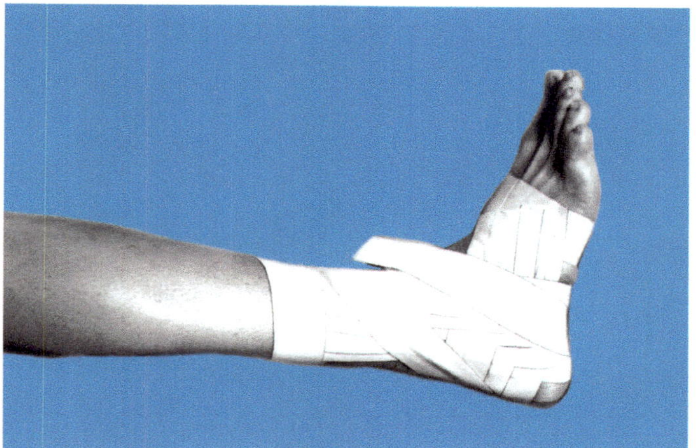

6. Apply the first heel lock strip. Begin on the anterior portion of the upper anchor, continuing down the outside of the leg, crossing the Achilles tendon around the medial aspect of the heel, angling underneath the foot, and moving up the lateral aspect of the leg. Apply proper tension to ensure stabilization of the calcaneus.

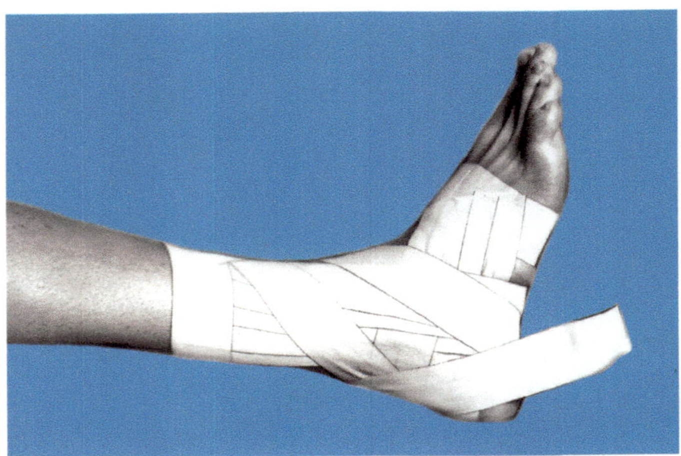

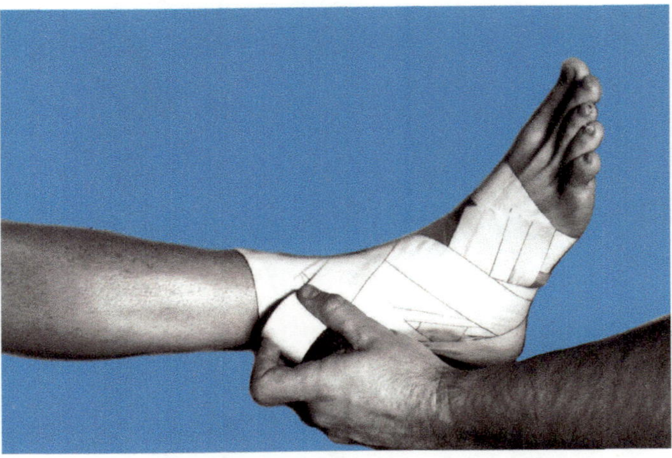

7. Apply the second heel lock strip. Begin on the anterior portion of the upper anchor, continuing down the inside of the leg, crossing the Achilles tendon around the lateral aspect of the heel, angling underneath the foot, and moving up the medial aspect of the leg.

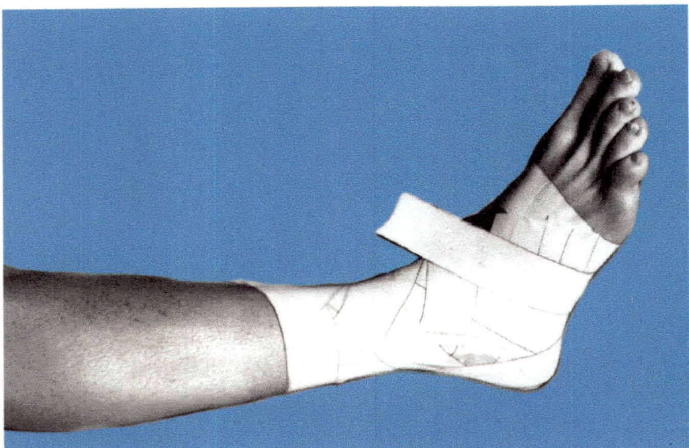

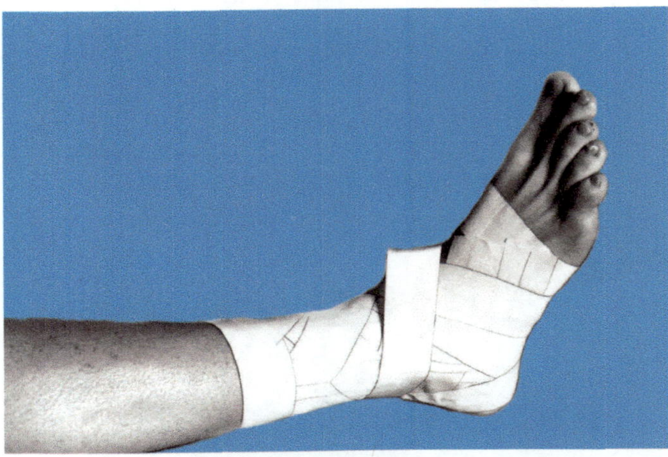

8. Apply a figure of 8. Starting on the dorsal aspect of the foot, move medially down the inside of the foot, across the plantar portion, up the outside of the foot to the starting point. Continue medially around the lower leg, crossing the Achilles tendon and finishing at the origin of this figure of 8 technique. By encircling the foot and leg, this technique will assist in dorsal flexion and eversion.

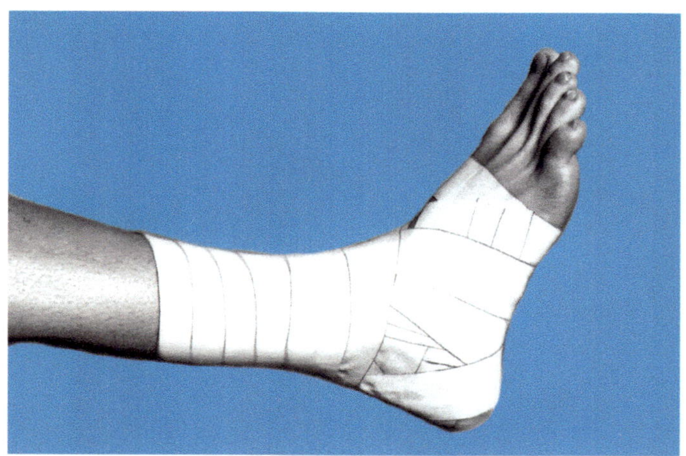

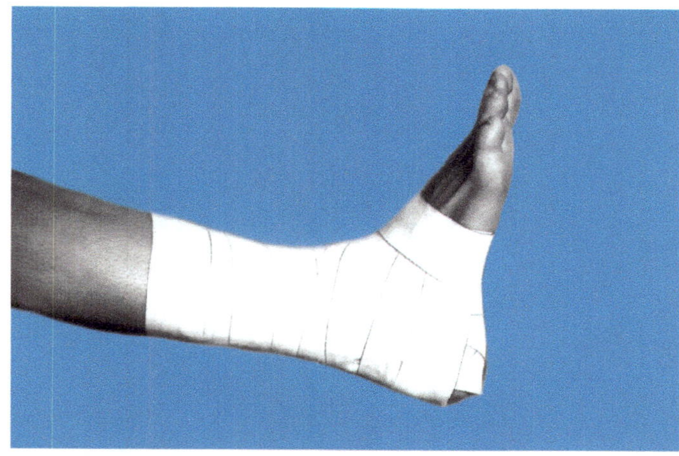

9. Apply final closure strips. Begin proximally and work distally. From the upper anchor, apply individual circular strips around the extremity to cover tape ends. Make sure you overlap the tape approximately one half of its width on each strip.

* *Upon completion of the procedure, make sure you check for neatness and gaps, adequate support, along with proper function of the affected area. In certain situations, the individual might be asked to perform function tests to establish appropriate technique application.*

Adjunct Taping Procedures: Ankle

These adjunct taping procedures can be used in conjunction with the basic technique presented.

Technique A. In conjunction with the stirrups, you can apply adhesive felt prior to the **adhesive tape** for additional support. It is recommended that the adhesive felt be placed on the plantar portion of the heel with equal tension applied both medially and laterally and/or tension bilaterally prior to attachment on the upper anchor.

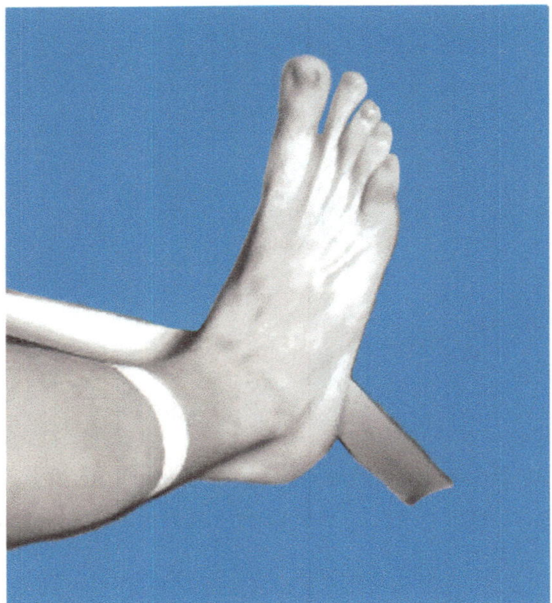

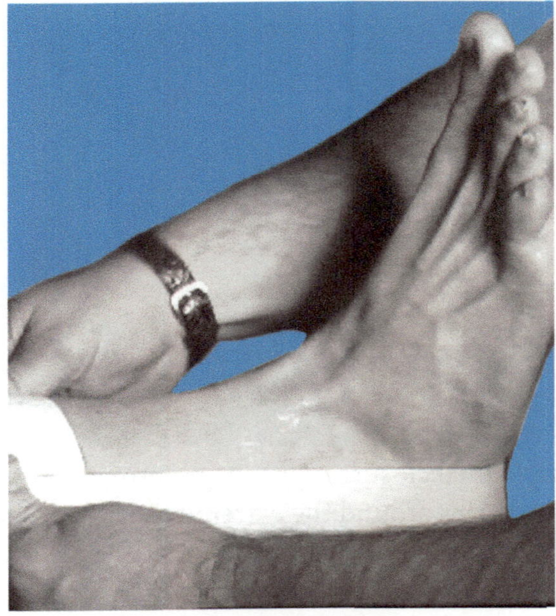

Technique B. In certain situations, joint trauma could be present on both the medial and lateral aspects of the ankle joint. It is recommended that the stirrups be placed on the plantar portion of the heel with equal tension applied both medially and laterally and/or tension bilaterally prior to attachment on the upper anchor.

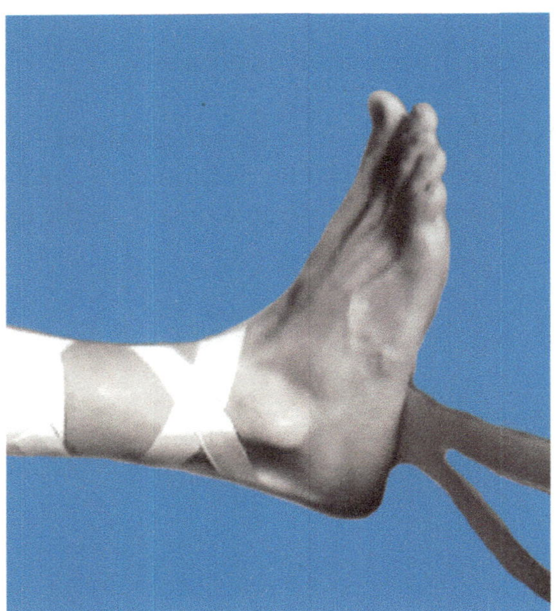

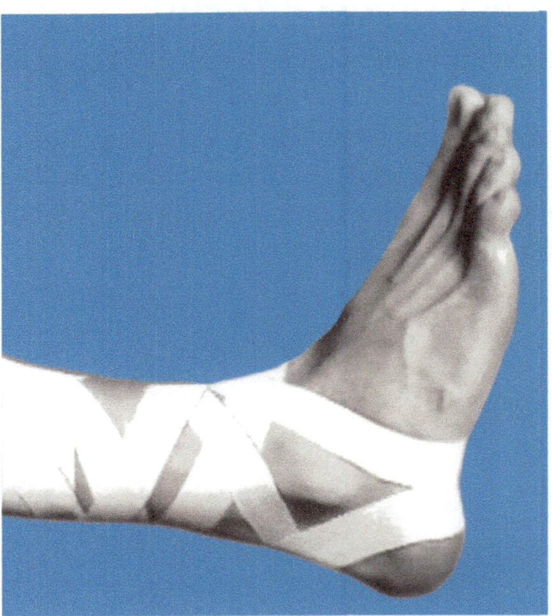

Technique C. This technique is known as the Spartan technique. Using 2-in. adhesive tape, approximately 24 in. to 30 in. in length, place the middle portion of this stirrup strip on the plantar portion of the heel. Split each end approximately 10 in. to 12 in. Starting on the medial side, place the first half strip below and in front of the medial malleolus and spiral up the leg. Place the second half of that strip below and behind the medial malleolus and spiral up the leg. Repeat this procedure on the lateral side. Two to three strips of adhesive tape with the Spartan technique can provide additional stability to ankle joint.

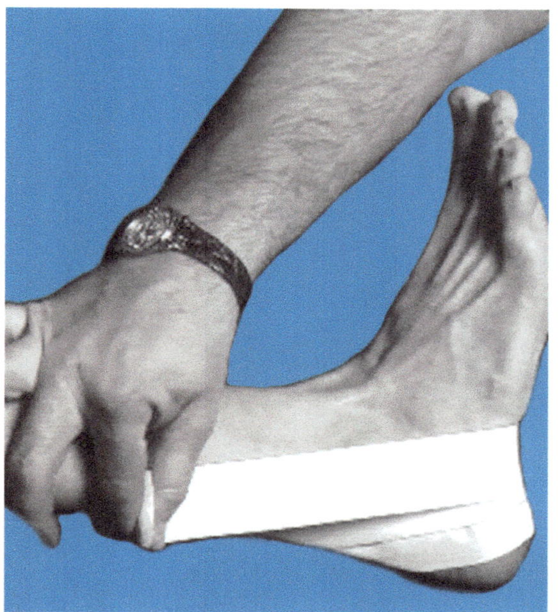

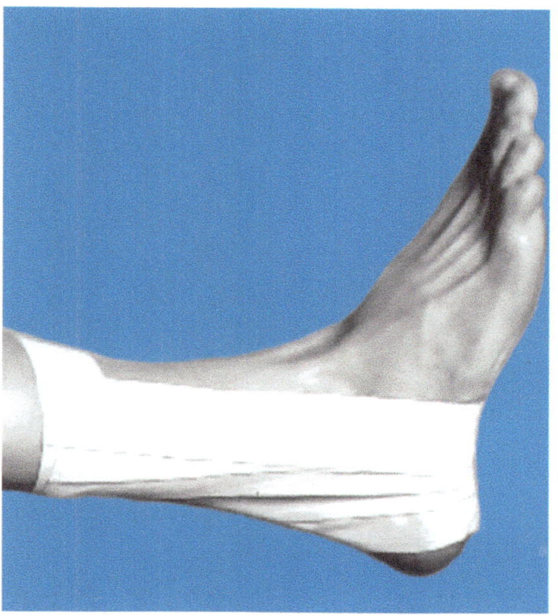

Technique D. The Side Bar technique will provide additional support to either the medial aspect or the lateral aspect of the ankle joint. Using 1½-in. adhesive tape, anchor lateral side bars on the medial aspect of the foot, angling underneath the foot, moving up the lateral aspect of the leg, and ending on the upper anchor. Depending on the size of the foot and severity of the injury, apply four to eight overlapping side bar strips.

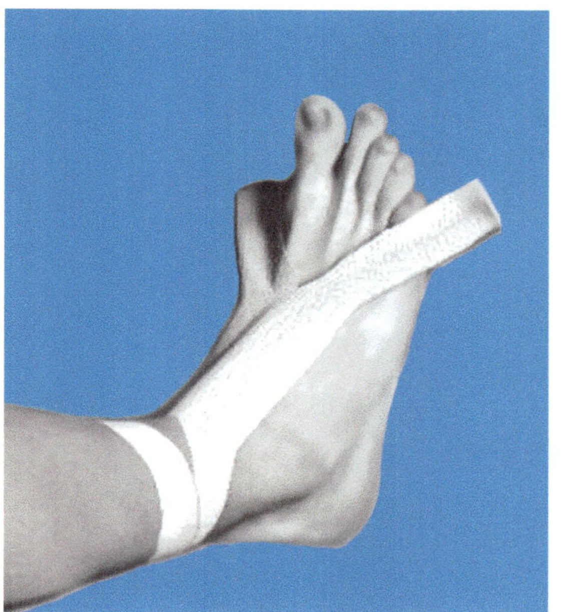

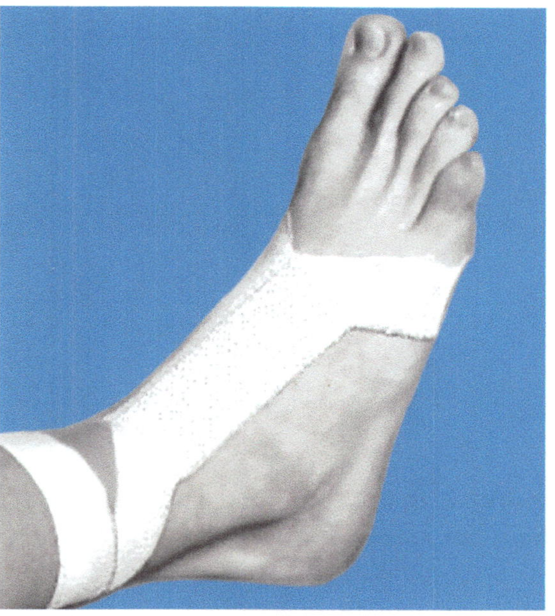

Technique E. The dorsal check rein aids in preventing the ankle joint from excessive plantar flexion. Using 3-in. elastic tape, cut a strip 12 in. to 15 in. in length, split both ends lengthwise approximately 4 in. With the ankle in neutral position, encircle the leg with one of the split ends, pulling the tape to full tension. Encircle the mid-foot region with the other split ends of the elastic tape.

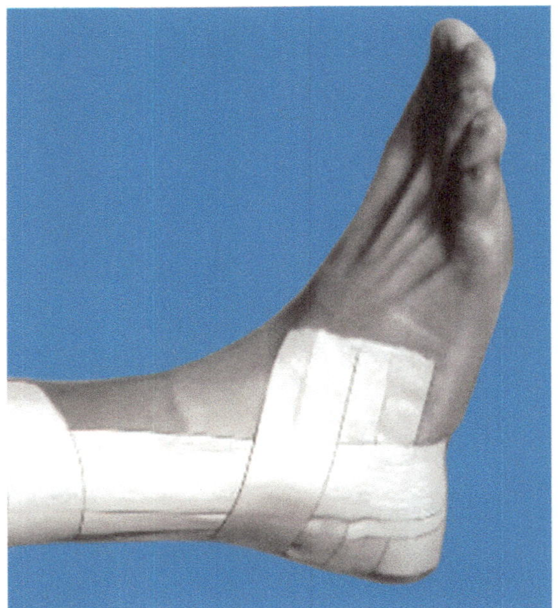

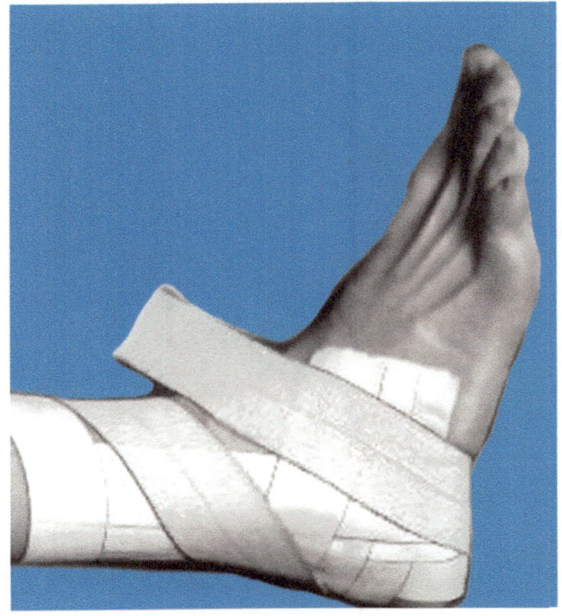

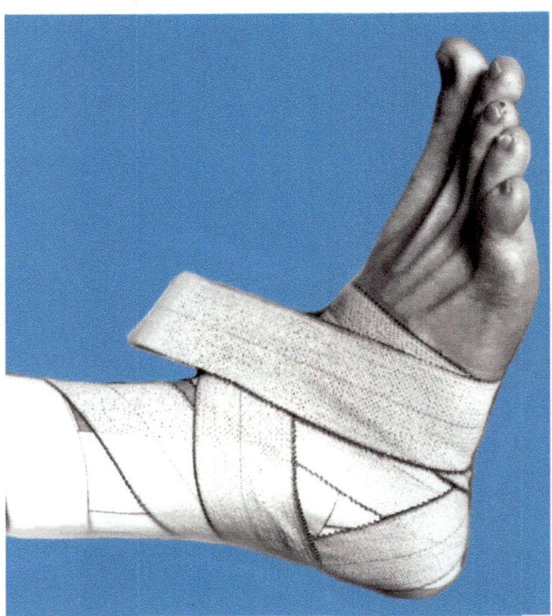

Technique F. In the combined elastic and adhesive tape technique, using 2-in. elastic tape, apply heel locks and figure of 8 in a continuous fashion.

*****High Ankle Sprain:*** Stabilizing the syndesmosis or high ankle ligaments and foot is critical when attempting to support an individual who has been evaluated by a health care professional with a *high ankle sprain.* The professional applying the taping techniques (*closed basket weave and their preferred adjunct taping procedures*), could provide additional support to the affected anatomical structures by using a protective device and/or properly fitted orthotics, which are displayed and/or described at the conclusion of this chapter.

ANKLE–OPEN BASKET WEAVE

Purpose: To provide compression and support to the ankle joint while allowing room for expansion due to swelling. This technique is commonly used for acute ankle injury treatment.

Clinical Application: Acute ankle sprain

Anatomical Structure: Ankle joint

Anatomical Position: Ankle joint in neutral position

Supplies: 1½-in. or 2-in. adhesive tape and 4-in. elastic wrap

Pre-taping Procedure: After hair removal, make sure the skin is clean and moisture free. Skin protection is important. Provide special care if the skin has allergies, infections, or open and closed wounds. Spray the affected area with an adherent to aid in the adhesive quality and provide stability to the supportive technique.

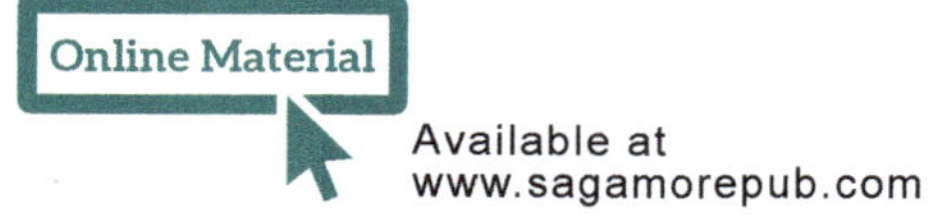

Available at www.sagamorepub.com

Taping Procedures

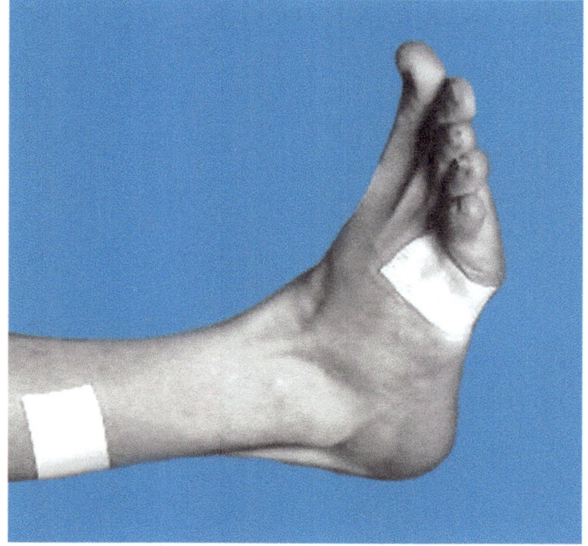

1. In this application, leave a 1-in. gap on the anterior aspect of the foot and ankle to allow for swelling. With the ankle joint in a neutral position, apply an adhesive tape anchor strip around the lower leg at approximately the musculo-tendon junction of the gastrocnemius. Because the leg at this site is not cylindrically shaped, apply the tape at a slight angle. Apply a distal anchor at the instep.

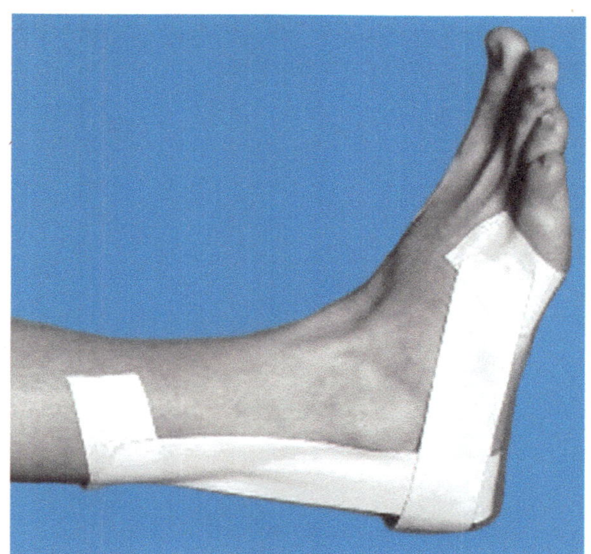

2. Apply the first stirrup strips. Beginning on the medial aspect of the upper anchor, continue this stirrup down the inside of the leg, over the medial malleolus, across the plantar aspect of the foot, and up the lateral aspect of the leg, ending at the lateral aspect of the upper anchor. Apply proper tension to prevent ankle inversion.

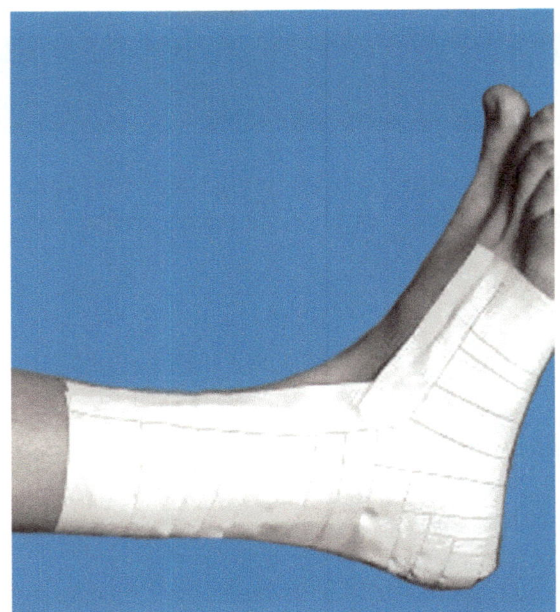

3. Apply the first horseshoe strips. The first horizontal strip is started on the medial aspect of the foot, continues toward the heel and below the medial malleolus, and crosses the Achilles tendon, ending on the lateral aspect of the foot. Remember to overlap the tape one half of its width, repeat steps 2 and 3. These interlocking strips provide additional support. Also, cohesive tape can be used to provide compression

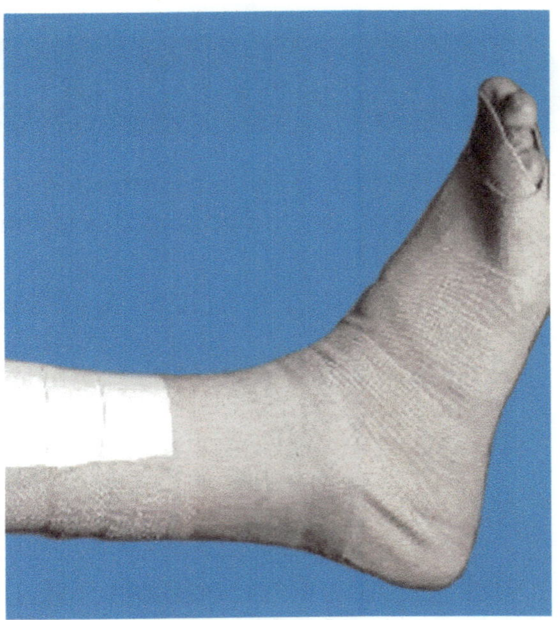

4 Using the 4-in. elastic wrap, begin the wrap at the distal part of the phalanges, spiral the wrap around the foot and ankle and up the leg. Secure the wrap with a small strip of adhesive tape. Also, cohesive tape can be used to provide compression.

**Upon completion of the procedure, make sure you check for neatness and gaps, adequate support, along with proper function of the affected area. In certain situations, the individual might be asked to perform function tests to establish appropriate technique.*

Adjunct Taping Procedures: Open Basket Weave

These adjunct taping procedures can be used in conjunction with the basic technique presented.

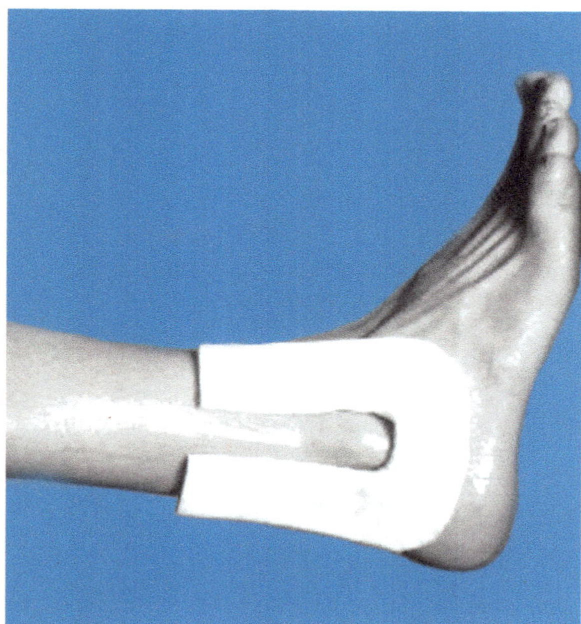

Technique A. Felt horseshoe. To apply additional compression to the lateral aspect of the ankle joint, construct a horseshoe out of ½-in. felt. Placement of this horseshoe is around the lateral malleolus, with the open ends of the horseshoe pointing upward and the curve of the horseshoe just distal to the malleolus. Then apply the open basket weave taping technique over the felt horseshoe.

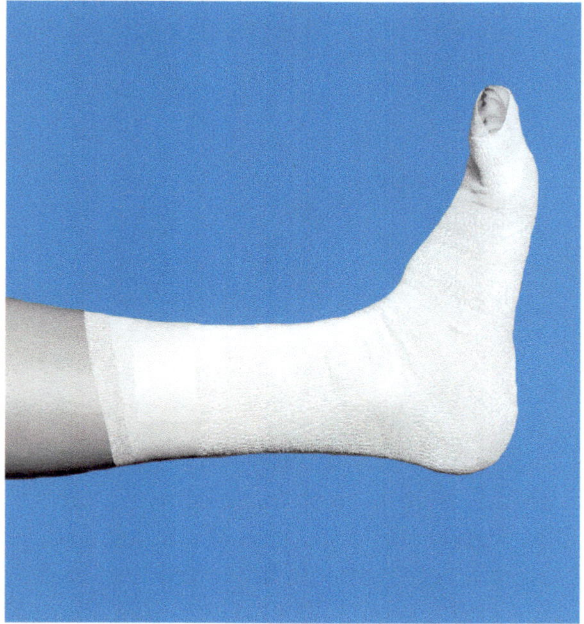

Technique B. Using cohesive tape, begin the wrap at the distal part of the phalanges, spiral the wrap around the foot and ankle and up the leg.

SHIN SPLINT

Purpose: To help reduce the pain associated with shin splints

Clinical Application: Shin splints (medial tibial stress syndrome)

Anatomical Structure: Lower leg, ankle, and foot

Anatomical Position: Knee should be fully extended and ankle joint slightly plantar flexed.

Supplies: ½-in. or ⅜-in. felt and 1½-in. adhesive tape

Pre-taping Procedure: Cut felt in 1-in. x 6-in. strip

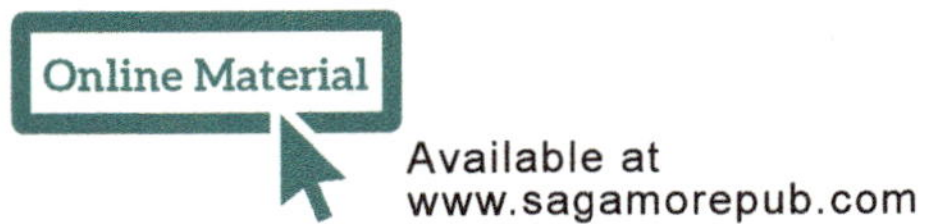

Taping Procedures

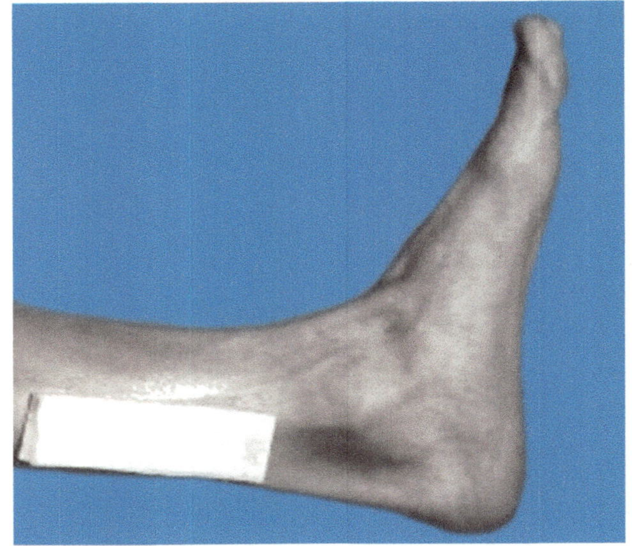

1. Place 1-in. x 6-in. felt strip over affected area.

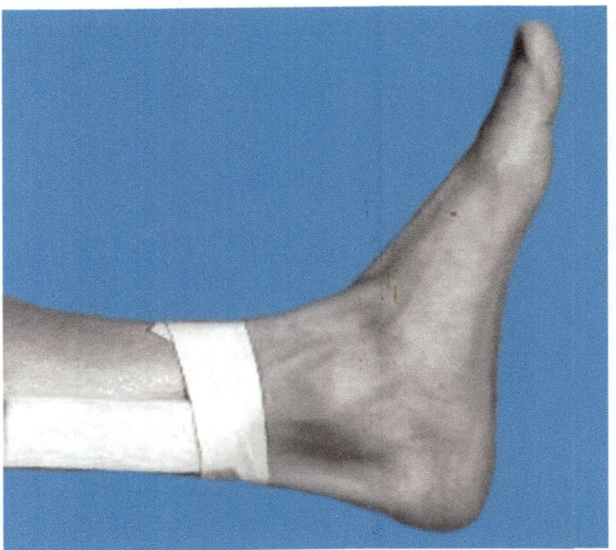

2. Apply an adhesive tape strip. Begin the tape 1 in. to 2 in. below the distal end of the felt pad, proceed laterally, cross the Achilles tendon, and pull the tape and felt back against the tibia. Tear the tape.

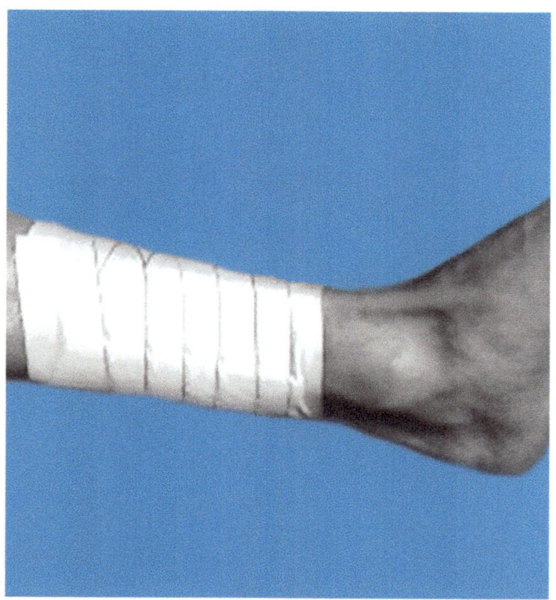

3. Apply four to six additional overlapping adhesive tape strips as applied in step 2.
Special Consideration: This taping technique is for pain on the medial aspect of the tibia. For pain on the lateral side of the tibia, pull the tape in the opposite direction.

**Upon completion of the procedure, make sure you check for neatness and gaps, adequate support, along with proper function of the affected area. In certain situations, the individual might be asked to perform function tests to establish appropriate technique.*

Adjunct Taping Procedures: Shin Splint

These adjunct taping procedures can be used in conjunction with the basic technique presented.

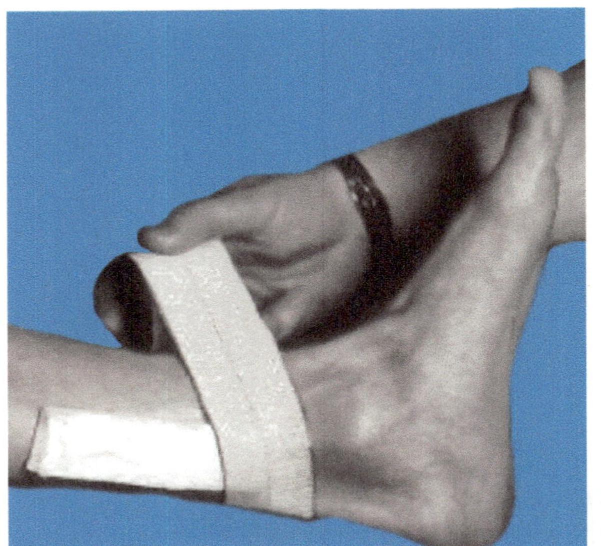

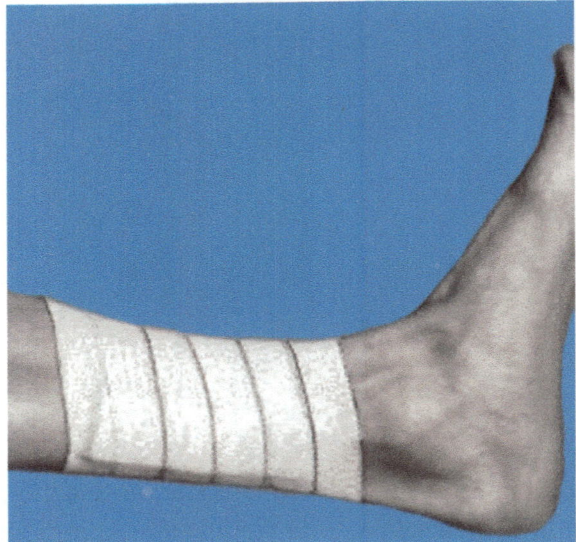

Technique A. Use 2-in. elastic tape in place of 1½-in. adhesive tape.

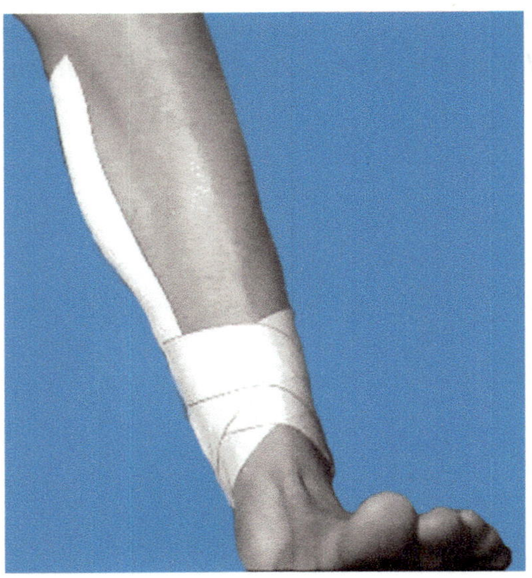

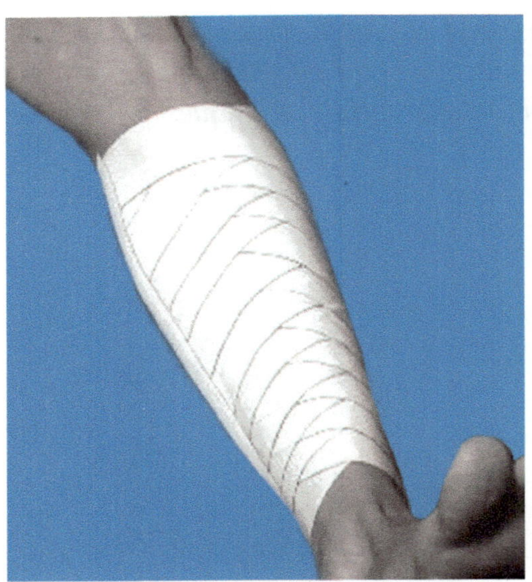

Technique B. X Pattern technique. Apply two vertical anchor strips, approximately 6 in. to 10 in. in length, over the medial and lateral aspects of the leg. Begin at the medial anchor, cross the anterior aspect at a 45-degree angle, and end on the lateral anchor. Apply the second strip from the lateral anchor, crossing the anterior aspect at a 45-degree angle and ending on the medial anchor. Repeat this step seven to nine times, overlapping the tape by one half of its width. Place a final anchor over each original anchor to help hold the tape in place. Do not cover the posterior aspect of the leg with adhesive tape.

ACHILLES TENDON

Purpose: To reduce the stress on the Achilles tendon

Clinical Application: Tendinitis and strains of Achilles tendon and posterior lower leg

Anatomical Structure: Achilles tendon, gastrocnemius, and soleus muscles

Anatomical Position: With individual in prone position, the ankle is placed in plantar flexion and knee in slight flexion.

Supplies: 1½-in. adhesive tape, 3-in. elastic tape, ½-in. felt, and heel and lace pads

Pre-taping Procedure: Apply heel and lace pads at high friction areas: one at the distal aspect of the Achilles tendon and the other at the dorsal aspect of the ankle joint.

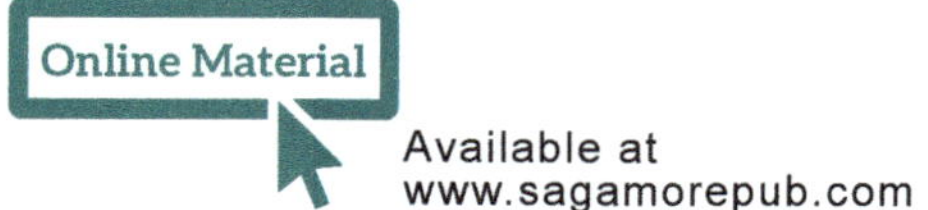

Available at
www.sagamorepub.com

Taping Procedures

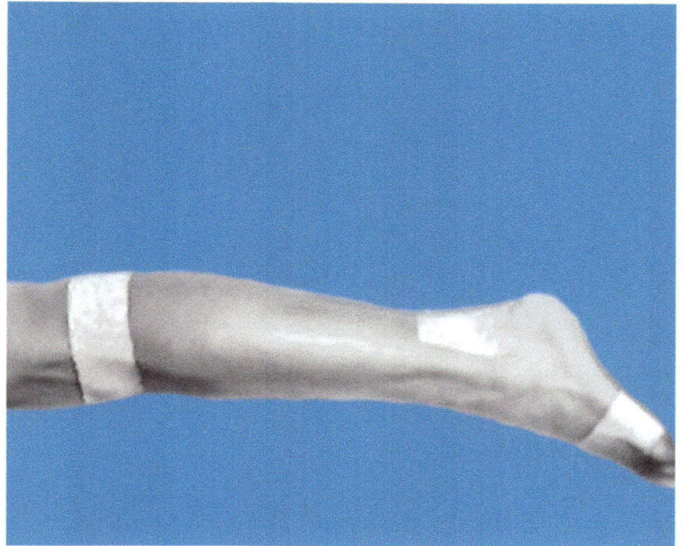

1. Apply two anchors using 3-in. elastic tape. Apply the proximal anchor on the proximal aspect of the gastrocnemius. Apply the distal anchor around the heads of the metatarsals (ball of the foot). It is preferred that this circular strip begin on the dorsal aspect, go laterally, and continue across the plantar aspect to medial side of the foot, crossing the tape ends.

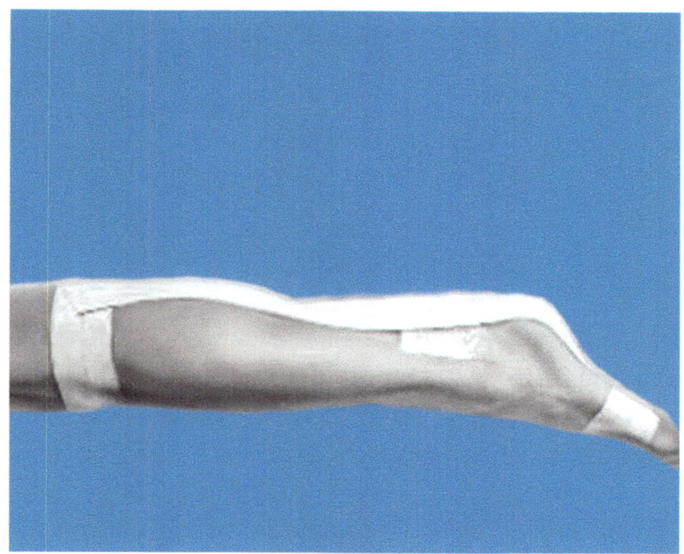

2. Using 3-in. elastic tape, measure on the posterior aspect the distance between the proximal and distal anchors. This will be the length required for your support strips. Apply the first support strip of elastic tape, going from the proximal anchor to the distal anchor. Upon application, apply full tension to the tape ends. Note that slight knee flexion and plantar flexion is maintained so that there is a small degree of tension across this first support strip.

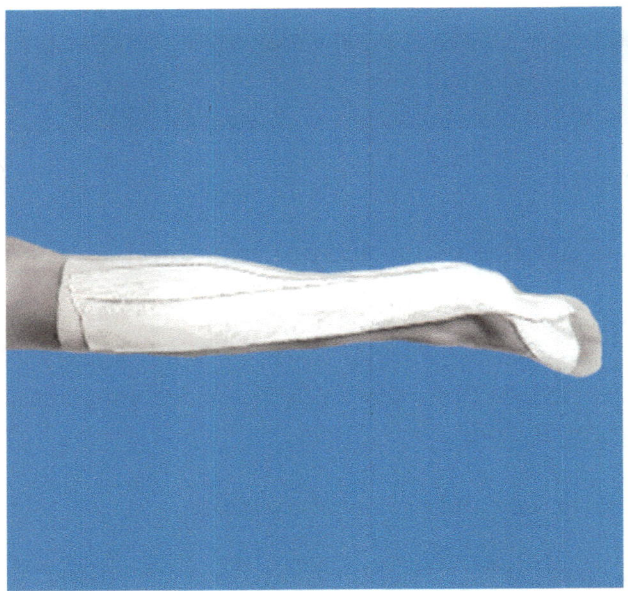

3. Apply additional strips of support in an angular fashion to cover the posterior aspect of the leg and the plantar aspect of the foot. For proper adherence, apply compression to the tape so that the tape conforms to the body parts.

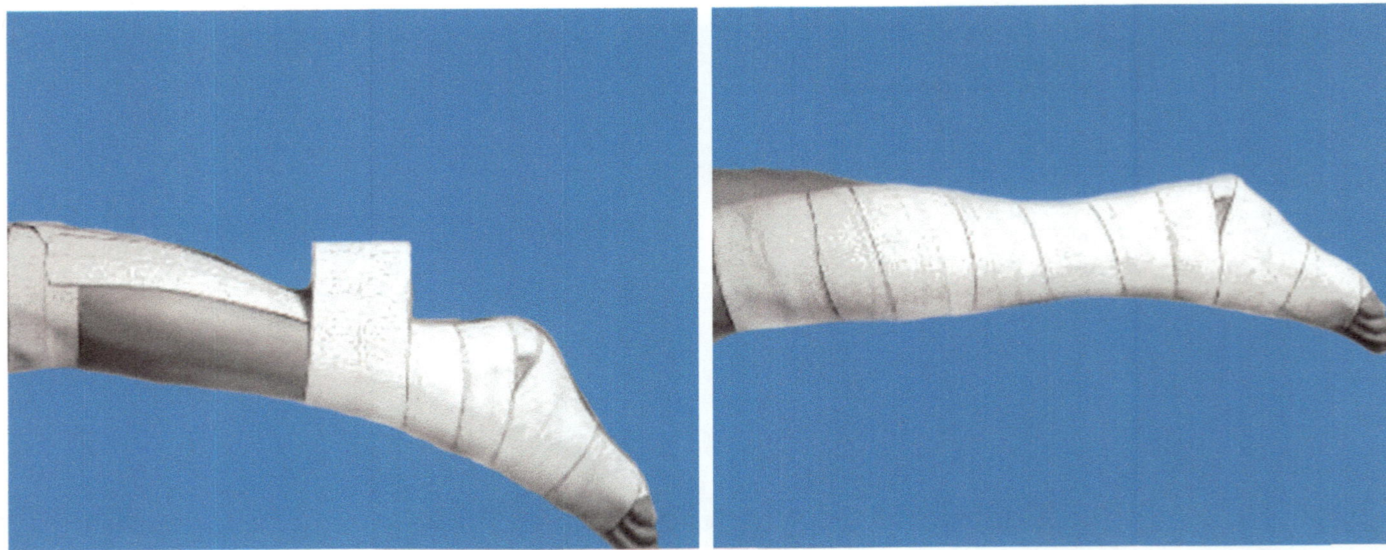

4. Using 3-in. elastic tape, close up the procedure by overlapping the tape by one half of its width on each revolution.
Comment: Secure the elastic tape ends with anchors of 1½-in. adhesive tape.

**Upon completion of the procedure, make sure you check for neatness and gaps, adequate support, along with proper function of the affected area. In certain situations, the individual might be asked to perform function tests to establish appropriate technique.*

Adjunct Taping Procedures: Achilles Tendon

This adjunct taping procedure can be used in conjunction with the basic technique presented.

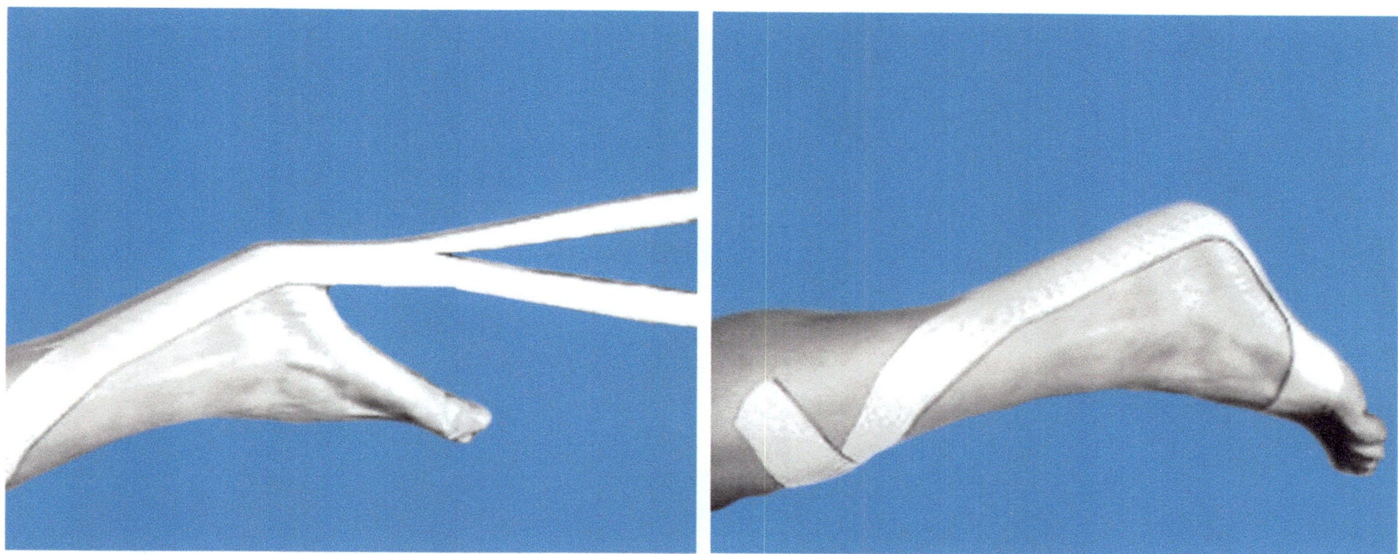

Technique A: Achilles tendon check rein. This technique will aid in preventing the ankle joint from excessive dorsiflexion. Using 3-in. elastic tape, cut a strip 15 in. to 20 in. in length, split both ends lengthwise approximately 5 in. to 7 in. With the ankle in plantar flexion, encircle the mid-portion of the lower leg with the split ends of the elastic tape. Pull the tape to full tension, crossing the heel and rear foot region. Encircle the mid-foot region with the other split ends of the elastic tape. Secure this technique with two anchors of 1½-in. adhesive tape.

Adjunct Padding Procedures: Achilles Tendon

These adjunct padding procedures can be used in conjunction with the basic technique presented.

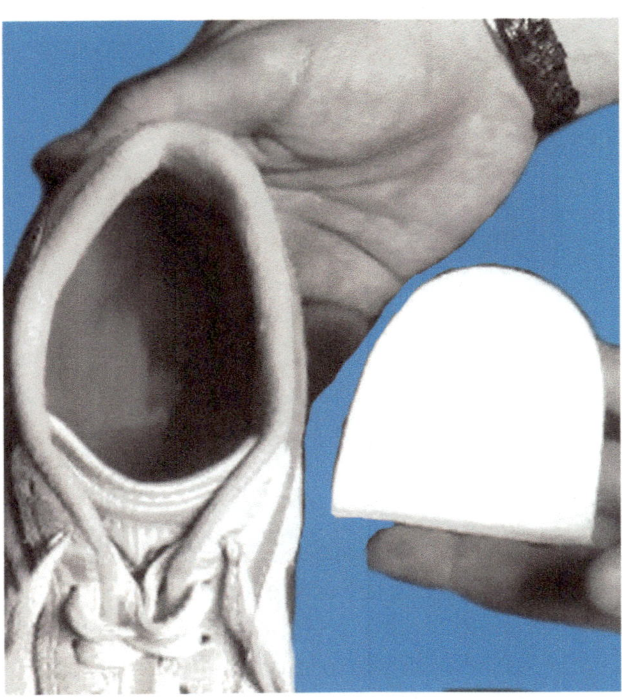

Special Padding Procedure A. Using 1/2-in. felt, cut a heel lift to be placed in the posterior aspect of the shoe. Place a similar felt heel lift in the shoe of the unaffected foot.

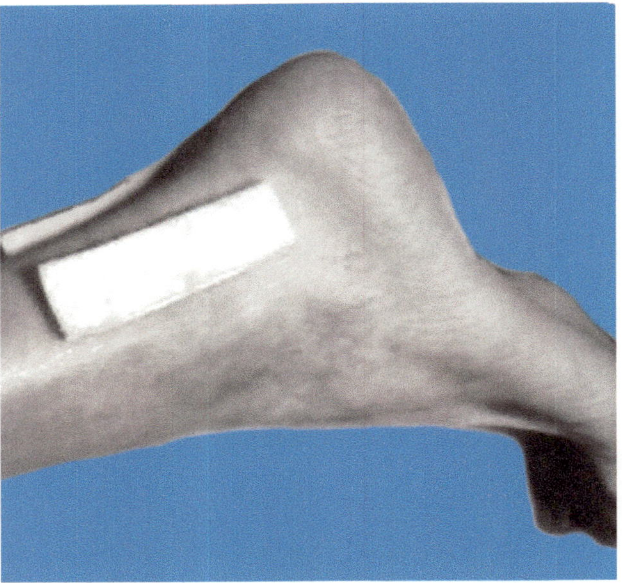

Special Padding Procedure B: Achilles tendon strips. To reduce pressure on the tendon, cut two strips of ½-in. felt, 1 in. x 3 in. Place one strip lateral and a second strip medial to the Achilles tendon. This will help reduce pressure on the Achilles tendon when the shoe is worn.

Wrapping Techniques for Support

During physical activity, supportive wraps are used to aid in muscle function and support and to reduce excessive range of motion. These applications are typically used in competition or practice. Spica wraps are traditionally employed at the hip and shoulder joints. Figure of eight wraps are placed over ankle, knee, elbow, wrist, and hand joints.

ANKLE WRAP–COHESIVE

Purpose: To provide support to the ankle joint

Clinical Application: Ankle sprains

Anatomical Structure: Ankle joint

Anatomical Position: Ankle in neutral position (90 degrees)

Supplies: Cohesive tape

Pre-wrapping Procedure: With the ankle in neutral position, instruct the individual to contract the muscles of the foot, ankle, and lower leg

Wrapping Procedures

A continuous wrap is used in this preventive technique and consists of a figure of 8 and medial and lateral heel locks and finishes with a figure of 8.

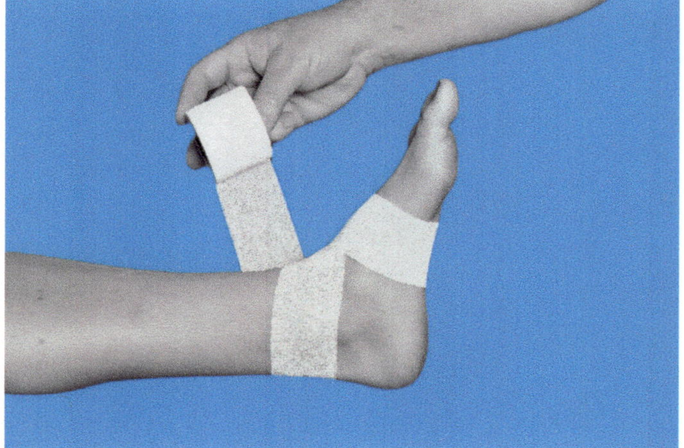

1. Figure of 8. Starting on the dorsal aspect of the foot, move medially down the inside of the foot, across the plantar portion, up the outside of the foot to the starting point. Continuation of the cohesive tape will proceed medially around the lower leg, crossing the Achilles tendon, returning to the origin of this figure of 8 technique.

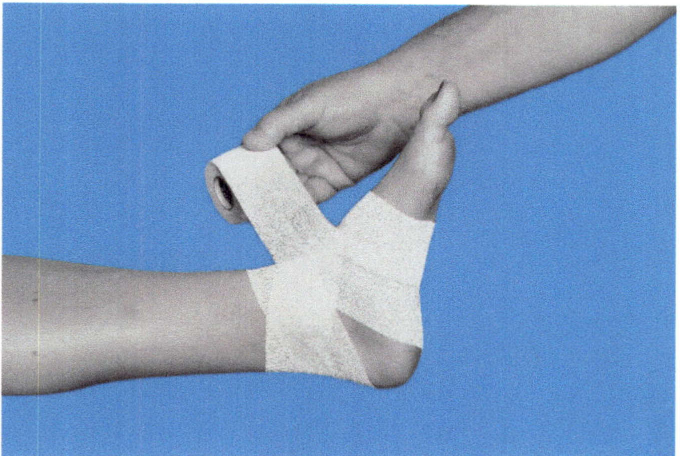

2. Apply the medial heel lock. This cohesive tape continues across the medial malleolus, crosses the Achilles tendon, goes around the lateral aspect of the heel, angles underneath the foot, and moves up to the dorsum of the foot.

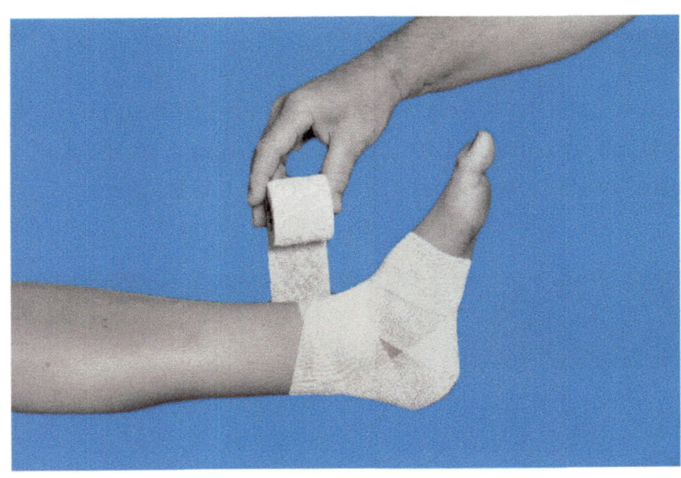

3. Continue the lateral heel lock across the lateral malleolus, cross the Achilles tendon, go around the medial aspect of the heel, angle underneath the foot, and move up to the dorsum of the foot.

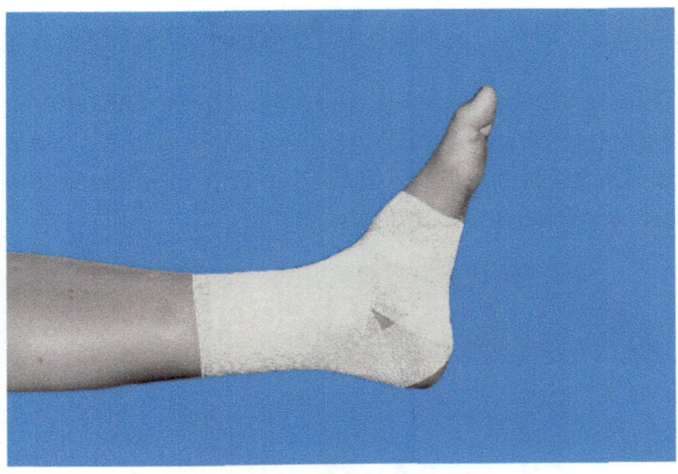

4. Repeat Step 1 (figure of 8 wrap).

**Upon completion of the procedure, make sure you check for neatness and gaps, adequate support, along with proper function of the affected area. In certain situations, the individual might be asked to perform function tests to establish appropriate technique.*

ANKLE WRAP–CLOTH

Purpose: To provide support to the ankle joint

Clinical Application: Ankle sprains

Anatomical Structure: Ankle joint

Anatomical Position: Ankle in neutral position (90 degrees)

Supplies: 2-in. cloth wrap (72 in. to 96 in.) and 1½-in. adhesive or elastic tape

Pre-wrapping Procedure: With the ankle in neutral position, apply the athletic sock. Instruct the individual to contract the muscles of the foot, ankle, and lower leg

Wrapping Procedures

A continuous wrap is used in this preventive technique and consists of a figure of eight and medial and lateral heel locks and finishes with a figure of 8.

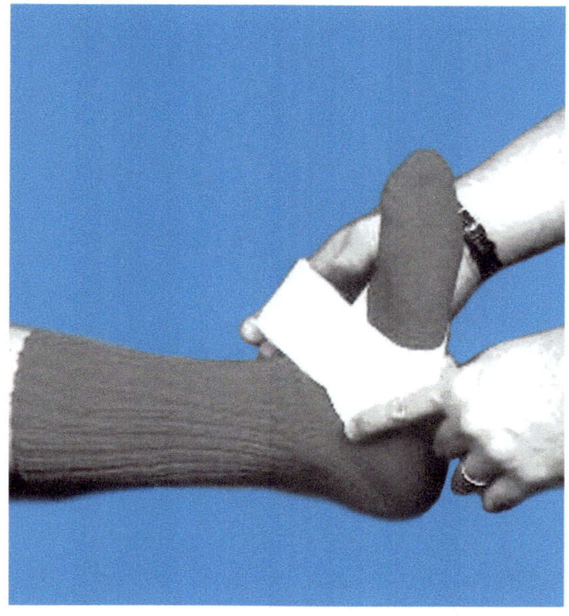

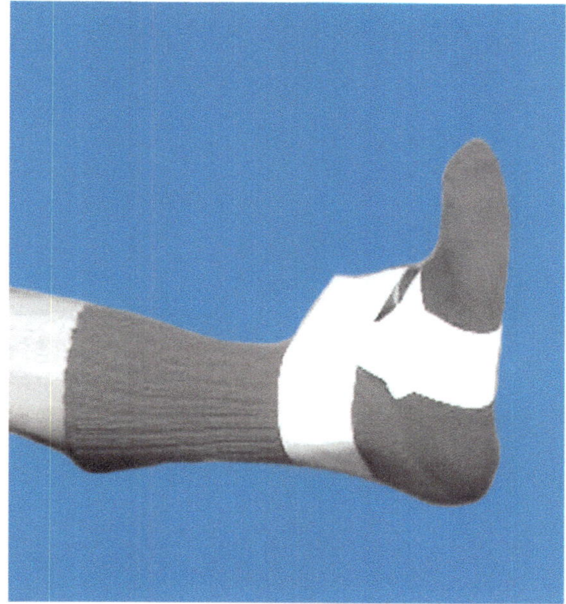

1. Figure of 8. Starting on the dorsal aspect of the foot, move medially down the inside of the foot, across the plantar portion, up the outside of the foot to the starting point. Continue the wrap medially around the lower leg, crossing the Achilles tendon, returning to the origin of this figure of 8 technique.

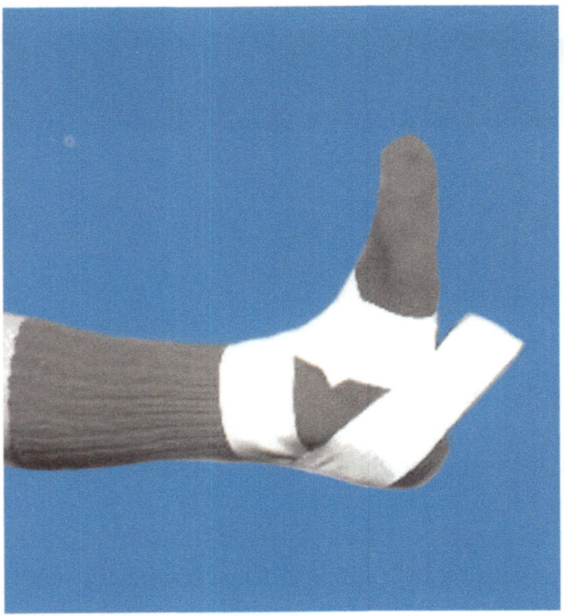

2. Apply the medial heel lock. This wrap continues across the medial malleolus, crosses the Achilles tendon, goes around the lateral aspect of the heel, angles underneath the foot, and moves up to the dorsum of the foot.

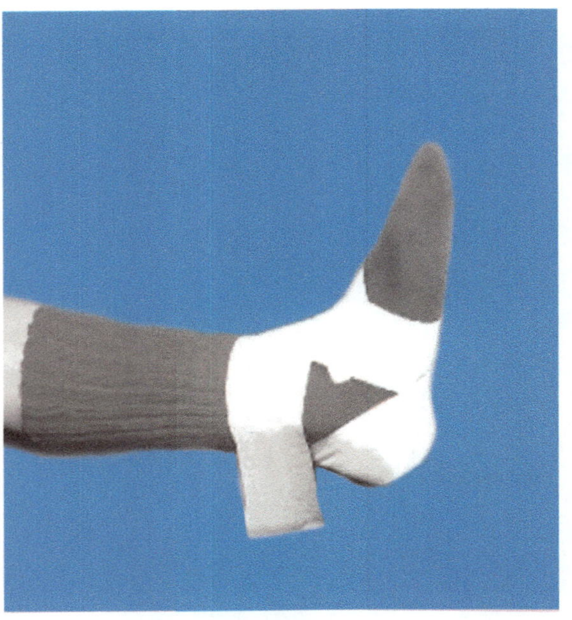

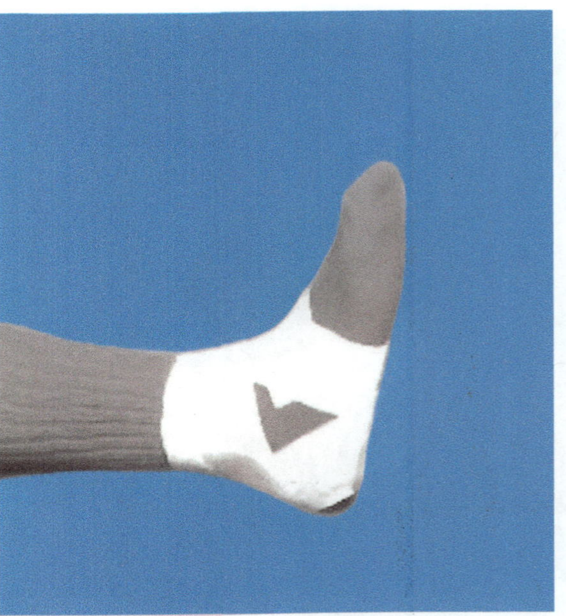

3. Continue the lateral heel lock wrap across the lateral malleolus, move across the Achilles tendon, go around the medial aspect of the heel, angle underneath the foot, and move up to the dorsum of the foot.

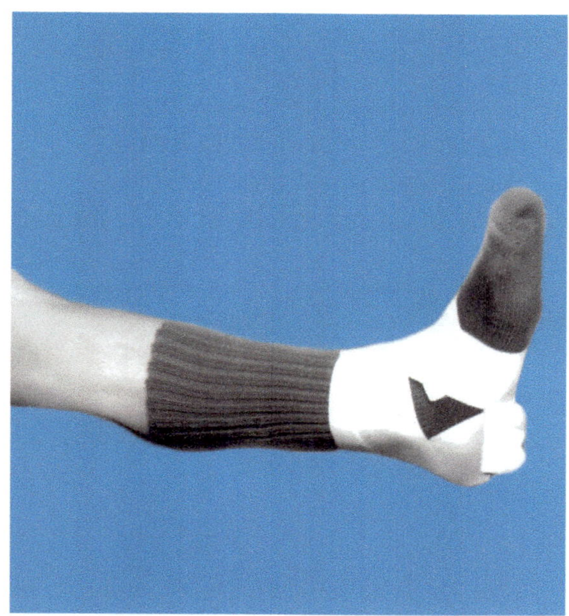

4. Repeat Step 1 (figure of 8 wrap).

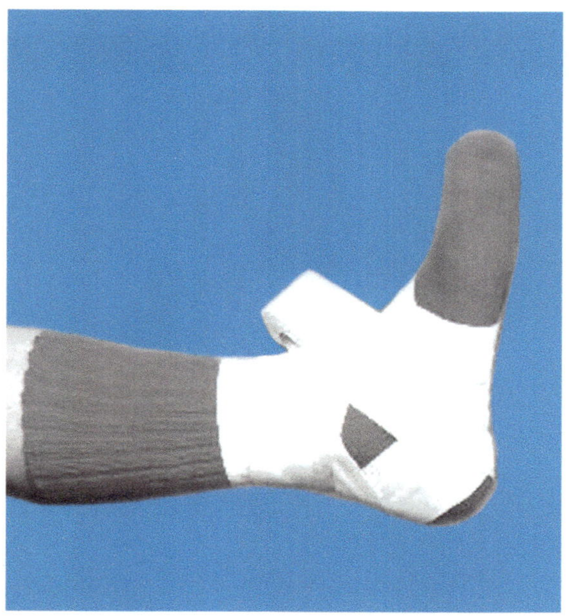

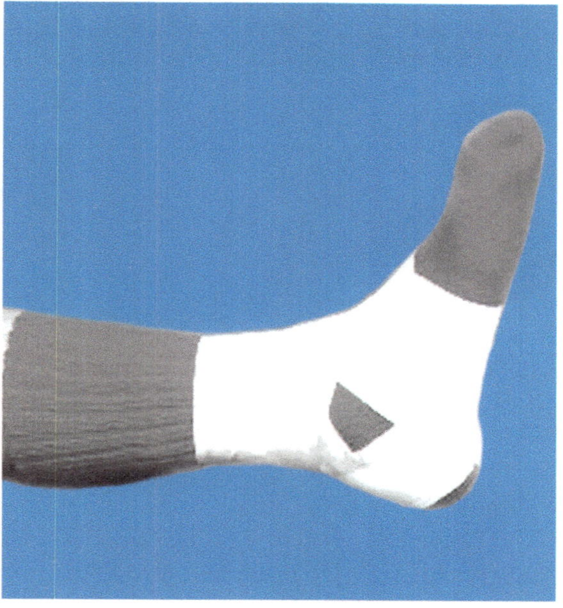

5. Reinforce this procedure by applying 1½-in. adhesive or elastic tape to construct extra figures of 8 and heel locks over the cloth wrap.

**Upon completion of the procedure, make sure you check for neatness and gaps, adequate support, along with proper function of the affected area. In certain situations, the individual might be asked to perform function tests to establish appropriate technique application.*

Protective Devices

The use of protective devices is beneficial if they are properly selected, used in the appropriate setting, correctly fitted, and follow the guidelines of the specific sport. Consultation with a medical equipment specialist is highly encouraged! In some cases, a prescription from a licensed physician may result in insurance reimbursement. Listed below are various protective devices that are commercially available for use in sports and/or physical activity.

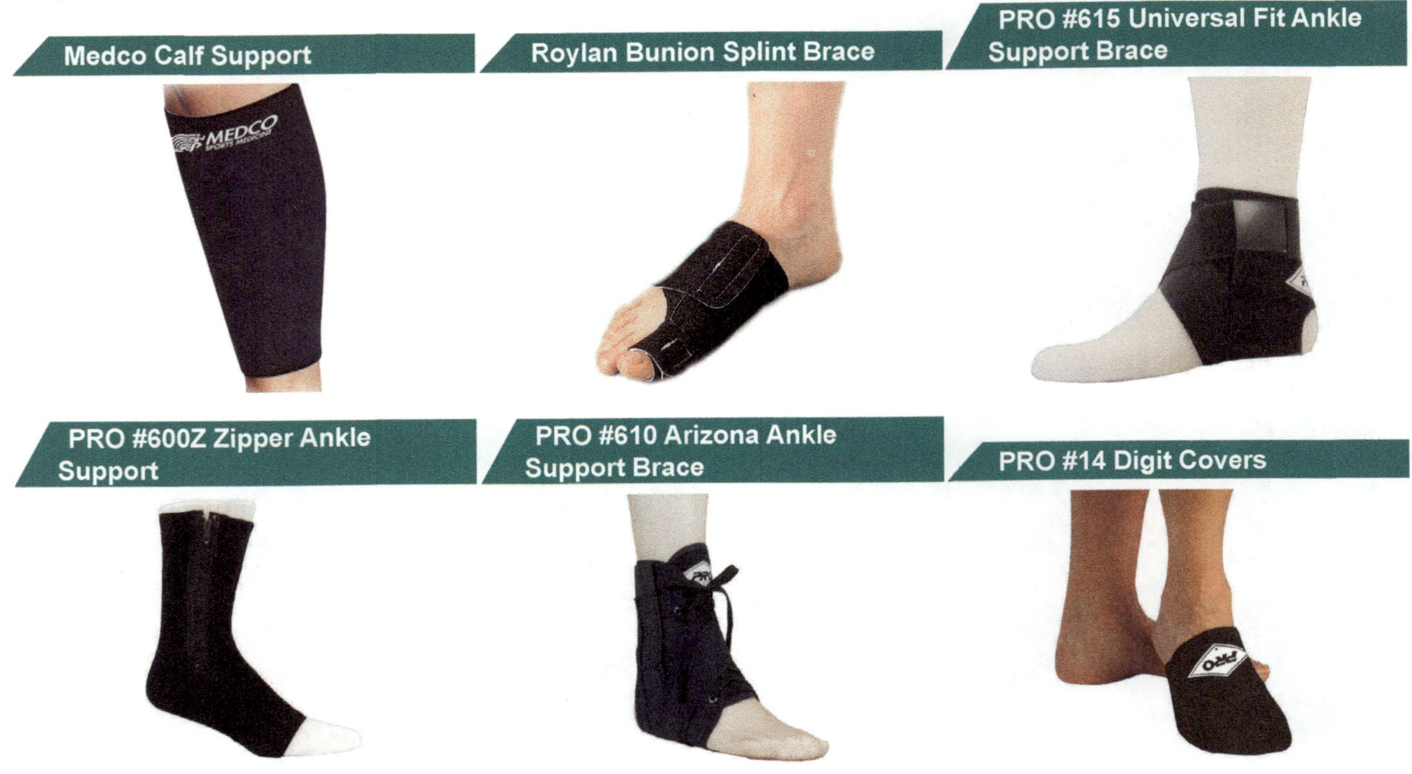

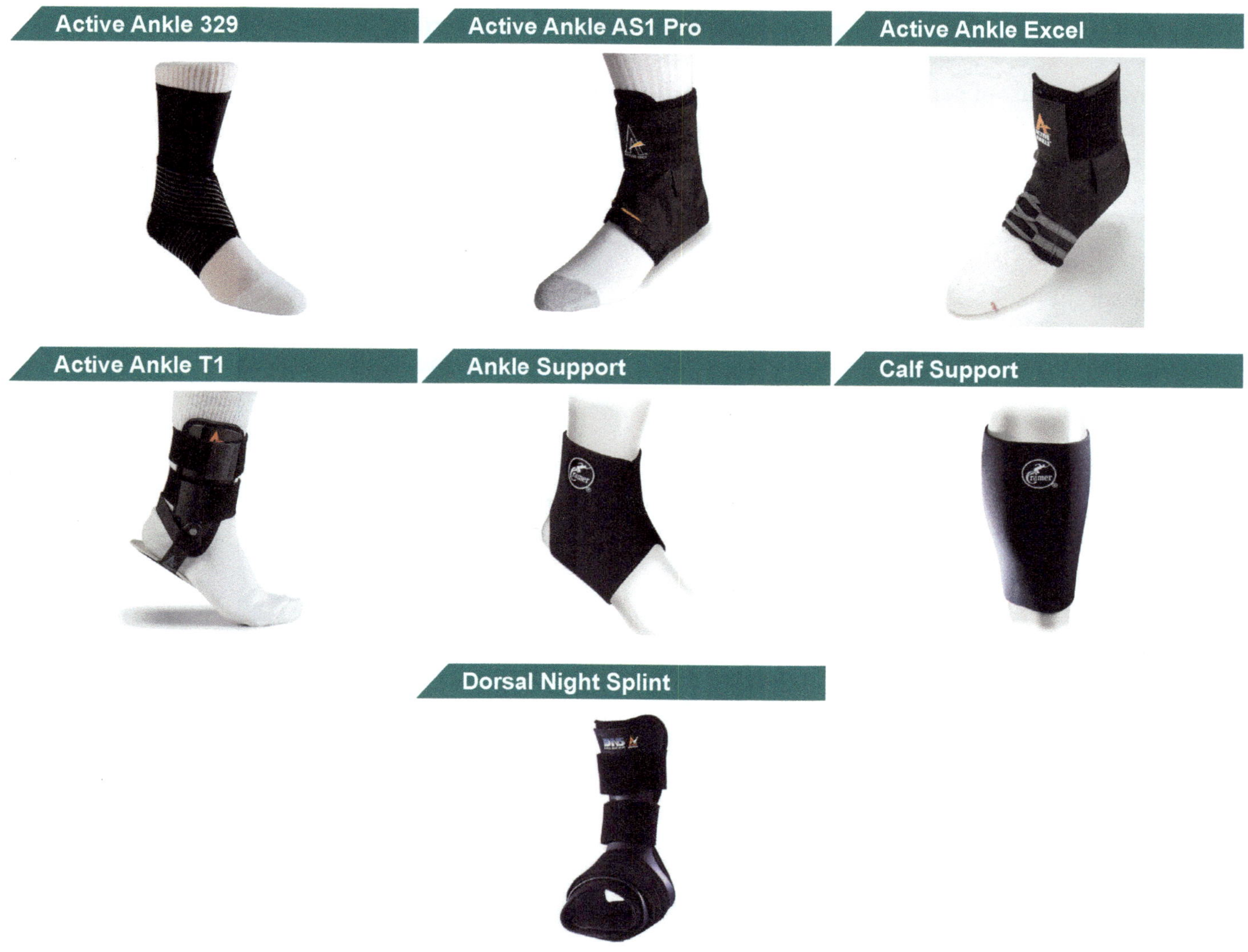

Listed below are various protective devices available to use in sport. Because a variety of protective devices are available, a qualified physician or qualified health care professional and medical equipment specialist can determine whether the individual is best suited for an off-the-shelf or custom brace.

- Achilles tendon strap
- Boots (hockey, ski, wrestling)
- Orthotics (soft, semirigid, rigid)
- Shin guards
- Turf toe brace
- Insoles and Orthotics (*Information to be added; Insite Orthotics - Matt Derringer)*

Musculoskeletal Disorders

The following is a list of common musculoskeletal disorders of the foot, ankle, and lower leg. For definitions of these terms, the authors encourage the learner to consult these medical references: *Taber's Medical Dictionary*, *Stedman's Medical Dictionary for the Health Professions and Nursing*, and/or *Signs and Symptoms of Athletic Injuries* (listed in Appendix B).

Foot, Ankle, and Lower Leg
Achilles tendinitis/tendinosis
Ankle sprain
Apophysitis calcaneus
Arch sprain
Bunion (Hallux Valgus)
Bunionette
Bursitis
Corn
Great toe sprain
Hallux rigidus
Hallux varus
Hammer toe
Heel spur
Interdigital neuroma
Mallet toe
Morton's neuroma
Plantar aponeurosis (Plantar fasciitis)
Plantar neuroma
Retrocalcaneal achilles bursitis
Sesamoiditis
Shin splints
Stone bruise
Talotibial exostosis
Tarsal tunnel syndrome
Tendinitis/tenosynovitis

Chapter 4

Knee, Thigh, and Hip

EDUCATIONAL OBJECTIVES

Upon completing this chapter, the reader will be able to do the following:

- Identify anatomical structures and landmarks critical for correct taping procedures
- Describe the purpose for the applications of adhesive and elastic tape
- Select the proper supplies and specialty items used for taping
- Explain the steps in preparing the body for taping, wrapping, or protective device
- Describe and demonstrate the purposes, clinical applications, anatomical structures, supplies needed, and pretaping and taping procedures for anatomical areas
- Identify the proper use and application of protective devices for the knee, thigh, and hip

Introduction

Techniques for lower extremities can be meaningful when injuries occur to the knee, thigh, and hip. Therefore, a basic foundation in understanding the area is important for injury care. This chapter will highlight the terminology, taping techniques, wrapping techniques, protective devices, and musculoskeletal disorders associated with the knee, thigh, and hip.

Terminology

Flexion. Movement around a transverse axis in an anterior–posterior plane with the angle between the anterior aspects of the displaced parts becoming smaller, as in bending the forearm toward the arm at the elbow joint; the act of drawing a body segment away from a straight line with its proximally conjoined body segment or toward smallest acute angle of that joint.

Extension. The reverse movement during which the angle between the anterior aspects of the displaced parts is increased, as in moving the forearm away from the upper arm; the act of drawing a body segment toward a straight line position with its proximally conjoined body segment or away from the body joint.

Abduction. Movement away from the median plane around an anterior–posterior axis with the angle between the displaced parts becoming greater, as in lifting the arm sideward away from the body; the act of drawing a body segment away from the median line of the body.

Adduction. Movement toward the median plane around an anterior–posterior axis with the angle between the displaced parts becoming lesser, as in bringing the arm sideward against the body; the act of drawing a body segment toward the median line of the body.

Rotation. Movement around a longitudinal axis that passes through a joint, as in turning the palm of the hand up or down with the arm abducted.

Valgus. Position of a body part that is bent outward.

Varus. Position of a body part that is bent inward.

Quadriceps. The muscle group in the anterior thigh consisting of the rectus femoris, vastus medialis, vastus intermedius, and vastus lateralis.

Hamstrings. A muscle group in the posterior thigh consisting of the semitendinosus, semimembranosus, and biceps femoris.

Popliteal space. Area behind the knee joint.

Anterior cruciate ligament (ACL). A ligament crossing through the knee joint that attaches from the anterior tibia to the posterior femur. It limits anterior movement of the tibia from the femur, as well as rotation of the tibia.

Taping Techniques and Protective Devices

Developing a thorough knowledge regarding the fundamentals of the application of taping/wrapping procedures is imperative. Review Chapter 1 before applying any technique.

Proper Assessment of Injury

Before applying a preventive technique (tape, wrap, and/or device), a qualified physician or qualified health care professional should complete a proper injury evaluation. Following injury evaluation, the professional can then recommend proper taping techniques. This ensures that proper taping techniques are applied for support and stabilization. Also, developing a thorough knowledge of taping application fundamentals is imperative.

Purpose and Application of Adhesive and Elastic Tape

The primary purpose for tape application is to provide additional support and stability for the affected body part. Through proper application, taping techniques can be applied to shorten the muscle's angle of pull; to decrease joint range of motion; to secure pads, bandages, and protective devices; and to apply compression to reduce swelling.

Medical Supplies and Specialty Items

Purchasing supplies depends on budget, philosophy of medical staff regarding taping techniques, and occurrence of injury. Review Chapter 1 before applying any technique.

Specific Rules on Taping, Wrapping, and/or Protective Device

If you apply supportive techniques to an individual, you should be aware of specific rules governing tape application in that particular sport or physical activity. Your application must fall within the guidelines established for each sport by appropriate governing bodies.

Special Techniques: Adjunct Taping Procedures

The taping techniques presented are the fundamental procedures. Adjunct techniques will be shown to provide additional support; however, you should still follow the fundamental procedures. Variations can be achieved by adapting these techniques to a particular injury situation. Always give special consideration to

- purpose of the taping procedure
- clinical application
- correct anatomical position
- supply selection
- tape/wrap technique or protective device

Preparation of Body Part for Taping

In preparing the body for tape application, consider these six items:

- removal of hair (optional)
- clean the area
- special considerations
- spray adherent (optional)
- skin lubricants
- underwrap or cohesive tape
- proper body positioning

Proper Body Positioning

Before beginning a taping procedure, select a comfortable table height and ask the individual to assume an anatomically correct and comfortable position.

Neutral Position of Knee: The knee should be in slight flexion (10 to 15 degrees).
Neutral Position of Hip Joint: The hip and knee joint should be placed in slight flexion.

When applying a technique, learn to stand at a comfortable and stationary position and place the body part to be taped at your elbow height.

Bones and Ligaments

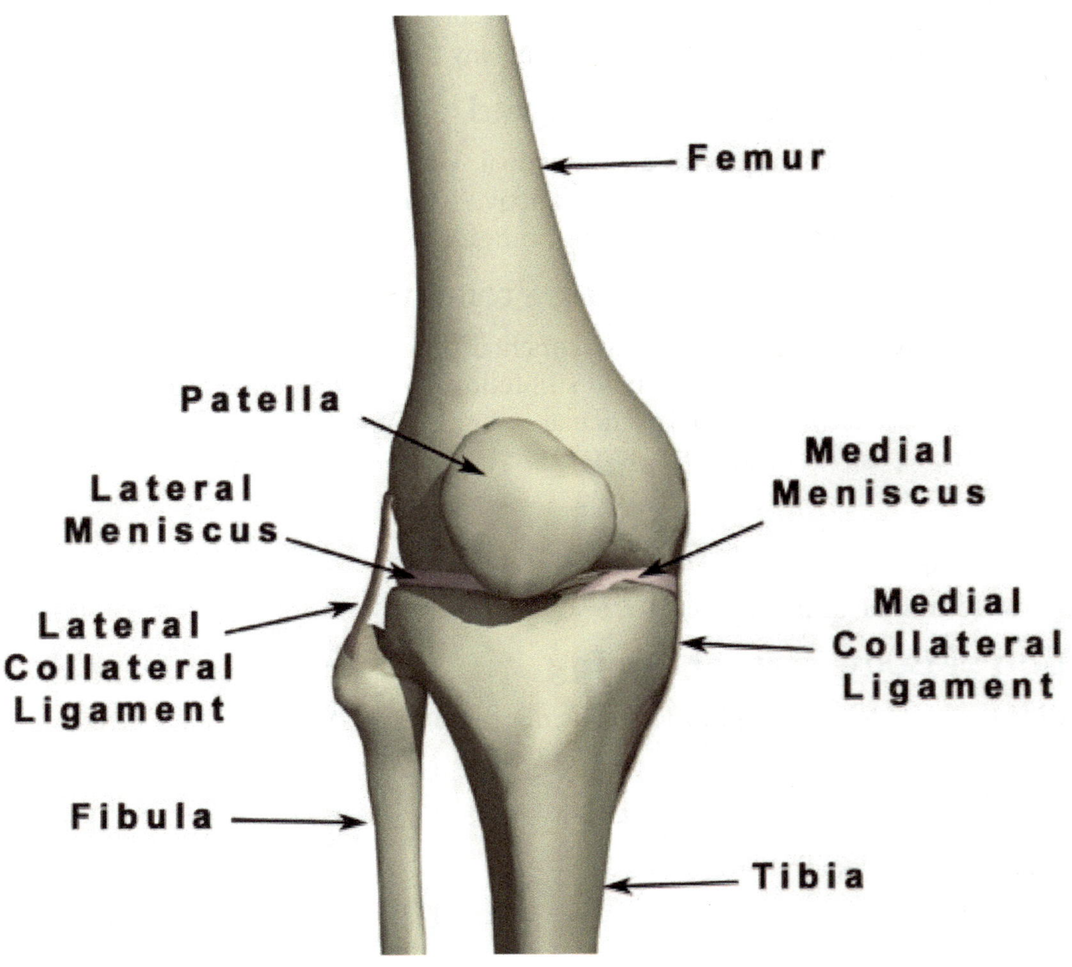

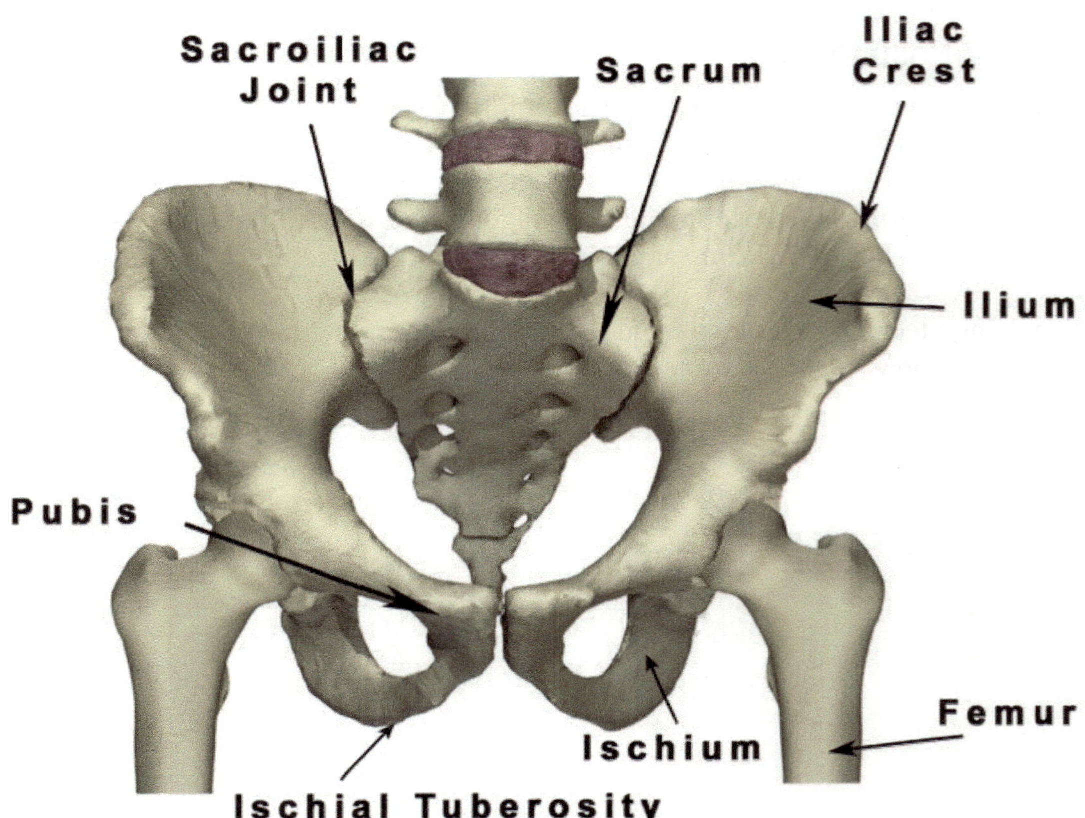

Muscles and Tendons

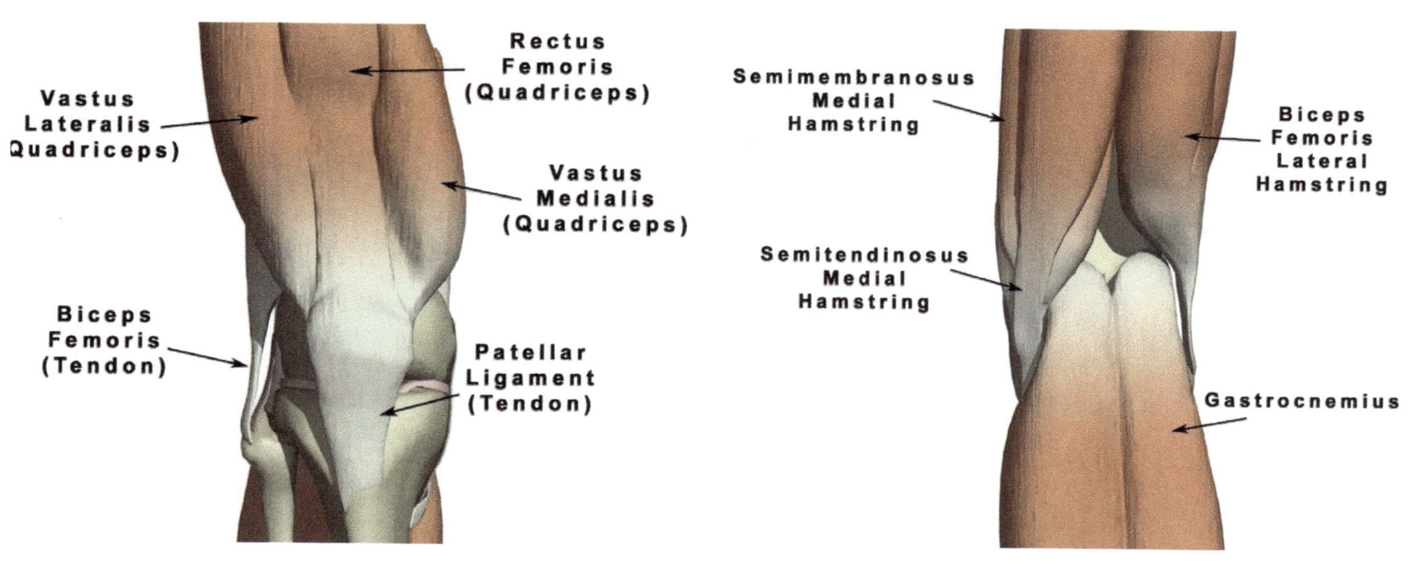

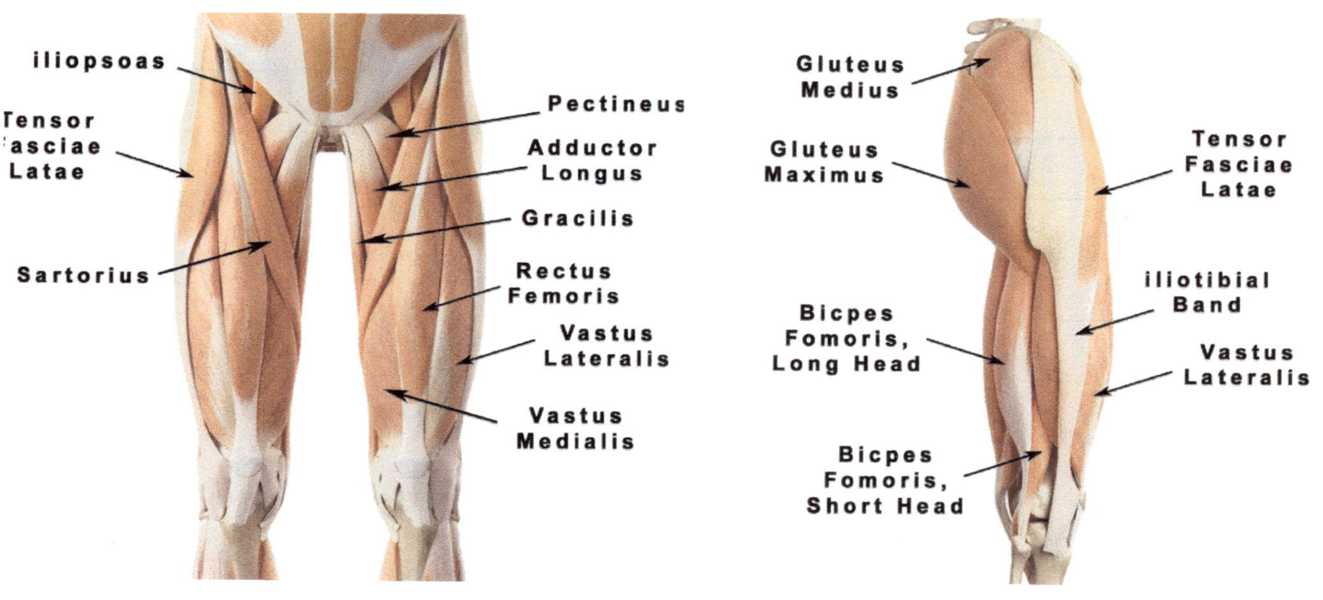

Taping Techniques

The taping techniques presented are the fundamental procedures. A strong knowledge of anatomy, physiology, biomechanics, and pathology is essential. Developing a thorough knowledge regarding the fundamentals about the application of taping/wrapping procedures is imperative. Review Section A - Chapter 1 before applying any technique.

The Kinesio® Taping Method is a therapeutic taping technique not only offering your patient the support they are looking for, but also rehabilitating the affected condition as well. Please consult Chapter 9 for specific application instructions.

NOTES:

COLLATERAL KNEE

Purpose: To provide support and stability to the collateral ligaments of the knee

Clinical Application: Sprains

Anatomical Structure: Knee joint

Anatomical Position: Knee joint in slight flexion (10 to 15 degrees)

Supplies: 1½-in. adhesive tape, 3-in. elastic tape, and gauze with lubricant (heel and lace pad)

Pre-taping Procedure

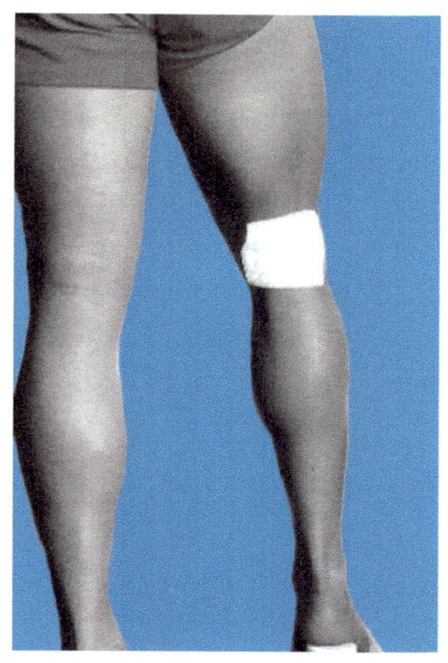

Apply gauze and lubricant to the posterior aspect (popliteal space) of the knee joint

Taping Procedures

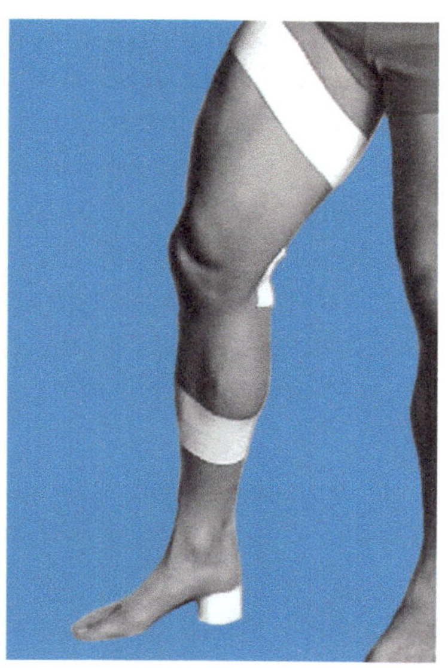

1. Apply two anchor strips of 3-in. elastic tape to the extremity. Place the proximal anchor strip at the mid-thigh or higher. Apply the distal anchor at the mid-gastrocnemius region or lower. Attach all collateral strips on these two anchors.

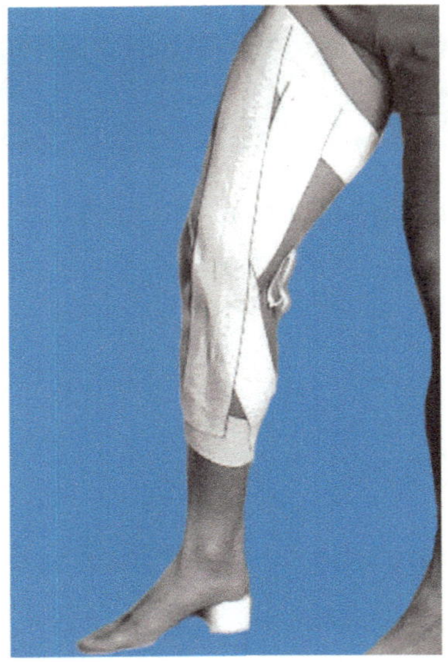

2. Apply collateral X pattern to the medial side of the knee. Using 3-in. elastic tape, start on the lateral aspect of the distal anchor, come below the patella, cross the medial joint line, and attach to the posteromedial aspect of the proximal anchor. Begin the second strip on the posterior aspect of the distal anchor, cross the medial joint line, and attach to the anterior portion of the proximal anchor. Apply a third strip vertically on the medial side. Begin this support strip on the distal anchor, cross the joint line, and attach to the proximal anchor.

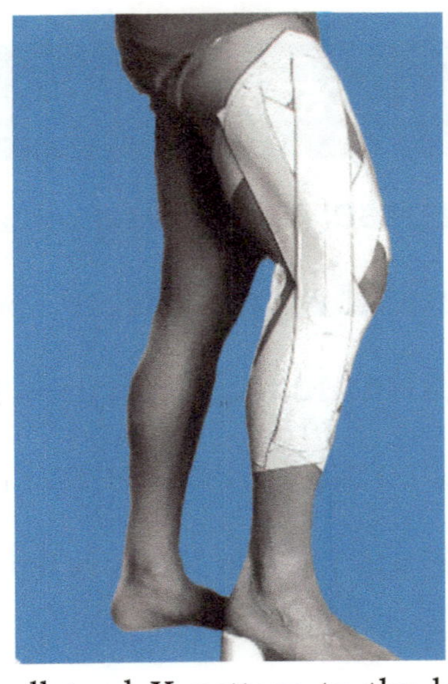

3. Apply collateral X pattern to the lateral side of the knee. Using 3-in. elastic tape, start on the medial aspect of the distal anchor, come below the patella, cross the lateral joint line, and attach to the posterolateral aspect of the proximal anchor. Begin the second strip on the posterior aspect of the distal anchor, cross the lateral joint line, and attach to the anterior portion of the proximal anchor. Apply a third strip vertically on the lateral side. Begin this support strip on the distal anchor, cross the joint line, and attach to the proximal anchor.

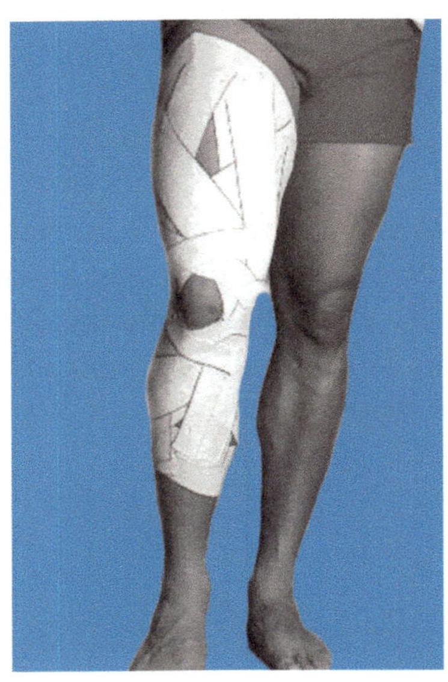

4. Apply a patella lock strip for support. Cut a strip of 3-in. elastic tape, 15 in. to 20 in. in length. Center this patella lock strip over the popliteal fossa. Split each end approximately 4 in. to 6 in. Cover the joint line and place the medial split ends inferior and superior to the patella. Apply the lateral split ends in the same manner. The four split ends should form a diamond shape near the patella.

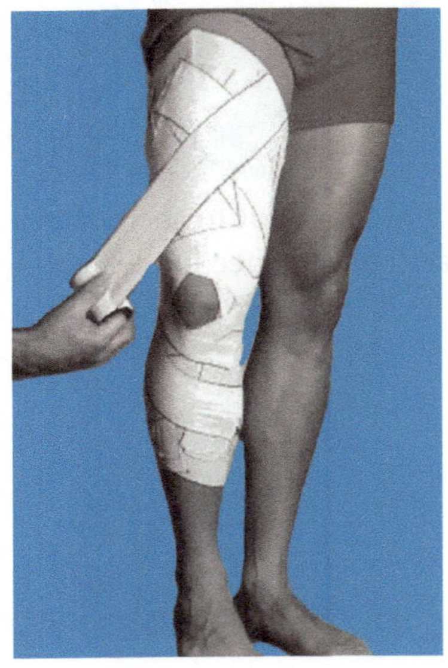

5. Apply two spiral strips to protect the popliteal fossa and to assist in preventing hyperextension. Using 3-in. elastic tape, begin on the anterior portion of the proximal anchor, and moving medially, spiral posteriorly, crossing the popliteal fossa, and complete the strip on the anterior portion of the distal anchor. Repeat this sequence a second time, applying the tape laterally.

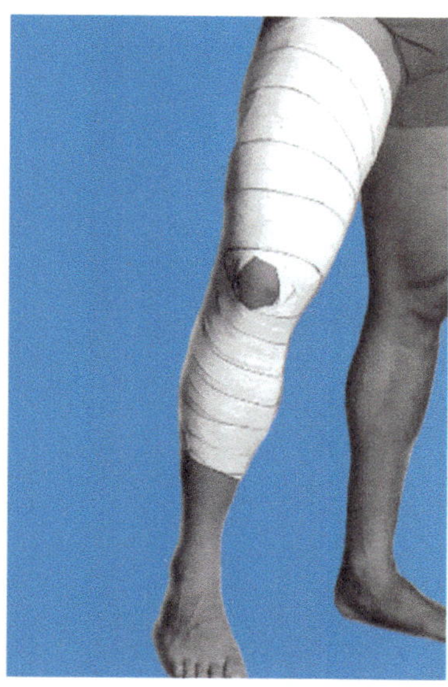

6. Apply final closure strips. Begin proximally and work distally. From the upper anchor, apply individual circular strips around the extremity to cover tape ends. Overlap the tape approximately one half of its width on each strip. Secure the elastic tape ends with anchors of 1½-in. adhesive tape.

**Upon completion of the procedure, make sure you check for neatness and gaps, adequate support, along with proper function of the affected area. In certain situations, the individual might be asked to perform function tests to establish appropriate technique application.*

Adjunct Taping Procedures: Collateral Knee

This adjunct taping procedure can be used in conjunction with the basic technique presented.

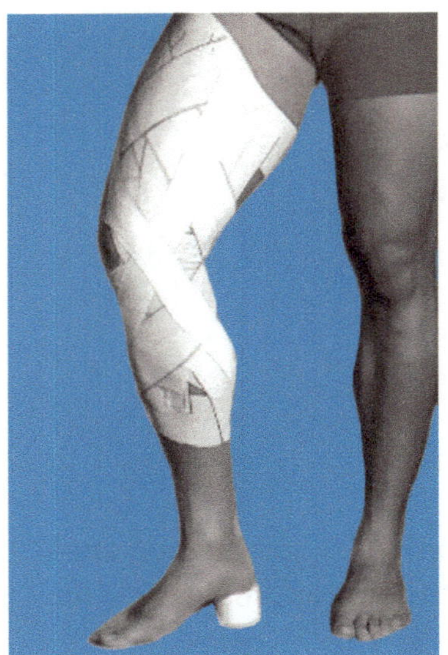

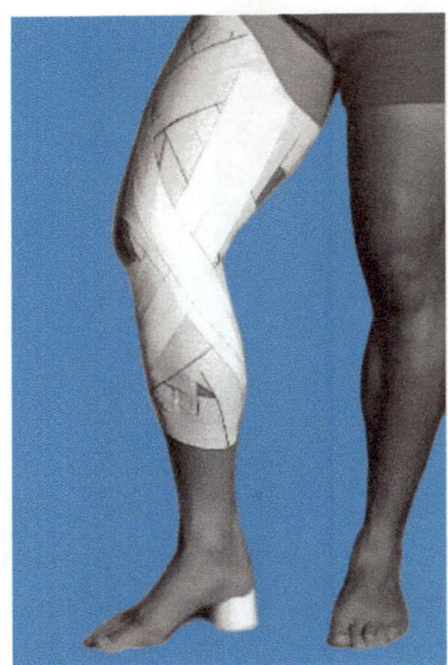

Technique A. Apply 1½-in. adhesive tape over the collateral X patterns to provide additional support.

HYPEREXTENDED KNEE

Purpose: To assist in prevention of knee joint hyperextension

Clinical Application: Hyperextension sprain

Anatomical Structure: Knee joint

Anatomical Position: Knee joint placed in slight flexion

Supplies: 1½-in. adhesive tape, 3-in. elastic tape, and gauze with lubricant

Pre-taping Procedure: Apply the gauze with lubricant to the popliteal fossa of the knee joint

Taping Procedures

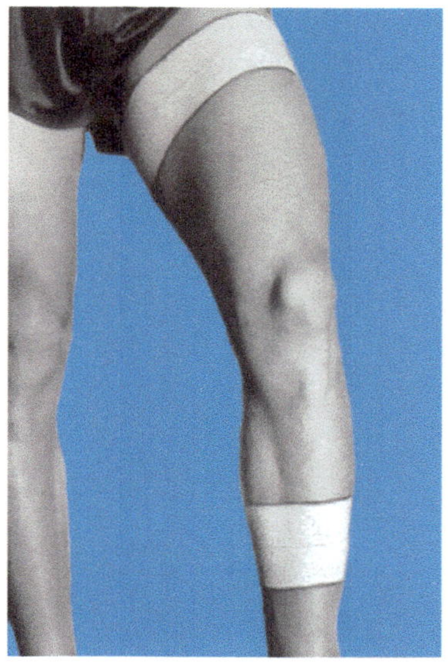

1. Apply two anchor strips of 3-in. elastic tape to the extremity. Place the proximal anchor strip at the mid-thigh or higher. Apply the distal anchor at the mid-gastrocnemius region or lower.

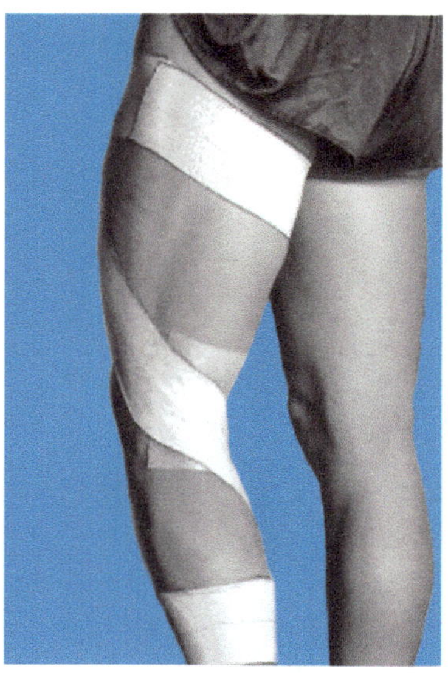

2. Using 3-in. elastic tape, begin on the anterior portion of the distal anchor, move laterally and spiral posteriorly, crossing the popliteal fossa, and complete the strip on the anterior portion of the proximal anchor.

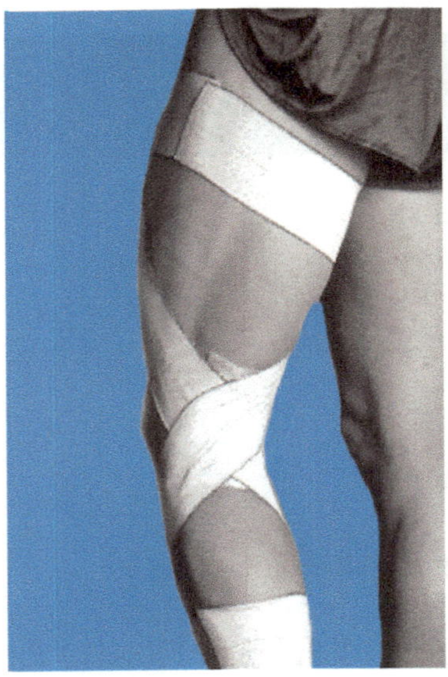

3. Using 3-in. elastic tape, begin on the anterior portion of the proximal anchor, and moving medially, spiral posteriorly, crossing the popliteal fossa, and complete this strip on the anterior portion of the distal anchor.

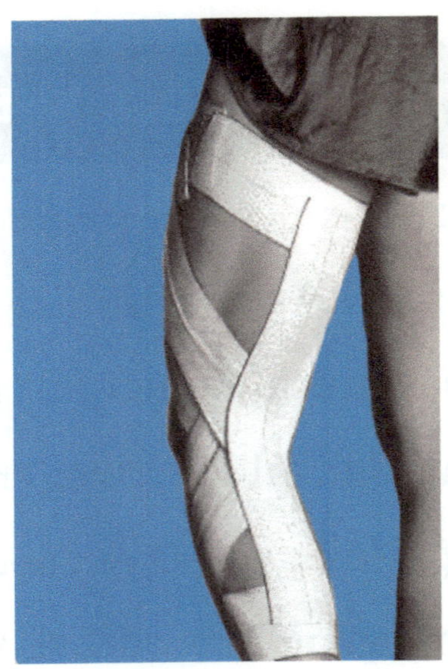

4. Apply a vertical strip starting on the proximal anchor, cross the popliteal fossa, and end on the distal anchor. Repeat steps 2, 3, and 4 a second time for additional support. Exercise caution when encircling the lower leg to avoid undue pressure on the musculature.

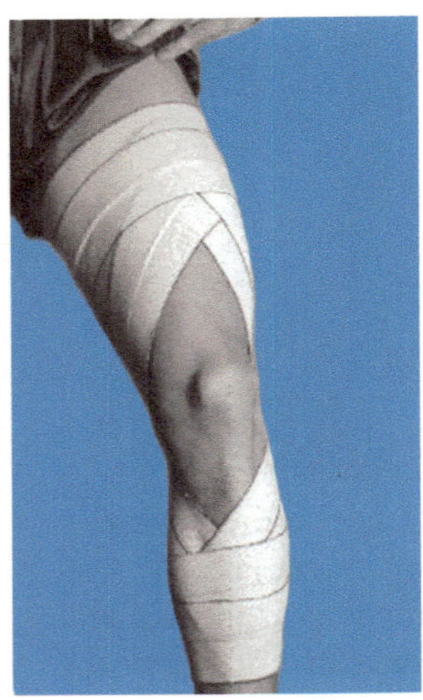

5. Apply final closure strips. Begin proximally and work distally. From the upper anchor, apply individual circular strips around the extremity to cover tape ends. Make sure you overlap the tape approximately one half of its width on each strip. Optional: secure the elastic tape ends with anchors of 1½-in. adhesive tape.

**Upon completion of the procedure, make sure you check for neatness and gaps, adequate support, along with proper function of the affected area. In certain situations, the individual might be asked to perform function tests to establish appropriate technique application.*

Adjunct Taping Procedures: Hyperextended Knee

This adjunct taping procedure can be used in conjunction with the basic technique presented.

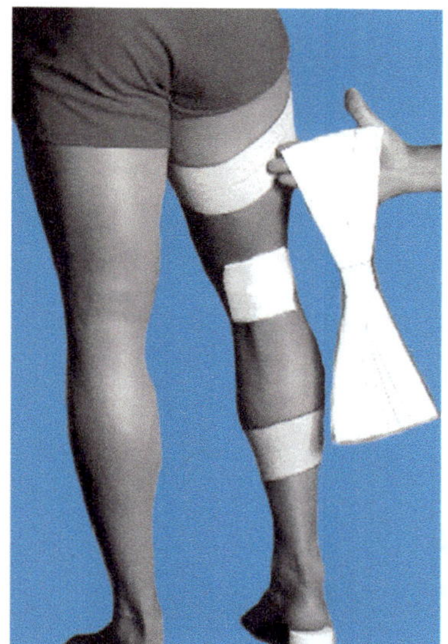

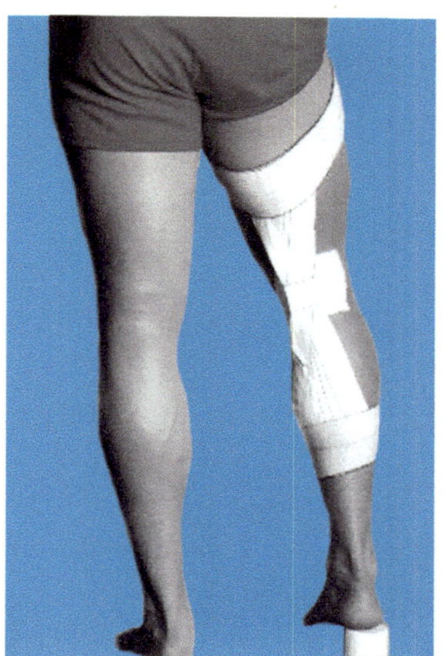

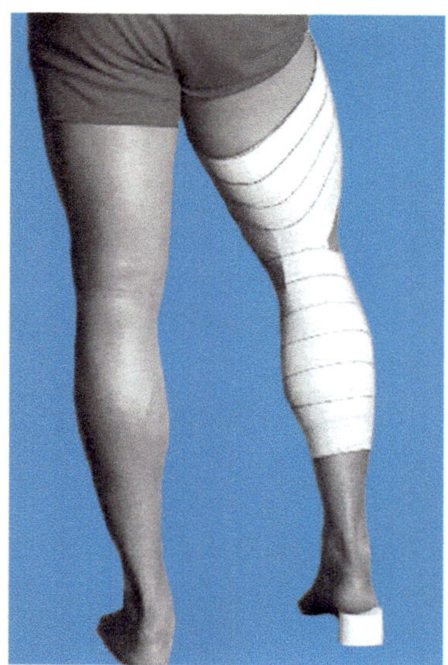

Technique A. Using either adhesive or elastic tape, construct a five- to seven-strip butterfly (hour glass) pattern that will extend from the proximal to the distal anchors. Prior to application, place a strip of tape around the mid-portion of this support pattern. Place the support on the proximal anchor, pull downward, and attach to the distal anchor. Secure this technique with strips of elastic tape over the proximal and distal anchor. This technique should help restrict hyperextension of the knee joint.

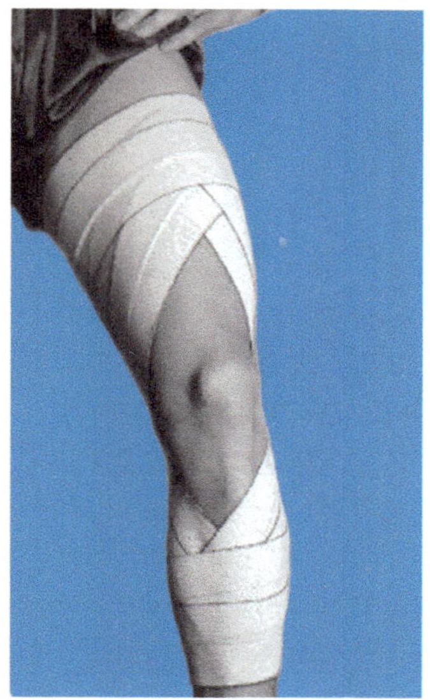

Technique B. Apply 1½-in. adhesive tape over the spiral strips to provide additional support.

ANTERIOR CRUCIATE

Purpose: To enhance support and stability to the anterior cruciate ligament of the knee

Clinical Application: Sprain to anterior cruciate ligament

Anatomical Structure: Knee

Anatomical Position: Knee and hip joints should be positioned in slight flexion

Supplies: 1½-in. adhesive tape, 3-in. elastic tape, and gauze with lubricant

Pre-taping Procedure

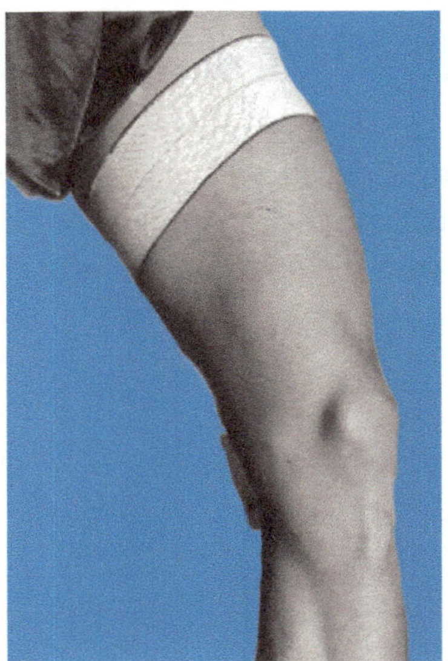

With the knee and hip joints in slight flexion, apply the gauze with lubricant to the posterior aspect of the knee joint. Also apply an anchor strip of 3-in. elastic tape around the upper third of the thigh. Comment: In this pretaping procedure, do not compress the popliteal fossa.

Taping Procedures

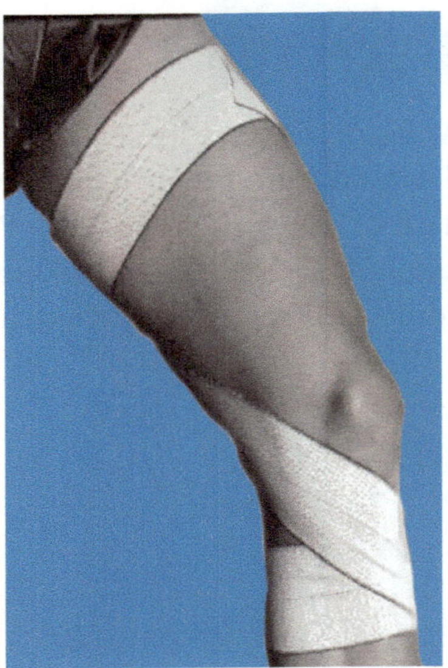

1. Using 3-in. elastic tape, begin on the lower lateral aspect of the leg, approximately 1 in. below the patella. Encircle the lower leg, moving anteriorly and then medially, continuing to the posterior aspect, and returning to the lateral side. Angle the tape below the patella, cross the medial joint line and popliteal fossa, and spiral up to anchor on the anterior portion of the upper thigh.

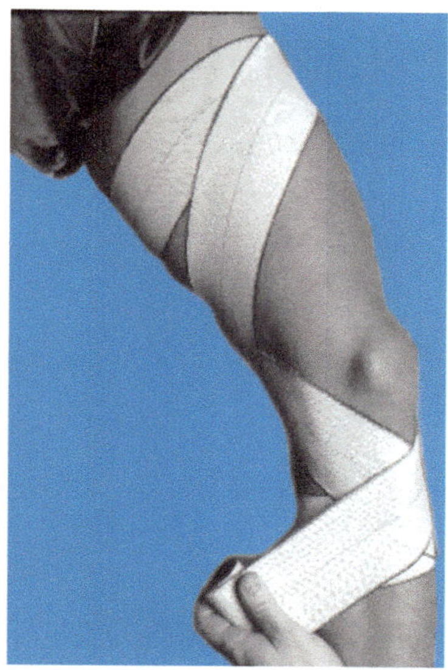

2. Begin the next strip of 3-in. elastic tape on the anterior aspect of the proximal anchor and cross medial portion of the thigh, covering the popliteal fossa, encircling the lower leg, and crossing the popliteal fossa again. Finish by spiraling up to anchor on the anterior aspect of the thigh.

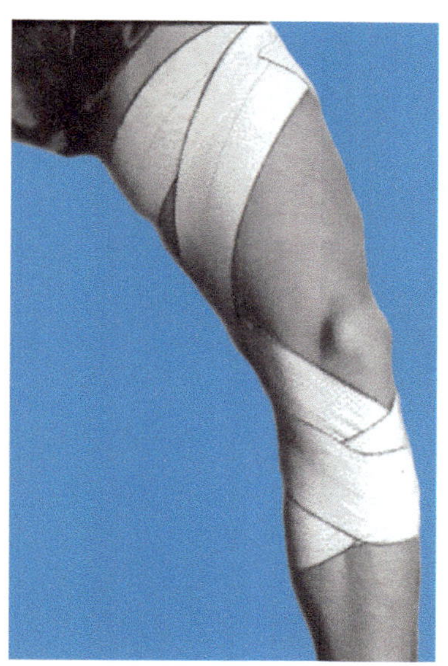

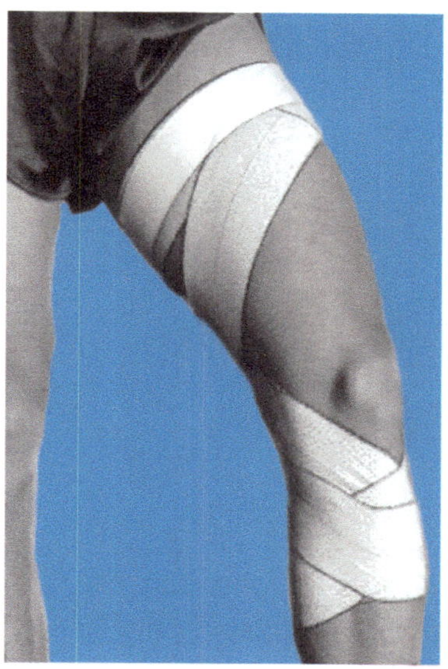

3. Repeat Step 2. Secure this technique by applying 11/2-in. adhesive tape over the anchor on the thigh.

**Upon completion of the procedure, make sure you check for neatness and gaps, adequate support, along with proper function of the affected area. In certain situations, the individual might be asked to perform function tests to establish appropriate technique application.*

PATELLA TENDON

Purpose: To reduce stress on the patella tendon

Clinical Application: Patella tendon strain and tendinitis

Anatomical Structure: Patella tendon

Anatomical Position: Knee joint slightly flexed and uscles of lower leg relaxed

Supplies: 1-in. adhesive or elaastic tape

Taping Procedures

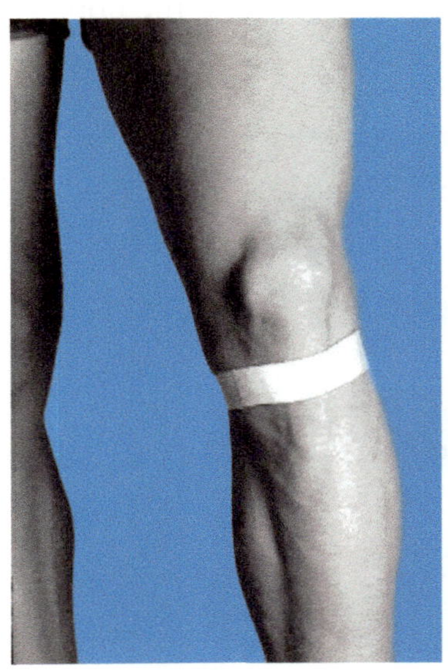

1. Apply tape with direct pressure between the distal end of the patella and superior aspect of the tibia tuberosity. Encircle the lower leg starting on the lateral side, move anteriorly and then to the medial side, continue to the posterior aspect, and return to the lateral side.

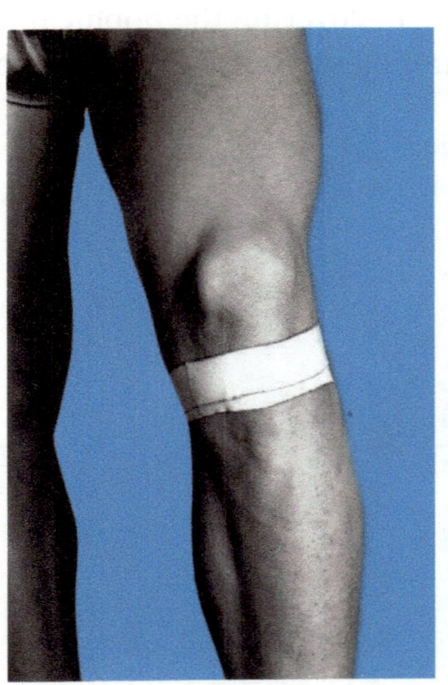

2. Repeat Step 1.

**Upon completion of the procedure, make sure you check for neatness and gaps, adequate support, along with proper function of the affected area. In certain situations, the individual might be asked to perform function tests to establish appropriate technique application.*

Adjunct Taping Procedures: Patella Tendon Taping

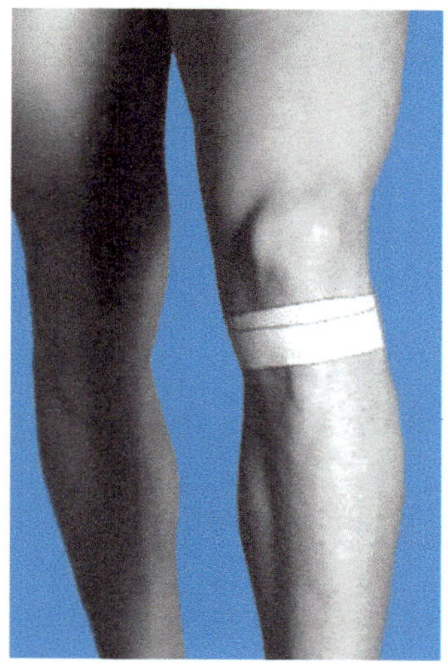

Technique A. In conjunction with the basic procedure, use 1-in. or 2-in. elastic tape in a continuous procedure for additional support.

HIP POINTER

Purpose: To provide support and protection to the contused tissue of the iliac crest

Clinical Application: Contusions and strains

Anatomical Structure: Iliac crest

Anatomical Position: Standing with slight lateral flexion of the waist to the affected side

Supplies: 1½-in. adhesive tape, 3-in. elastic tape, ½-in. foam pad, and 6-in. extra long elastic wrap

Pre-taping Procedure: Cut a foam pad that will cover the affected area. In certain situations, construct a doughnut pad that will relieve pressure on the affected area.

Taping Procedures

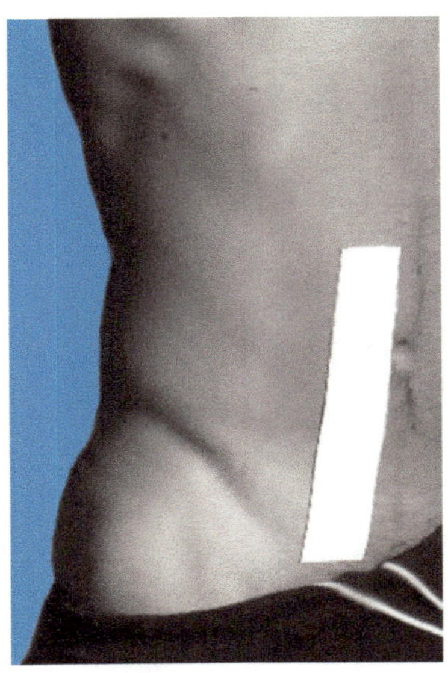

1. Apply two vertical anchor strips approximately 4 in. to 6 in. anteriorly and posteriorly to the affected area.

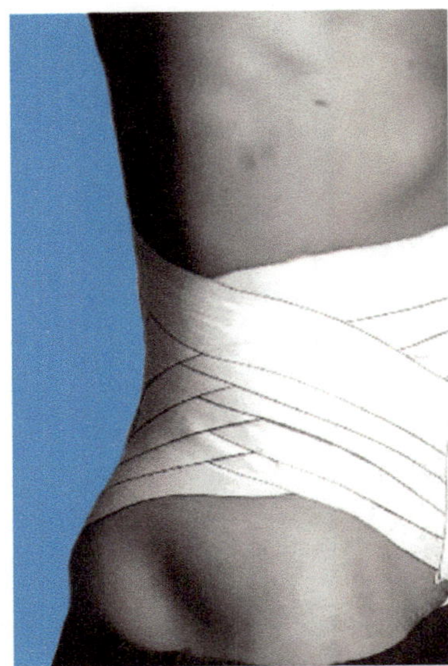

2. Apply the X pattern technique, overlapping by one half, beginning at the anterior aspect of the anchors, and moving posteriorly until the entire crest of the hip is covered.

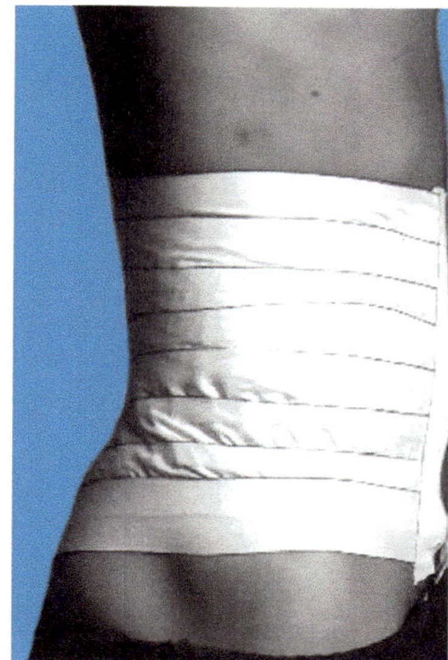

3. Apply horizontal strips, beginning on the superior anchor, and moving inferiorly, overlap by one half until the entire area is covered.

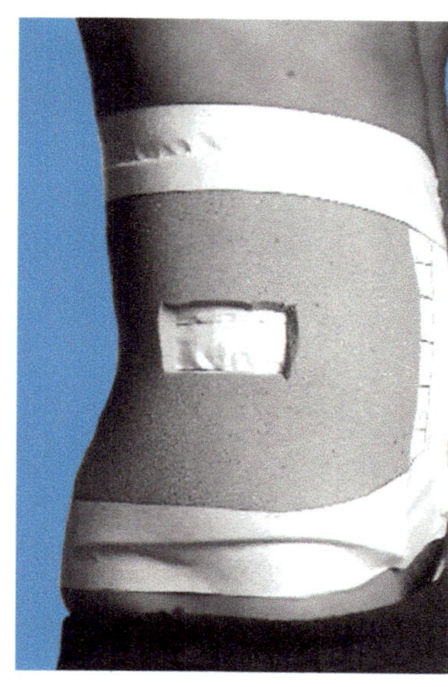

4. Place the foam pad over the affected area. This pad is held in place with two strips of adhesive tape.

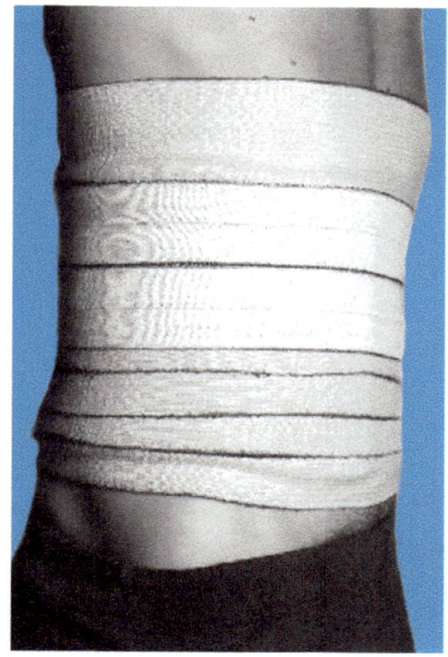

5. Have the individual inhale to expand the thorax when applying the elastic wrap. Then apply a strip of elastic tape over the wrap to secure the ends.

**Upon completion of the procedure, make sure you check for neatness and gaps, adequate support, along with proper function of the affected area. In certain situations, the individual might be asked to perform function tests to establish appropriate technique application.*

***In certain situation, a hard shell pad can be placed over the foam rubber to provide better protection. Consultation with physician and sports official prior to use.*

Adjunct Taping Procedures: Hip Pointer

This adjunct taping procedure can be used in conjunction with the basic technique presented.

Technique A. Under certain situations, the application of this hip flexor wrap is preferred. This wrap will encircle the complete thigh and waist region of the body. (Refer to Hip Flexor Wrap)

Wrapping Techniques for Support

During physical activity, supportive wraps are used to aid in muscle function and support and to reduce excessive range of motion. These applications are typically used in competition or practice. Spica wraps are traditionally employed at the hip and shoulder joints. Figure of eight wraps are placed over ankle, knee, elbow, wrist, and hand joints.

KNEE JOINT WRAP

Purpose: To provide compression and support to the knee joint

Clinical Application: Sprains to the knee joint

Anatomical Structure: Knee joint

Anatomical Position: Knee joint places in slight flexion, through a heel lift under the heel

Supplies: 4-in. double length elastic wrap and 1½-in. adhesive tape

Pre-wrapping Procedure: The individual should stand with the affected knee in slight flexion. Instruct the individual to contract the muscles around the knee joint.

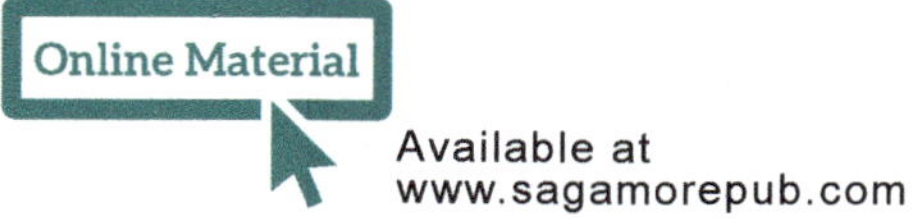

Wrapping Procedures

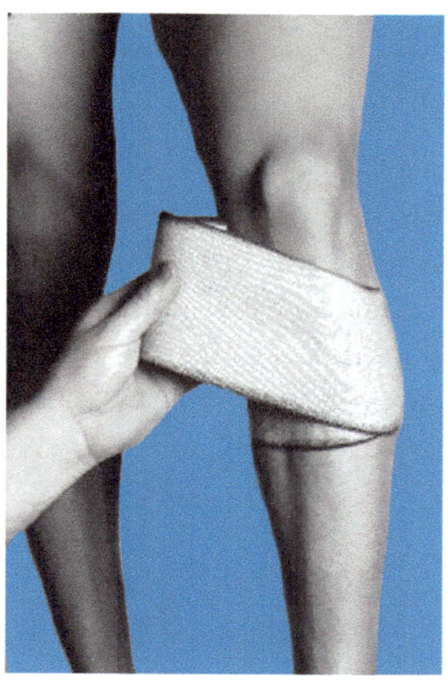

1. Begin the wrap on the lateral/posterior aspect of the lower leg. Encircle the lower leg, moving medially to laterally.

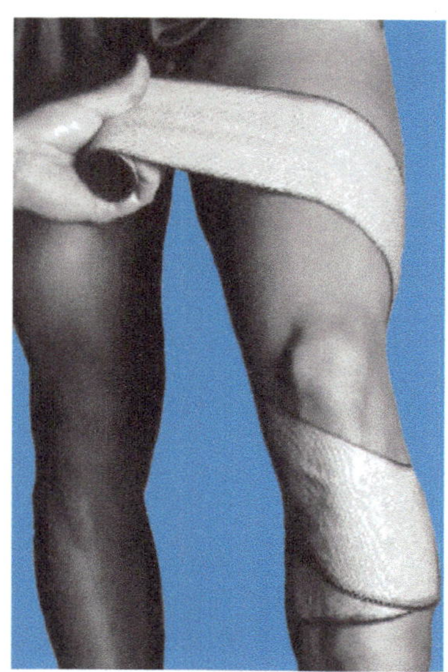

2. Angle the wrap below the patella and cross the medial joint line. Cover the posterior and lateral aspects of the thigh.

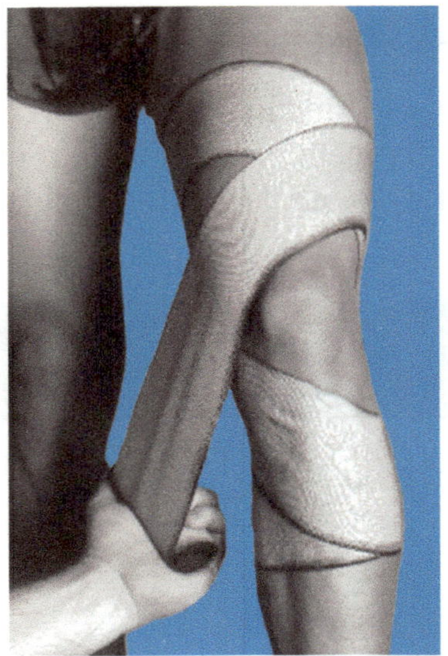

3. Encircle the thigh, moving medially to laterally. Angle the wrap downward, staying above the patella and crossing the medial joint line.

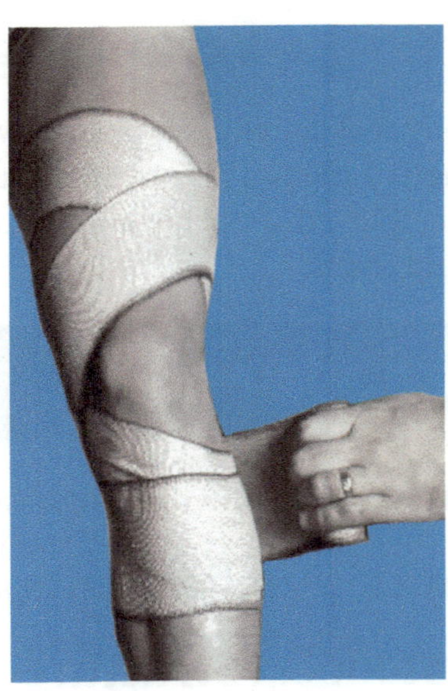

4. Cross the popliteal space and encircle the lower leg.

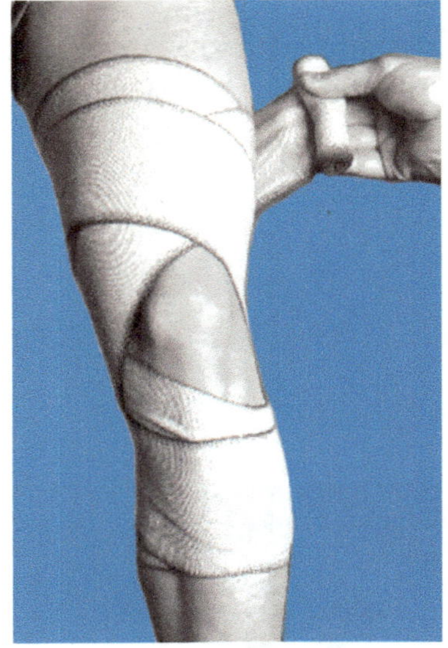

5. Proceed with the wrap, crossing the lateral joint line and angling above the patella.

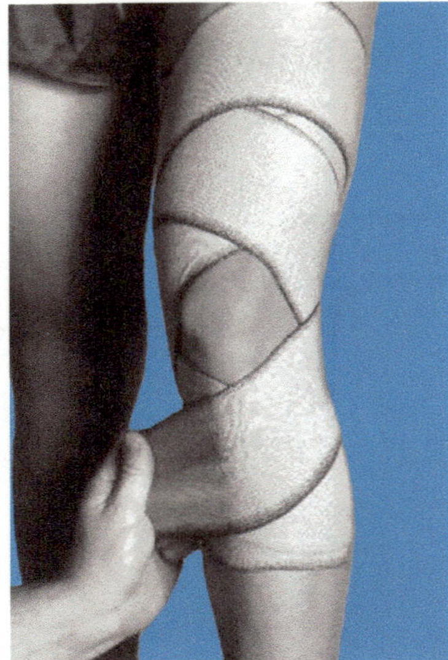

6. Encircle the thigh, and on the posterior aspect, angle across the lateral joint line of the knee, staying below the patella. This configuration should resemble a diamond shape around the patella and cover from mid-thigh to the gastrocnemius belly.

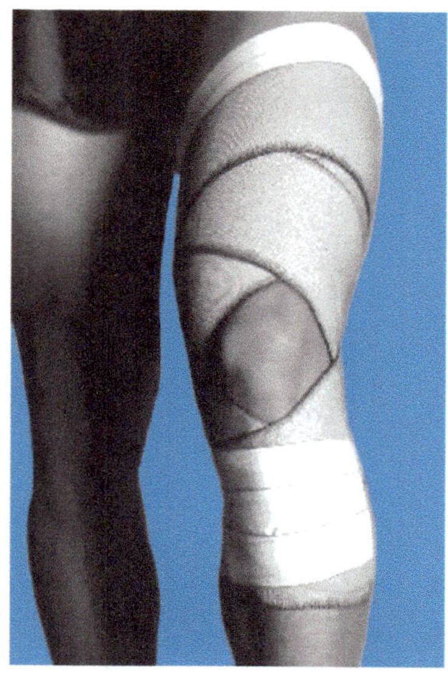

7. To secure this wrap, apply 1½-in. adhesive tape to the loose end of the wrap.

**Upon completion of the procedure, make sure you check for neatness and gaps, adequate support, along with proper function of the affected area. In certain situations, the individual might be asked to perform function tests to establish appropriate technique application.*

Adjunct Taping Procedures: Knee Wrap

This adjunct taping procedure can be used in conjunction with the basic technique presented.

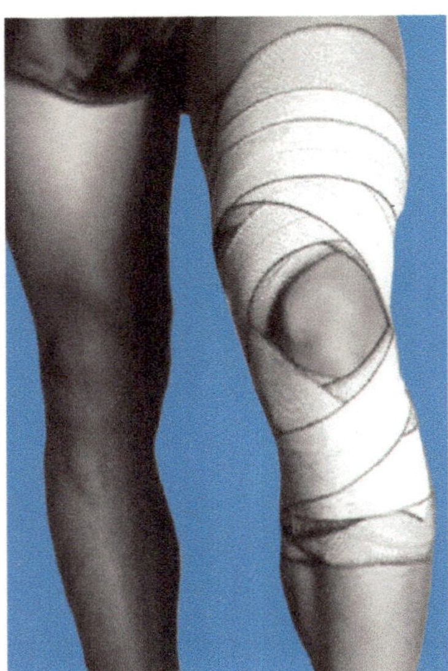

Technique A. In conjunction with the elastic wrap, you can use 2-in. or wider elastic tape in a continuous method.

HAMSTRING WRAP

Purpose: To provide support to the hamstring muscle group

Clinical Application: Strain to hamstring muscles

Anatomical Structure: Posterior aspect of the thigh

Anatomical Position: In standing position, affected extremity is in hip extension

Supplies: 1½-in. adhesive tape and 6-in. elastic wrap

Pre-wrapping Procedure: The individual should stand with the affected extremity placed in hip extension and the individual should contract the hamstring muscles

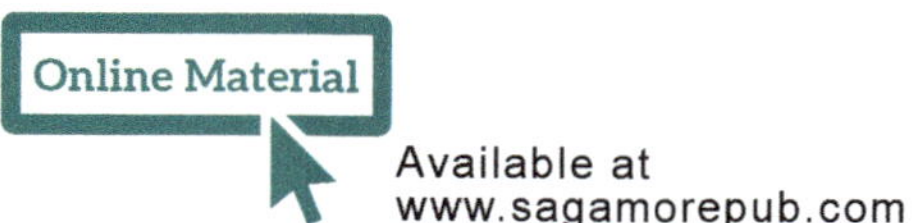

Wrapping Procedures

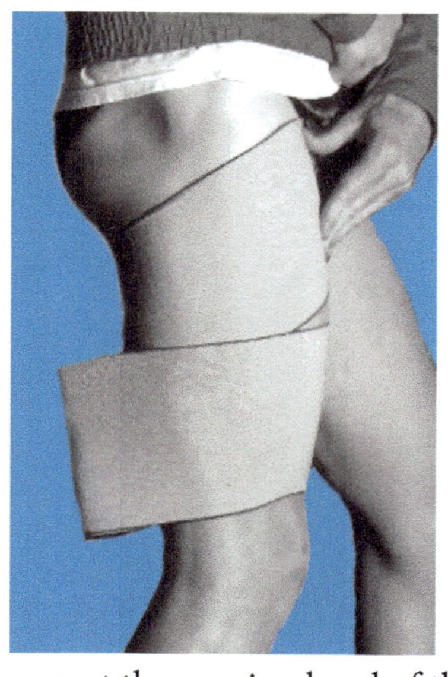

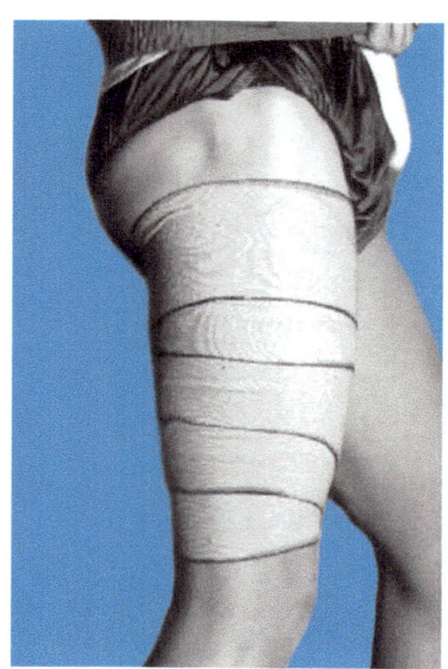

1. Begin the wrap at the proximal end of the thigh. Angle diagonally to the distal aspect of the hamstrings. At this point, begin an upward spiral supportive procedure with the wrap. Overlap each layer by one half of its width, ending at the proximal end of the thigh.

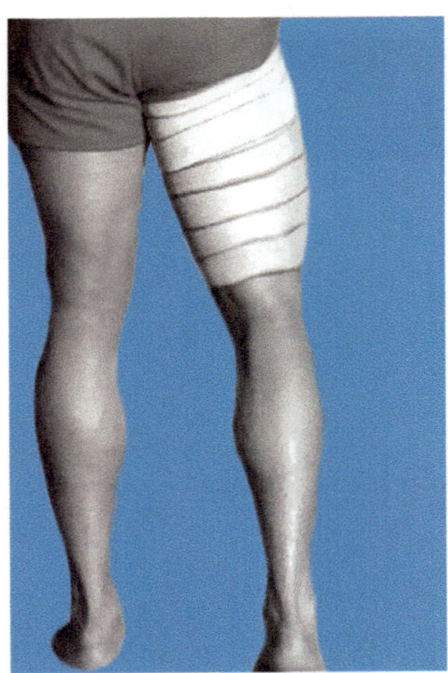

2. Secure the wrap in place by applying an anchor strip of 1½-in. adhesive tape.

**Upon completion of the procedure, make sure you check for neatness and gaps, adequate support, along with proper function of the affected area. In certain situations, the individual might be asked to perform function tests to establish appropriate technique application.*

Adjunct Taping Procedures: Hamstring Wrap

This adjunct taping procedure can be used in conjunction with the basic technique presented.

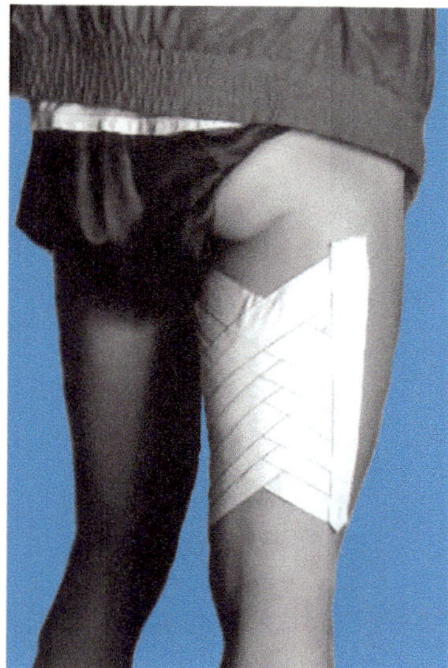

Technique A: The X pattern technique. Apply the wrap over this technique for additional support. Apply two vertical anchor strips approximately 4 in. to 6 in. anteriorly and posteriorly to the affected area. Overlap by one half, beginning at the anterior aspect of the anchors and moving posteriorly until the entire area is covered.

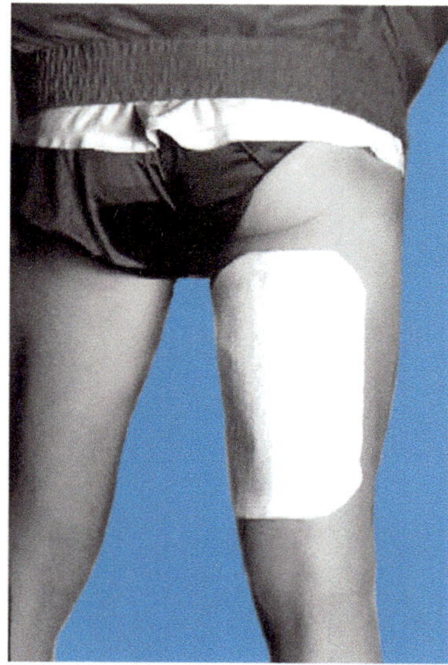

Technique B: Felt pad. Apply a 3-in. x 5-in. (or larger) felt pad over the affected area. Using ½-in. felt, apply the wrap over this technique for additional support and compression.

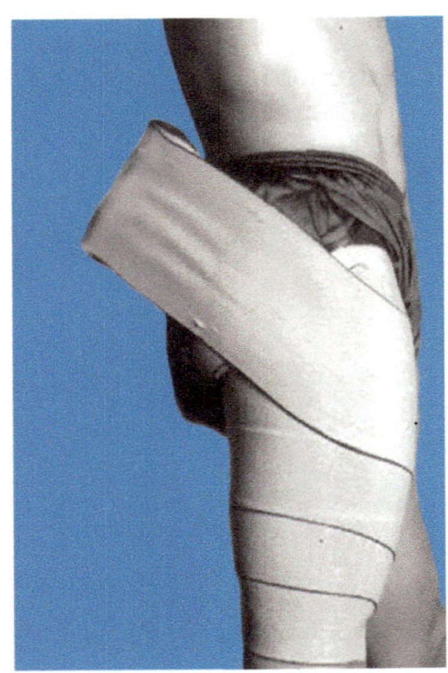

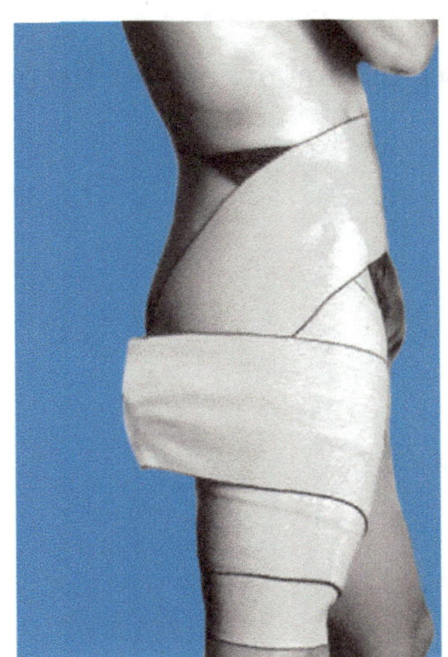

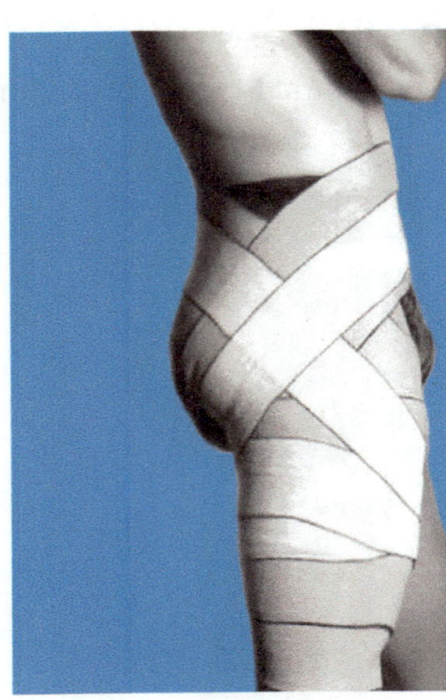

Technique C: Hip extension wrap. Using a 6-in. double length elastic wrap, apply a hip spica wrap, encircling the complete thigh and waist region of the body.

QUADRICEPS WRAP

Purpose: To provide support to the hamstring muscle group

Clinical Application: Strain to hamstring muscles

Anatomical Structure: Posterior aspect of the thigh

Anatomical Position: In standing position, affected extremity is in hip extension

Supplies: 1½-in. adhesive tape and 6-in. elastic wrap

Pre-wrapping Procedure: The individual should stand with the affected extremity placed in hip extension and the individual should contract the hamstring muscles

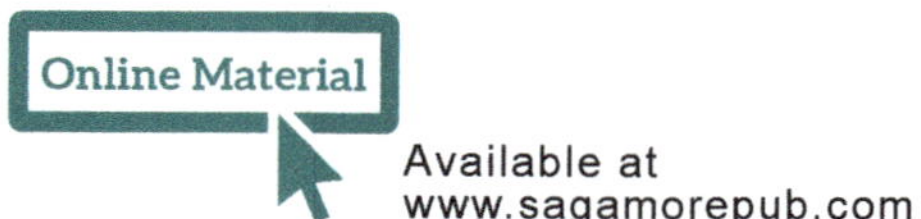

Wrapping Procedures

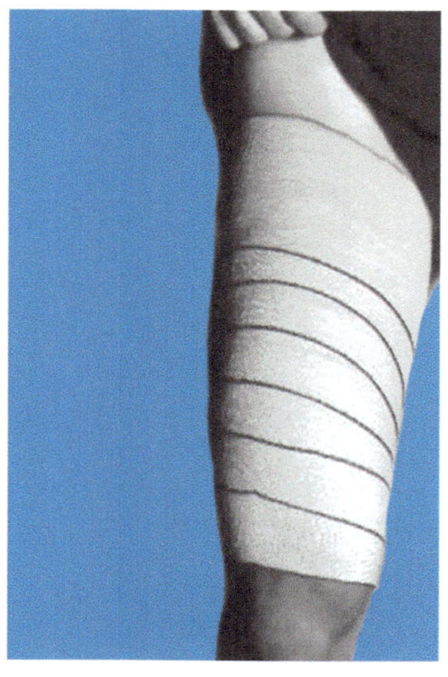

1. Begin the wrap at the proximal end of the thigh. Angle diagonally to the distal aspect of the quadriceps. At this point, begin an upward spiral supportive procedure with the wrap. Overlap each layer by one half of its width, ending at the proximal end of the thigh.

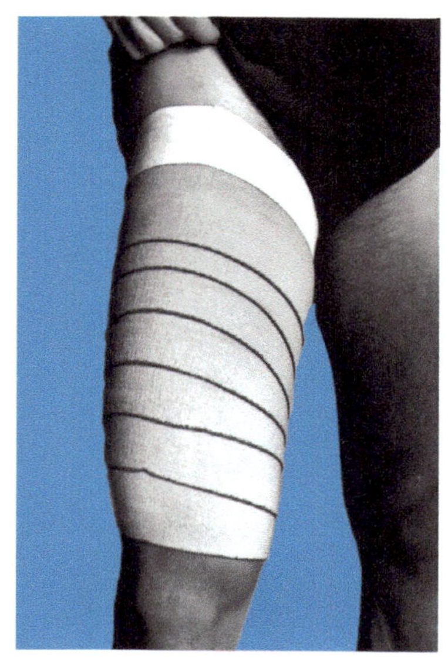

2. Secure the wrap in place by applying an anchor strip of 1½-in. adhesive tape.

**Upon completion of the procedure, make sure you check for neatness and gaps, adequate support, along with proper function of the affected area. In certain situations, the individual might be asked to perform function tests to establish appropriate technique application.*

Adjunct Taping Procedures: Quadriceps Wrap

These adjunct taping procedures can be used in conjunction with the basic technique presented.

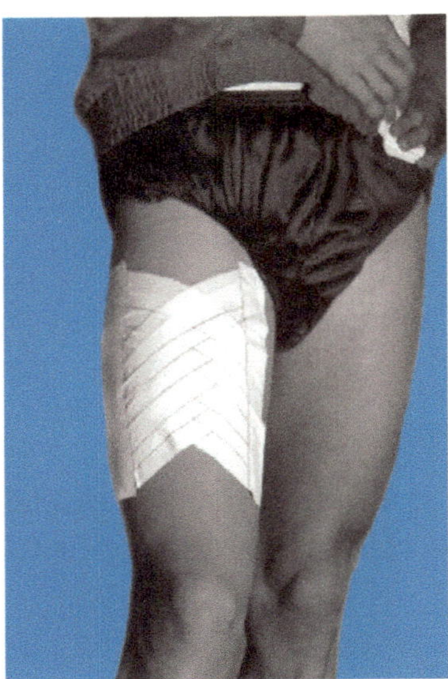

Technique A: The X pattern technique. Apply the wrap over this technique for additional support.

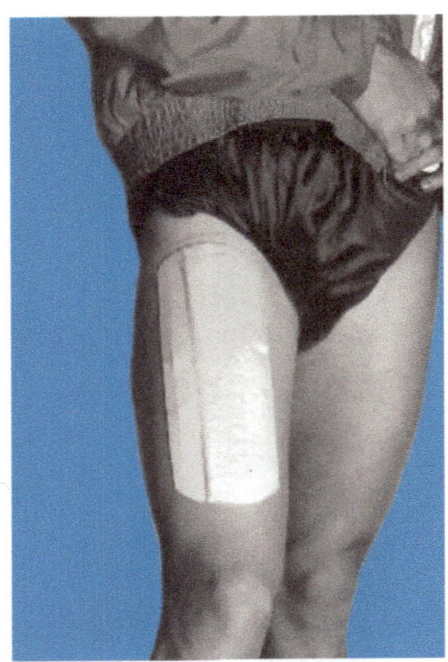

Technique B: Adhesive felt. Apply adhesive felt over the affected area of the anterior thigh.

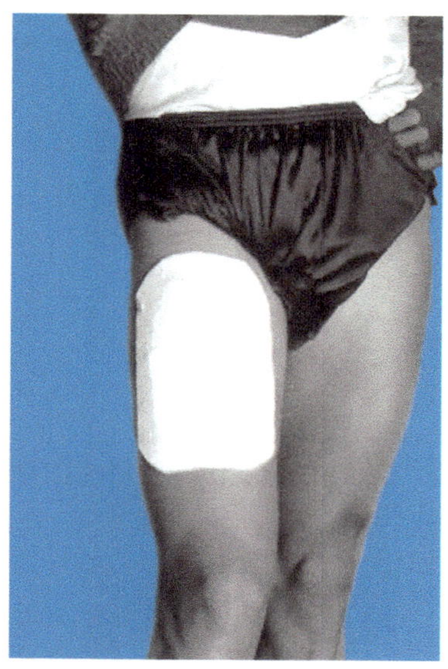

Technique C: Felt pad. Apply a 3-in. x 5-in. (or larger) felt pad (½ in. thick) over the affected area. Apply the wrap over this technique for additional support and compression.

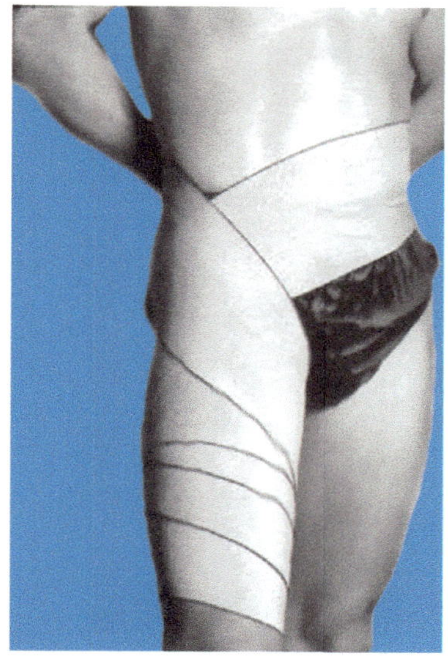

Technique D: Thigh/hip flexion wrap. Under certain situations, the application of this hip flexor wrap is preferred. This wrap will encircle the complete thigh and waist region of the body.

HIP FLEXOR WRAP

Purpose: To provide support to the hip flexor

Clinical Application: Strain to hip flexors

Anatomical Structure: Hip and thigh

Anatomical Position: The individual should stand with the affected extremity placed in hip flexion and the foot in slight internal rotation. The elastic wrap is continually applied in a hip spica method, abducting the thigh in the process.

Supplies: 6-in. extra long elastic wrap and 1½-in. adhesive tape

Pre-wrapping Procedure: The individual should contract the muscles around the hip joint

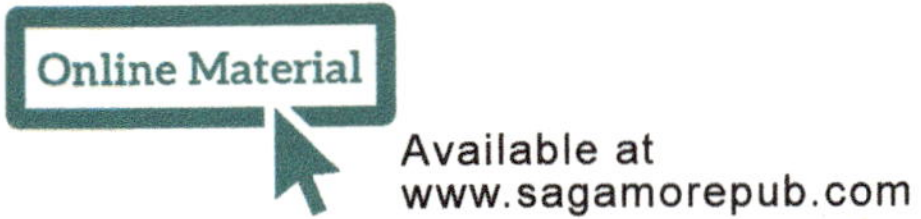

Wrapping Procedures

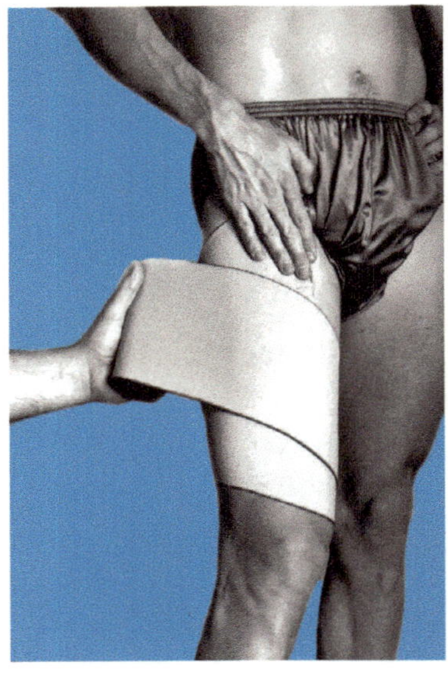

1. Begin the wrap at the proximal end of the thigh. From the anterior surface, angle diagonally to the distal lateral aspect of the quadriceps. Above the knee, begin an upward spiral supportive procedure with the wrap. Overlap each layer by one half of its width.

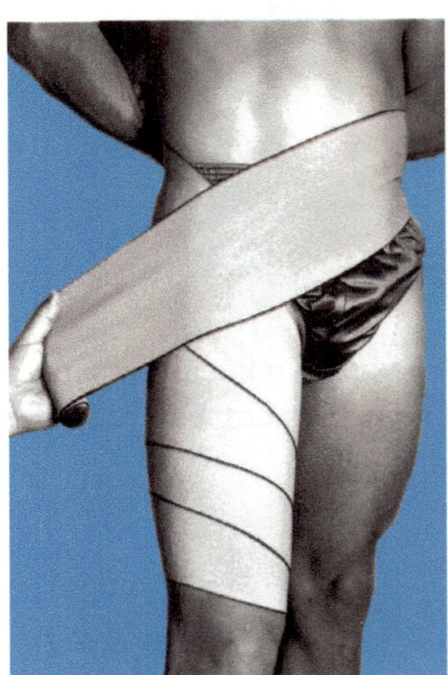

2. At the proximal end of the thigh, continue the wrap around the waist, pulling to the lateral and posterior aspect.

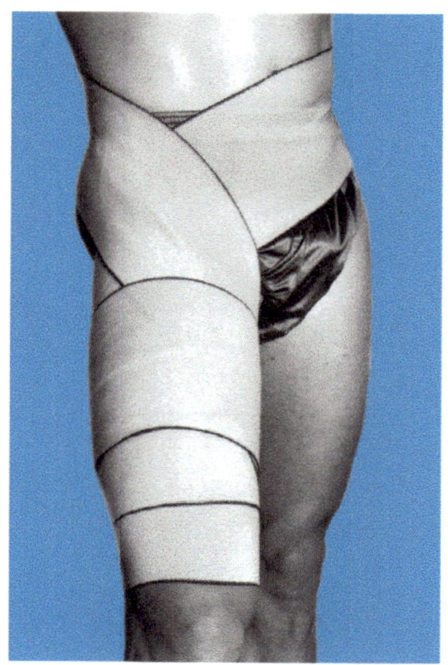

3. Once the waist has been encircled, continue the wrap around the thigh two to three times.

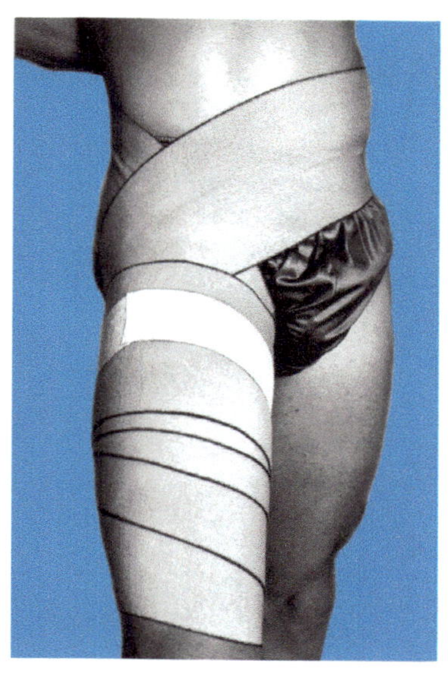

4. At this point, continue the wrap around the waist. This upward and outward pull should assist in hip flexion and limit hip extension. End the wrap on the thigh. Secure the wrap in place by applying an anchor strip of 1½-in. adhesive tape.

**Upon completion of the procedure, make sure you check for neatness and gaps, adequate support, along with proper function of the affected area. In certain situations, the individual might be asked to perform function tests to establish appropriate technique application.*

Adjunct Taping Procedures: Hip Flexor Wrap

This adjunct taping procedure can be used in conjunction with the basic technique presented.

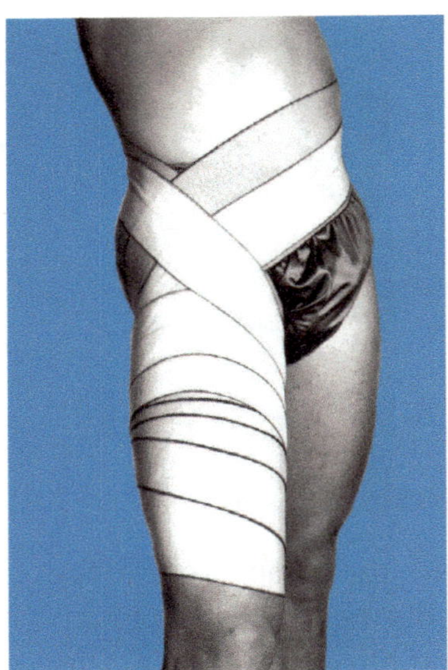

Technique A. Using 3-in. elastic tape, apply the tape over the wrap following the same pattern.

HIP ADDUCTOR WRAP

Purpose: To provide support to the hip adductors

Clinical Application: Strain to hip adductors

Anatomical Structure: Hip and thigh

Anatomical Position: The individual should stand with the affected extremity placed in hip flexion and the foot in slight internal rotation. The elastic wrap is continually applied in a hip spica method, abducting the thigh in the process.

Supplies: 6-in. extra long elastic wrap and 1½-in. adhesive tape

Pre-wrapping Procedure: The individual should contract the muscles around the hip joint.

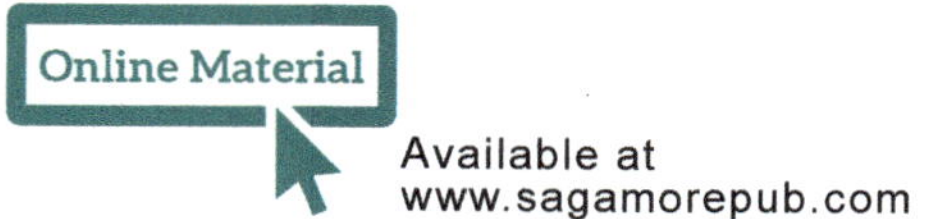

Wrapping Procedures

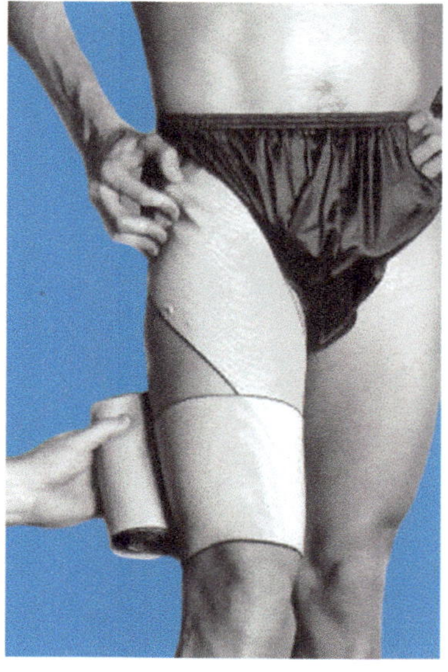

1. Begin the wrap at the proximal end of the thigh. From the anterior surface, angle diagonally to the distal medial aspect of the quadriceps. Above the knee, begin an upward spiral supportive procedure with the wrap. Overlap each layer by one half of its width.

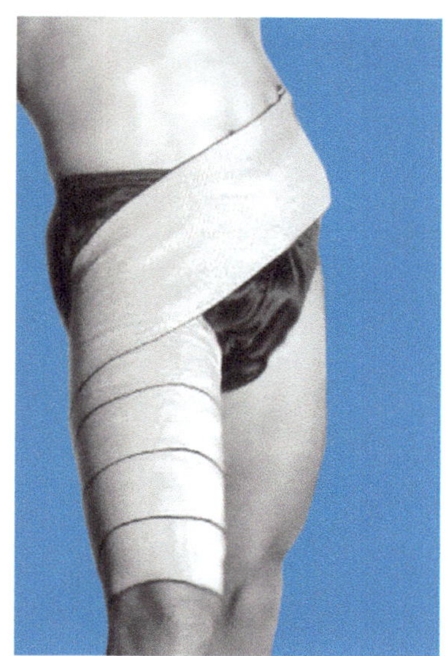

2. At the proximal end of the thigh, continue the wrap around the waist, pull across the abdomen to the lateral aspect and then to the posterior aspect. This upward and anterior pull should assist in hip adduction and limit hip abduction.

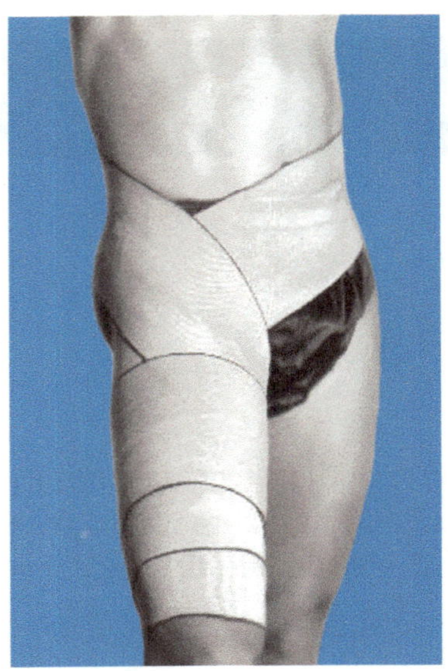

3. Once the waist has been encircled, continue the wrap downward and around the quadriceps muscle group two to three times.

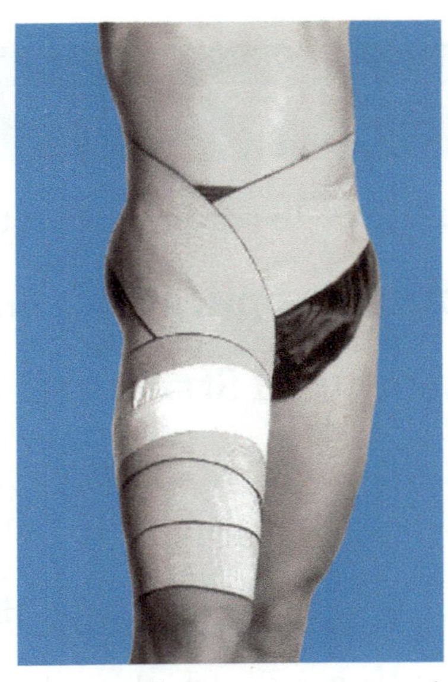

4. At this point, pull the wrap around the waist, crossing the abdomen, lateral, and posterior aspects. End the wrap on the thigh. Secure the wrap in place by applying an anchor strip of 1½-in. adhesive tape.

**Upon completion of the procedure, make sure you check for neatness and gaps, adequate support, along with proper function of the affected area. In certain situations, the individual might be asked to perform function tests to establish appropriate technique application.*

Adjunct Taping Procedures: Hip Adductor Wrap

This adjunct taping procedure can be used in conjunction with the basic technique presented.

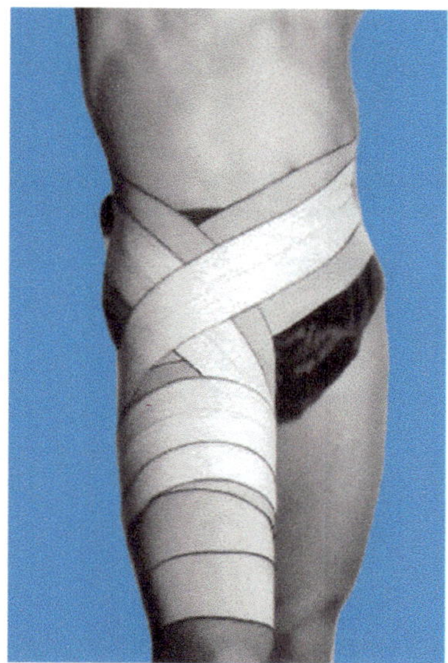

Technique A. Using 3-in. elastic tape, apply the tape over the wrap following the same pattern.

Protective Devices

The use of protective devices is beneficial if they are properly selected, used in the appropriate setting, correctly fitted, and follow the guidelines of the specific sport. Consultation with a medical equipment specialist is highly encouraged! In some cases, a prescription from a licensed physician may result in insurance reimbursement. Listed below are various protective devices that are commercially available for use in sports and/or physical activity.

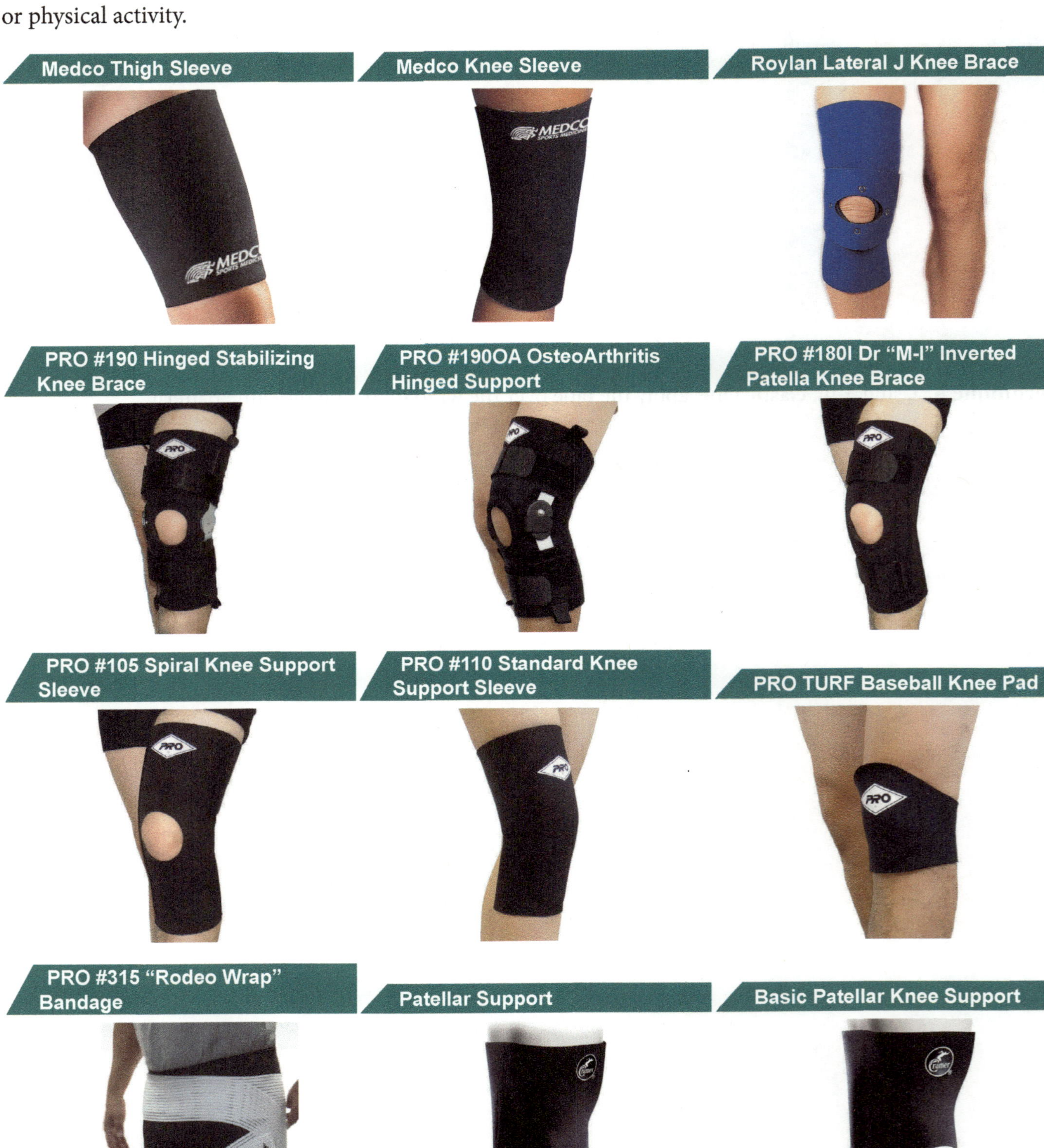

Patellar Tendon Strap

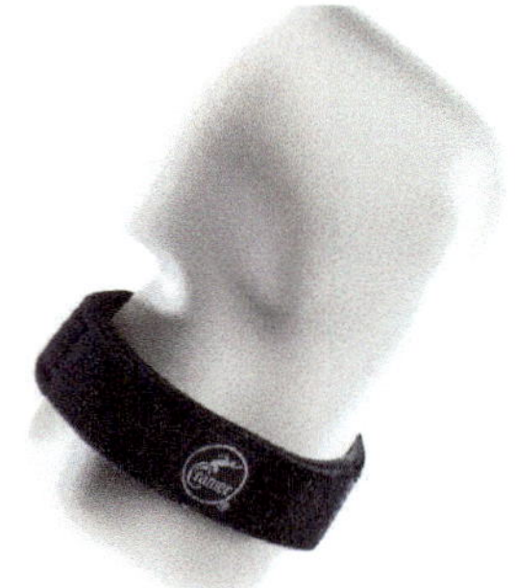

Groin Stain Support

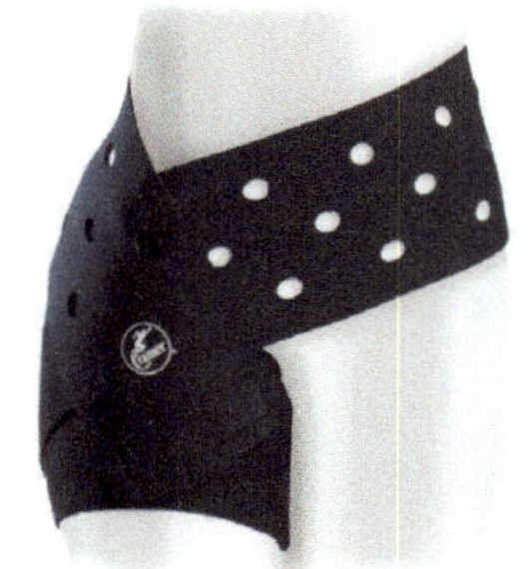

GH2 Support System

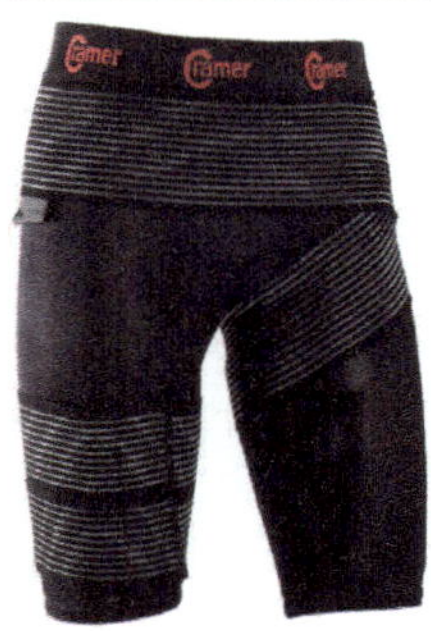

Listed below are various protective devices available to use in sport. Because a variety of protective devices is available, a qualified physician or qualified health care professional and medical equipment specialist can determine whether the individual is best suited for an off-the-shelf or custom brace.

Osgood Schlatter condition brace
Patella tendon strap
Sports compression girdle

Musculoskeletal Disorders

The following is a list of common musculoskeletal disorders of the knee, thigh, and hip. For definitions of these terms, the authors encourage the learner to consult these medical references: Taber's Medical Dictionary, Stedman's Medical Dictionary for the Health Professions and Nursing, and/or Signs and Symptoms of Athletic Injuries (listed in Appendix B).

Knee
Anterior cruciate ligament sprain
Bursitis
Lateral collateral ligament sprain
Medial collateral ligament sprain
Meniscal tear
Myositis ossificans
Popliteal cyst
Posterior cruciate ligament sprain
Tendinitis

Thigh and Hip
Bursitis
Hip pointer
Iliotibial ossificans
Quadriceps contusion
Sprain
Strain

PART III
Techniques for Upper Extremities

Chapter 5
Shoulder and Upper Arm

EDUCATIONAL OBJECTIVES

Upon completing this chapter, the reader will be able to do the following:

- Identify anatomical structures and landmarks critical for correct taping procedures
- Describe the purpose for the applications of adhesive and elastic tape
- Select the proper supplies and specialty items used for taping
- Explain the steps in preparing the body for taping, wrapping, or protective device
- Describe and demonstrate the purposes, clinical applications, anatomical structures, supplies needed, and pretaping and taping procedures for anatomical areas
- Identify the proper use and application of protective devices for the shoulder and upper arm

Introduction

The shoulder and upper arm can be complex to understand due to multiple movements. The occurrence of an injury to the area can compound the complexity. In this chapter, terminology, taping techniques, wrapping techniques, protective devices, and musculoskeletal disorders to the shoulder and upper arm will be discussed to provide greater clarity.

Terminology

External rotation. Turning outwardly or away from the midline of the body.

Internal rotation. Turning inwardly or toward the midline of the body.

Abduction. Lateral movement of a limb away from the median plane of the body; movement away from the median plane around an anterior–posterior axis with the angle between the displaced parts becoming greater, as in lifting the arm sideward away from the body.

Adduction. Lateral movement of a limb toward the median plane of the body; movement toward the median plane around an anterior–posterior axis with the angle between the displaced parts becoming lesser, as in bringing the arm sideward against the body.

Circumduction. Movement around an axis such that the proximal end of a limb is fixed and the distal end traces a circle.

Shoulder and Upper Arm

Taping and Wrapping Techniques and Protective Devices

Developing a thorough knowledge regarding the fundamentals about the application of taping/wrapping procedures is imperative. Review Chapter 1 before applying any technique.

Proper Assessment of Injury

Before applying a preventive technique (tape, wrap, and/or device), a qualified physician must complete a proper injury evaluation. Following the injury evaluation, a qualified health care professional can then recommend proper taping techniques. This ensures that proper taping techniques are applied for support and stabilization. Also, developing a thorough knowledge of taping application fundamentals is imperative.

Purpose and Application of Adhesive and Elastic Tape

The primary purpose for tape application is to provide additional support and stability for the affected body part. Through proper application, taping techniques can be applied to shorten the muscle's angle of pull; to decrease joint range of motion; to secure pads, bandages, and protective devices; and to apply compression to reduce swelling.

Medical Supplies and Specialty Items

Purchasing supplies depends on budget, philosophy of medical staff regarding taping techniques, and occurrence of injury. Review Chapter 1 before applying any technique.

Specific Rules on Taping, Wrapping, and/or Protective Device

If you apply supportive techniques to an individual, you should be aware of specific rules governing tape application in that particular sport or physical activity. Your application must fall within the guidelines established for each sport by appropriate governing bodies.

Special Techniques: Adjunct Taping Procedures

The taping techniques presented are the fundamental procedures. Adjunct techniques will be shown to provide additional support; however, you should still follow the fundamental procedures. Variations can be achieved by adapting these techniques to a particular injury situation. Always give special consideration to

- purpose of the taping procedure
- clinical application
- correct anatomical position
- supply selection
- tape/wrap technique or protective device

Preparation of Body Part for Taping

In preparing the body for tape application, consider these items:

- removal of hair (optional)
- clean the area
- special considerations
- spray adherent (optional)
- skin lubricants
- underwrap or cohesive tape
- proper body position

Proper Body Position

Before beginning a taping procedure, select a comfortable table height and ask the individual to assume an anatomically correct and comfortable position.

- Neutral Position of Shoulder—Acromioclavicular Joint: The individual should be in a standing position with shoulder abducted, elbow flexed, hand set on waist, and chest slightly expanded.
- Neutral Position of Shoulder—Glenohumeral Joint: The individual should stand with should abducted, elbow flexed, and bicep muscles contracts, hand set on low back and chest expanded.
- When applying a technique, learn to stand at a comfortable and stationary position and place the body part to be taped at your elbow height.

Bones and Ligaments

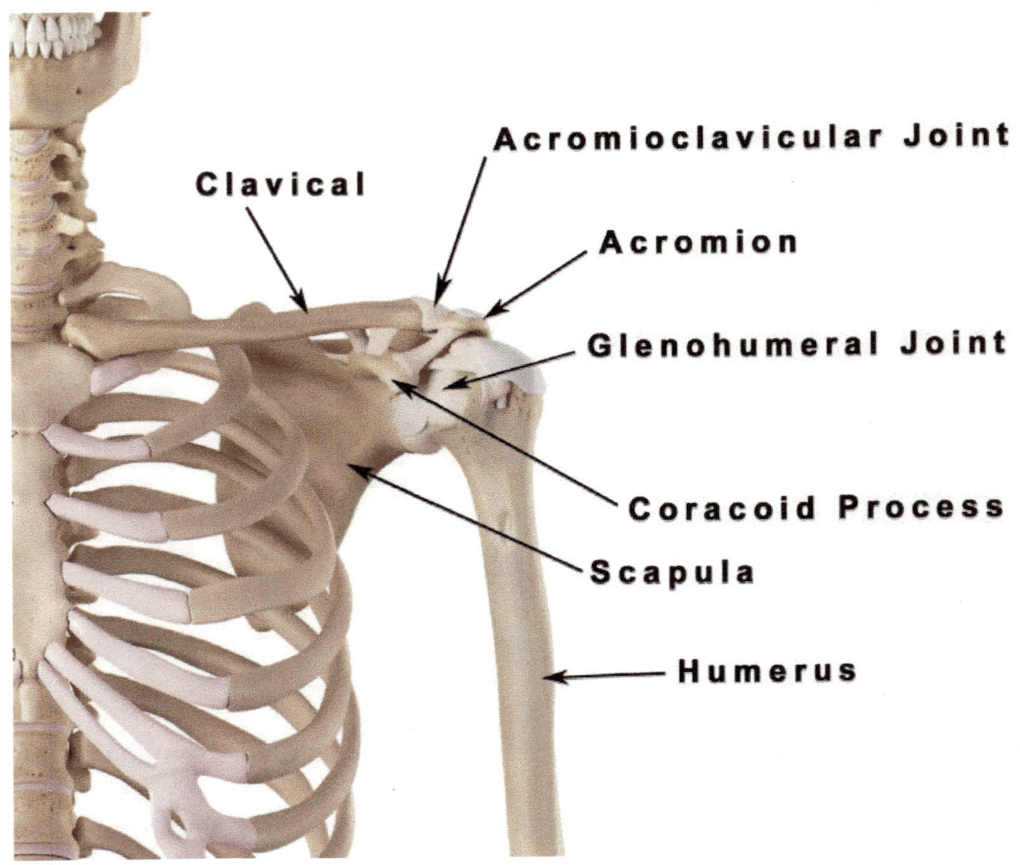

Muscles and Tendons

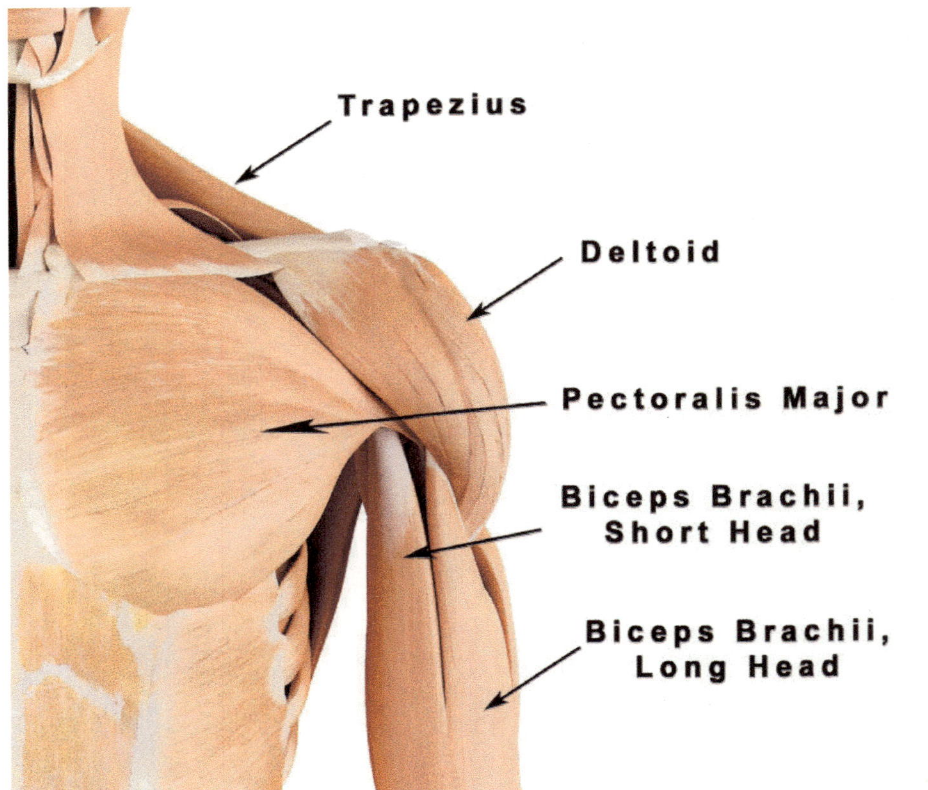

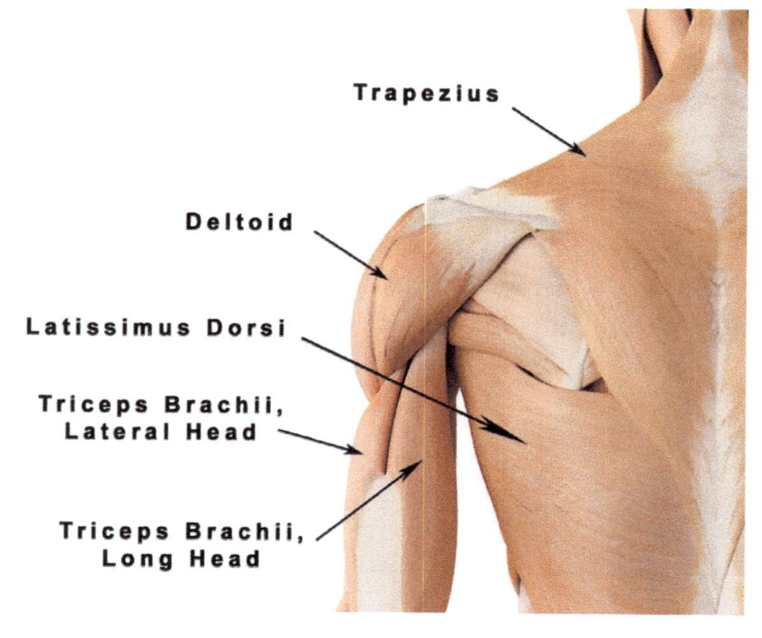
Trapezius
Deltoid
Latissimus Dorsi
Triceps Brachii,
Lateral Head
Triceps Brachii,
Long Head

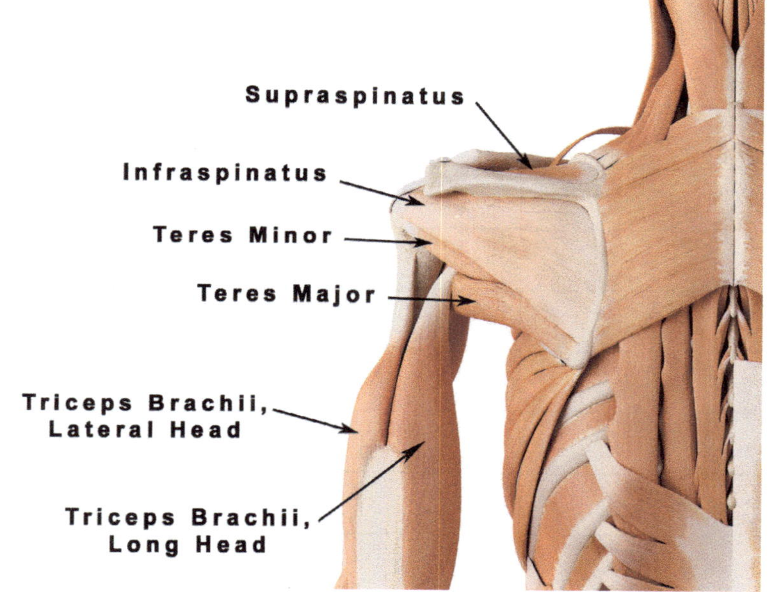
Supraspinatus
Infraspinatus
Teres Minor
Teres Major
Triceps Brachii,
Lateral Head
Triceps Brachii,
Long Head

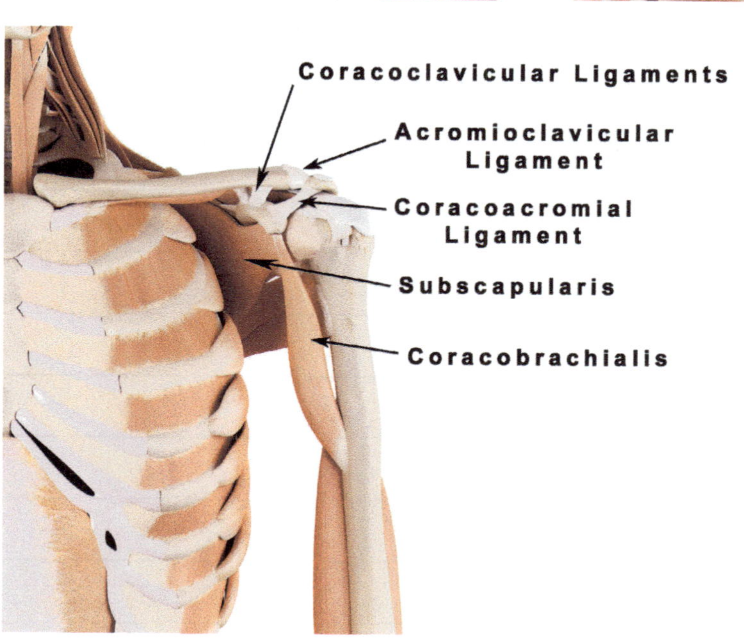
Coracoclavicular Ligaments
Acromioclavicular
Ligament
Coracoacromial
Ligament
Subscapularis
Coracobrachialis

Taping Techniques

The taping techniques presented are the *fundamental procedures*. A strong knowledge of anatomy, physiology, and biomechanics is essential. Developing a thorough knowledge regarding the fundamentals about the application of taping/wrapping procedures is imperative. Review Section A–Chapter 1 before applying any technique. When applying tape to the foot or ankle, pull the tape lateral to avoid excessive tension/compression on the fifth metatarsal.

The Kinesio® Taping Method is a therapeutic taping technique not only offering your patient the support they are looking for, but also rehabilitating the affected condition as well. Please consult Chapter 9 for specific application instructions.

NOTES:

ACROMIOCLAVICULAR (AC) JOINT

Purpose: To provide support and stabilization to the acromioclavicular (AC) joint

Clinical Application: Sprains and contusions

Anatomical Structure: Acromioclavicular joint of the shoulder

Anatomical Position: The individual should be in a standing position with shoulder abducted, elbow flexed, hand set on waist, and chest slightly expanded.

Supplies: 2-in. elastic tape, 1½-in. adhesive tape, and gauze pad or large Band-Aid

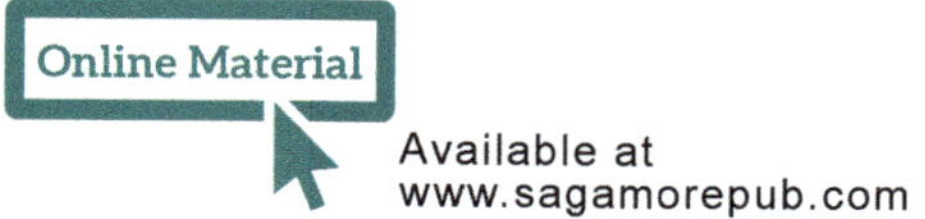

Pre-taping Procedure

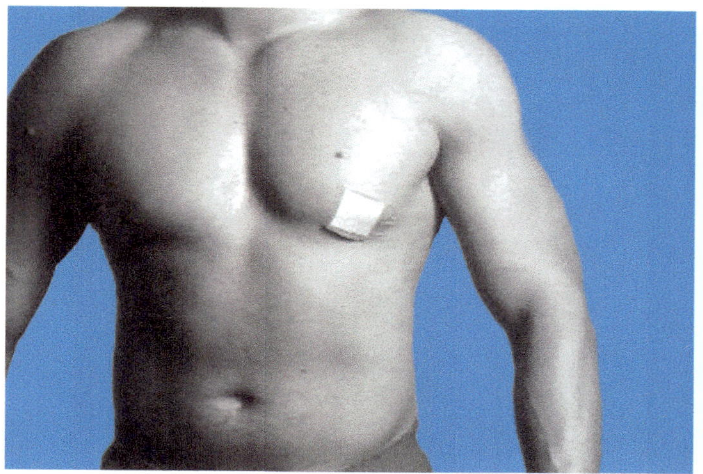

Place the gauze pad or Band-Aid over the nipple of the affected side.

Taping Procedures

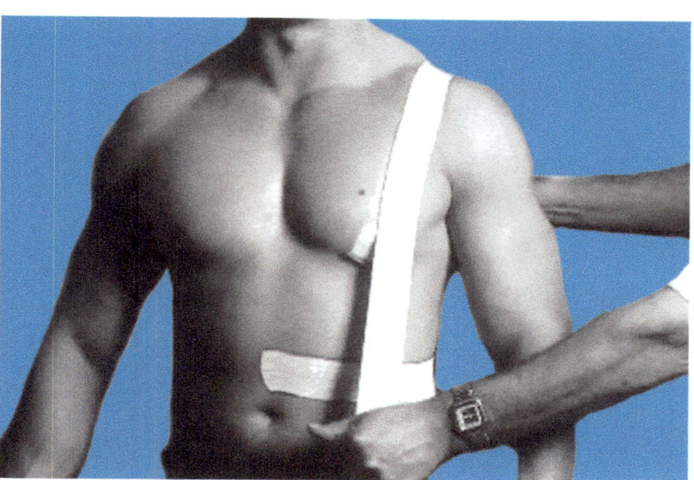

1. Using 2-in. elastic tape, place a horizontal anchor strip from the anterior to the posterior body midline. This anchor strip should cover the mid- or lower portion of the rib cage.

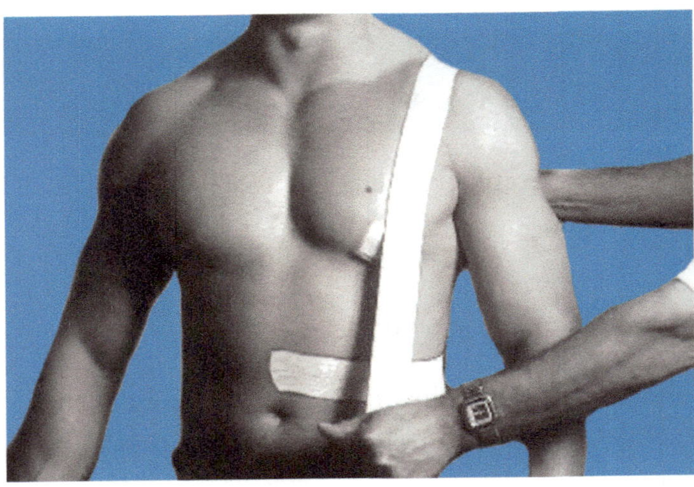

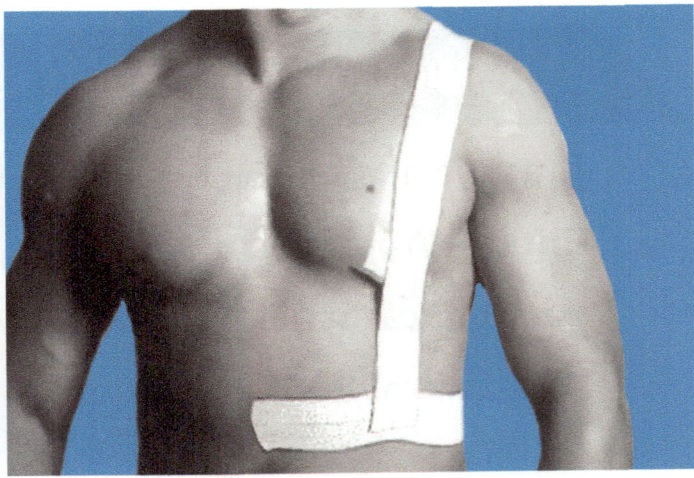

2. Measure the distance from the anterior portion of the anchor across the AC joint and end on the posterior anchor. Apply a strip of 1½-in. adhesive tape to this area. With the middle of the tape placed on the AC joint, apply equal tension toward both the anterior end and the posterior end and attach tape to the anchor.

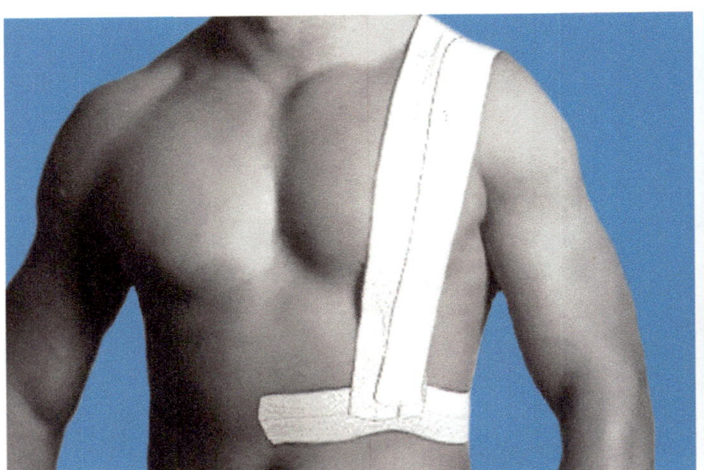

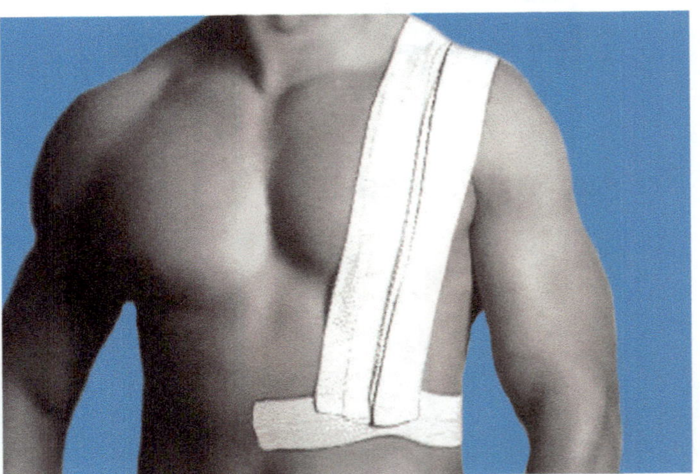

3. Repeat step 2 three times.

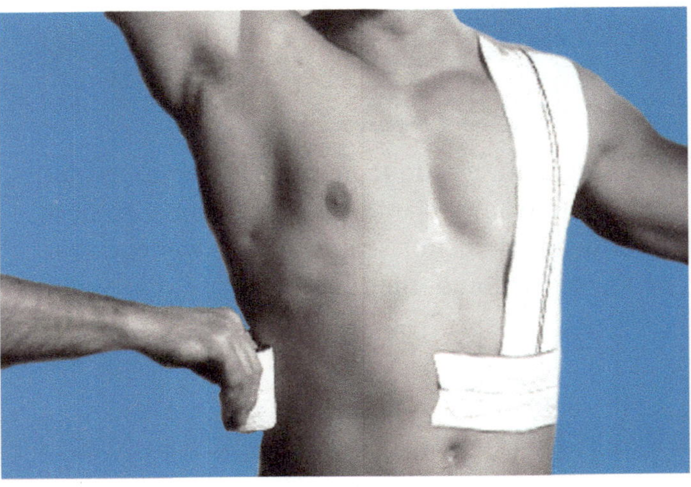

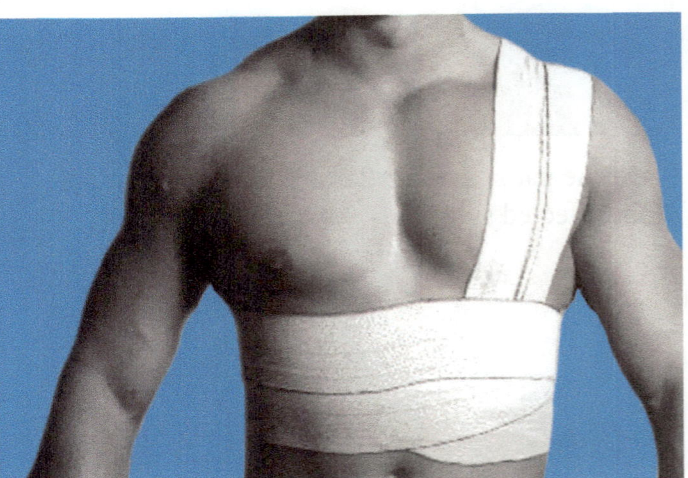

4. To add additional support, encircle a second horizontal anchor strip around the torso.

**Upon completion of the procedure, make sure you check for neatness and gaps, adequate support, along with proper function of the affected area. In certain situations, the individual might be asked to perform function tests to establish appropriate technique application.*

Adjunct Taping Procedures: Acromioclavicular Joint

These adjunct taping procedures can be used in conjunction with the basic technique presented.

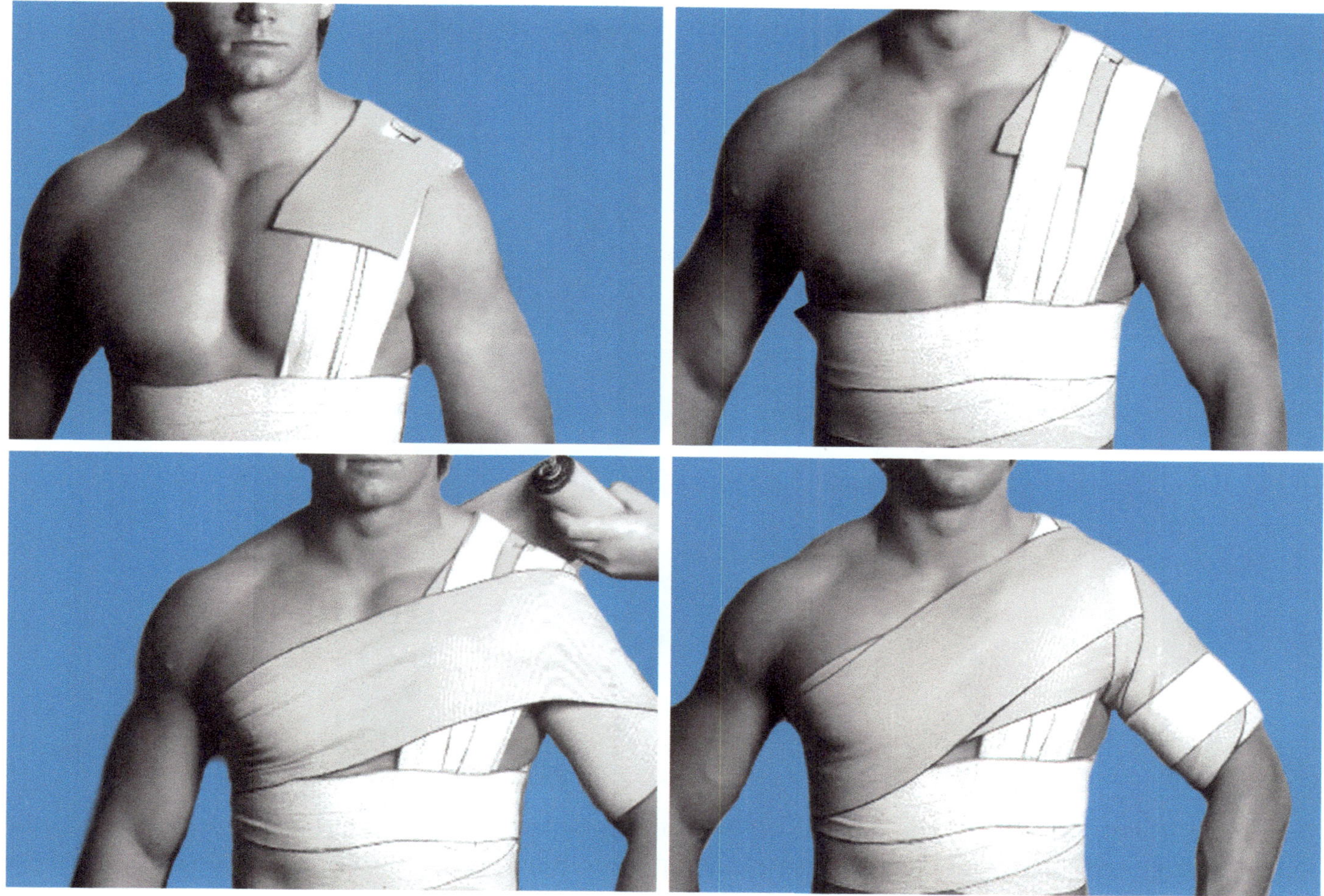

Technique A. For additional protection to the AC joint, construct a felt or foam rubber pad that is at least 1/2 in. thick. Also, a "thermoplastic" pad may be used! The pad must be large enough to cover the affected superior aspect of the shoulder. Cut a hole in this protective pad and place over the affected AC joint. To secure this pad, apply 2-in. elastic tape over the AC joint. Using a 6-in. extra long elastic wrap, apply a shoulder spica wrap to this area to hold in place. Begin on the posterior aspect of the upper arm, move anteriorly, encircle the arm, continue across the anterior aspect of the chest, go under the opposite arm, go across the posterior aspect of the torso angling upward and over the affected AC joint, and encircle the upper arm. Repeat this procedure a second time. Secure the wrap with 2-in. elastic tape. *When taping the FEMALE INDIVIDUAL, apply this procedure the same; however, the horizontal strips should end above the breast.*

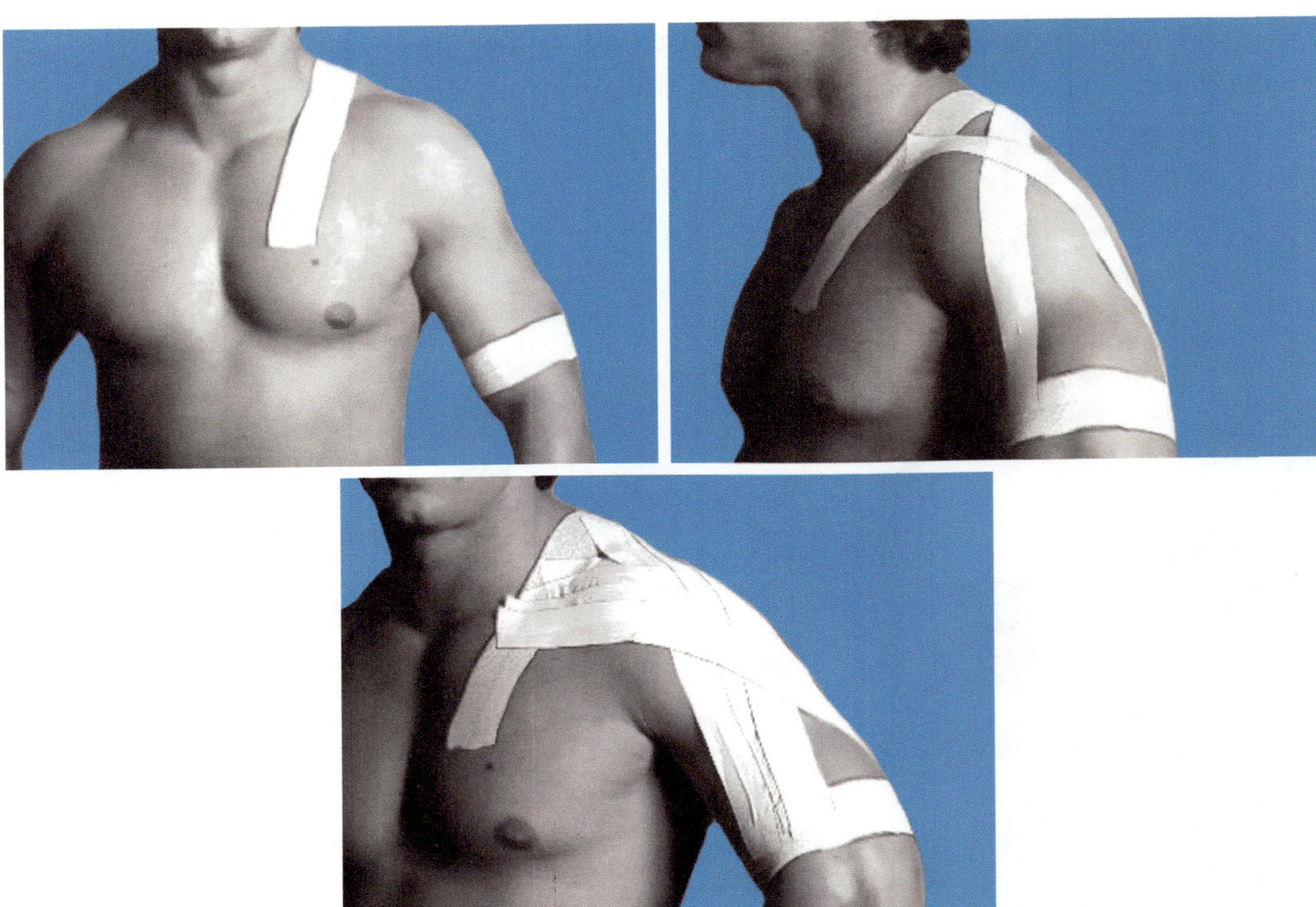

Technique B. For individuals who have difficulty in the complete application of this technique around the shoulder girdle and torso, a modified version can be applied. After placing the horizontal anchor strip in the mid-region of the chest, apply stability strips with equal tension toward the anterior and posterior anchors strips. Repeat this step four times, and then anchor for stability.

GLENOHUMERAL JOINT

Purpose: To provide support and stability to the glenohumeral joint of the shoulder. A continuous strip of elastic tape is applied in a shoulder spica method. This supportive technique should restrict abduction and external rotation of the glenohumeral joint.

Clinical Application: Sprains and strains

Anatomical Structure: Glenohumeral joint

Anatomical Position: The individual should stand with shoulder abducted, elbow flexed, biceps muscles contracted, hand set on low back, and chest expanded

Supplies: 3-in. elastic tape and gauze pads or Band-Aid

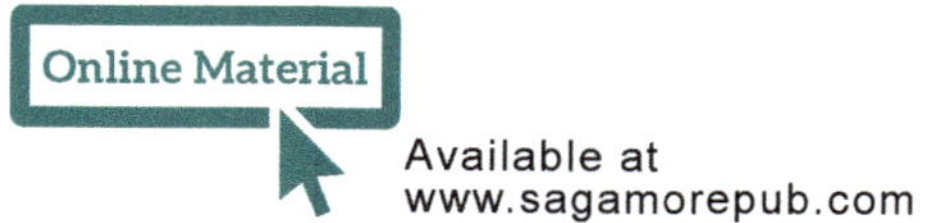

Pre-taping Procedure

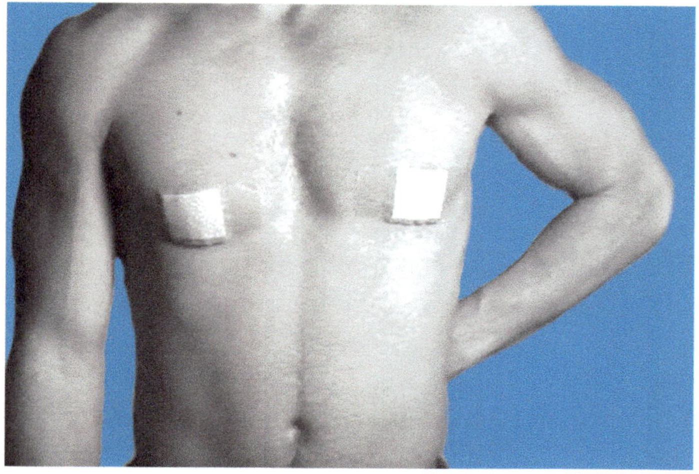

Cover both nipples with gauze pads or Band-Aid

Taping Procedures

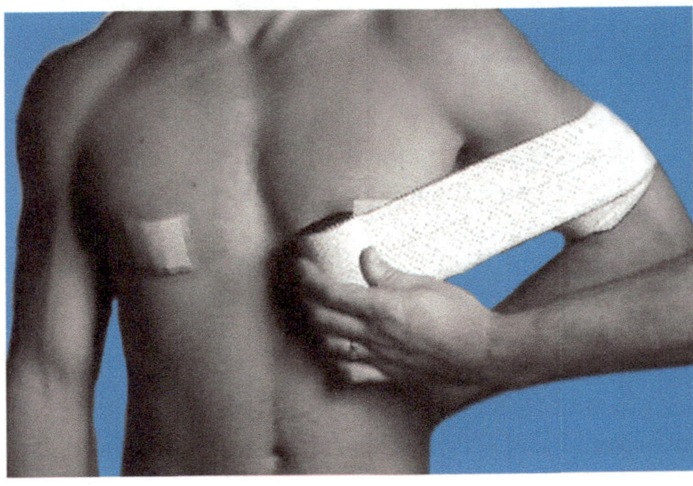

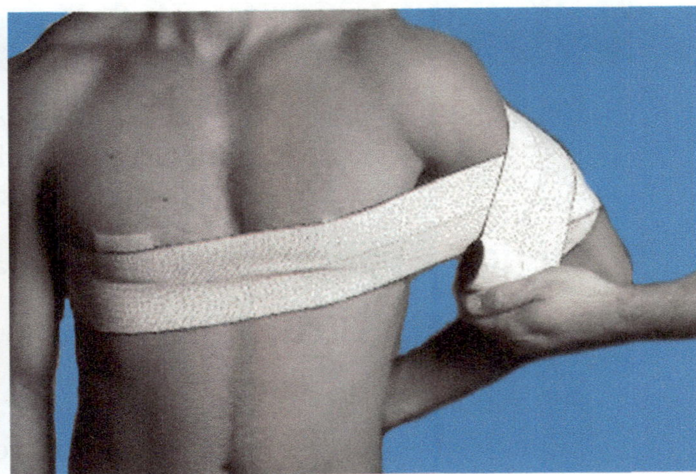

1. Begin on the distal aspect of the affected upper arm, move anteriorly, encircle the arm, continue across the anterior aspect of the chest, go under the opposite arm, go across the posterior aspect of the torso, and encircle the distal aspect of the upper arm.

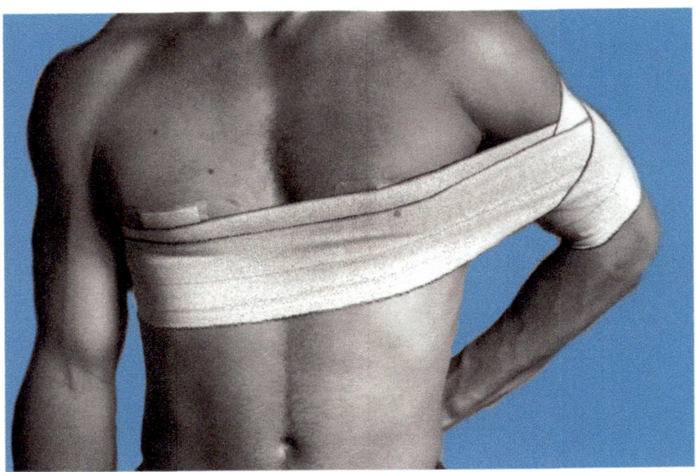

2. Repeat this procedure a second time. *Comment:* In certain situations, a check rein can be applied between the torso and upper arm. This technique will aid in preventing the glenohumeral joint from excessive abduction and external rotation.

**Upon completion of the procedure, make sure you check for neatness and gaps, adequate support, along with proper function of the affected area. In certain situations, the individual might be asked to perform function tests to establish appropriate technique application.*

Adjunct Taping Procedures: Glenohumeral Joint

These adjunct taping procedures can be used in conjunction with the basic technique presented.

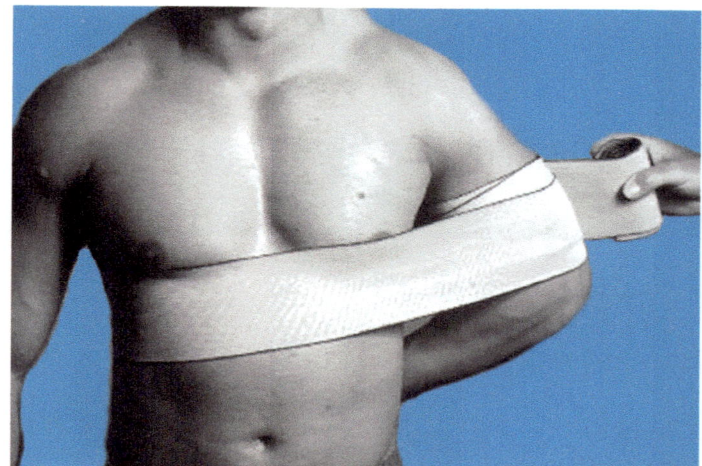

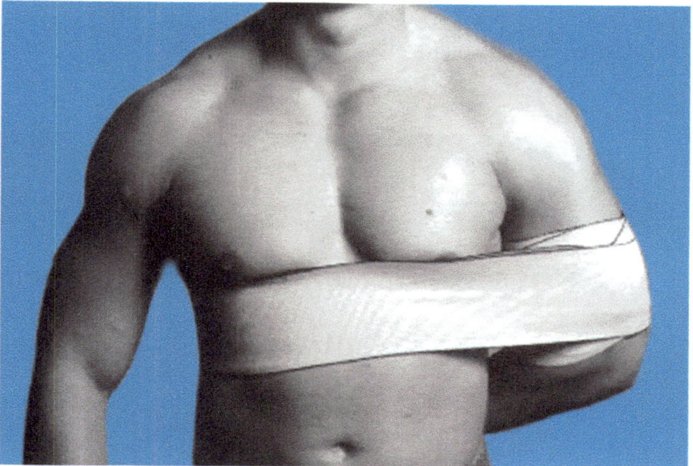

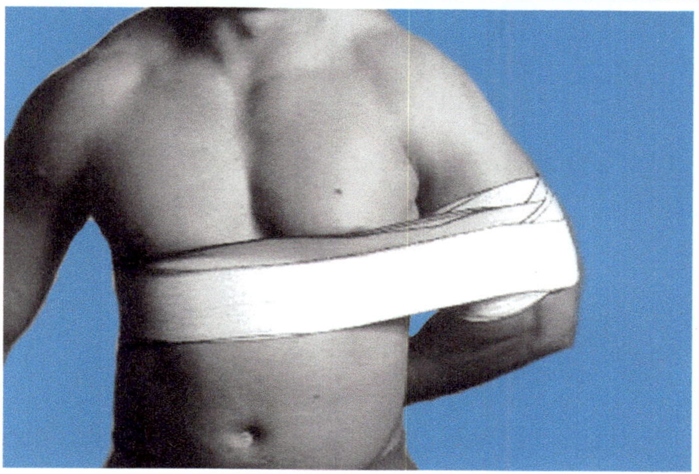

Technique A. Using a 6-in. extra long elastic wrap, apply a shoulder spica wrap to this area. This support wrap should restrict abduction and external rotation of the shoulder. Begin on the posterior aspect of the upper arm, move anteriorly, encircle the arm, continue across the anterior aspect of the chest, go under the opposite arm, go across the posterior aspect of the torso angling upward, go over the affected joint, and then encircle the upper arm. Repeat this procedure a second time. Secure the wrap by using a continuous strip of elastic tape in the same pattern as the wrap.

Wrapping Techniques for Support

During physical activity, supportive wraps are used to aid in muscle function and support and to reduce excessive range of motion. These applications are typically used in competition or practice. Spica wraps are traditionally employed at the hip and shoulder joints. Figure of 8 wraps are placed over ankle, knee, elbow, wrist, and hand joints.

GLENOHUMERAL JOINT WRAP

Purpose: To provide support to the glenohumeral joint of the shoulder

Clinical Application: Sprains of the glenohumeral joint

Anatomical Structure: Glenohumeral joint

Anatomical Position: The individual should stand with shoulder abducted, elbow flexed, biceps muscle contracted, hand set on hip or low back, and chest expanded

Supplies: 6-in. extra long elastic wrap and 2-in. adhesive tape

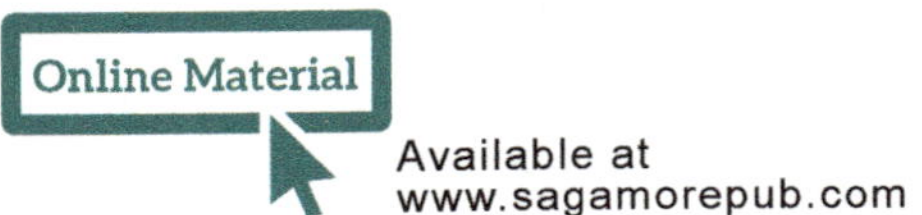

Wrapping Procedures

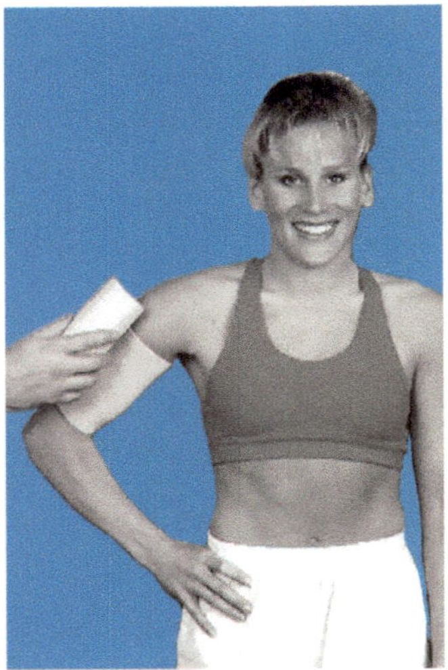

1. Apply a continuous strip of 6-in. elastic wrap in a shoulder spica method. This supportive technique should restrict abduction and external rotation of the glenohumeral joint. Begin on the distal aspect of the biceps muscle of the affected arm, move anteriorly, and encircle the arm.

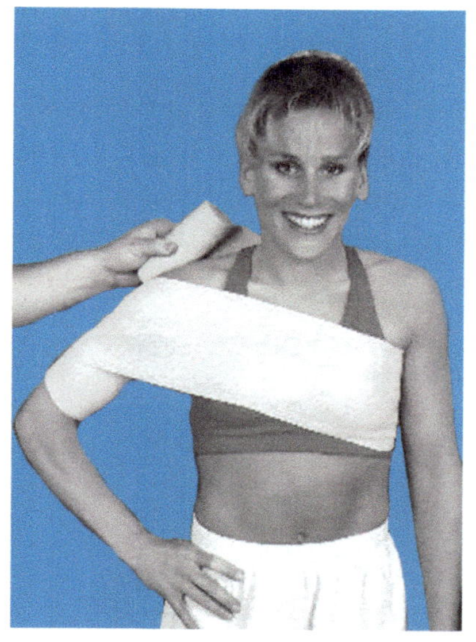

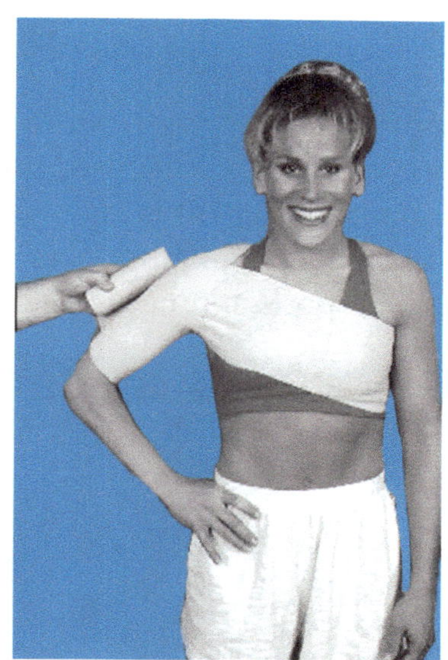

2. Continue the wrap across the anterior aspect of the chest, go under the opposite arm, go across the posterior aspect of the torso, and encircle the distal aspect of the upper arm.

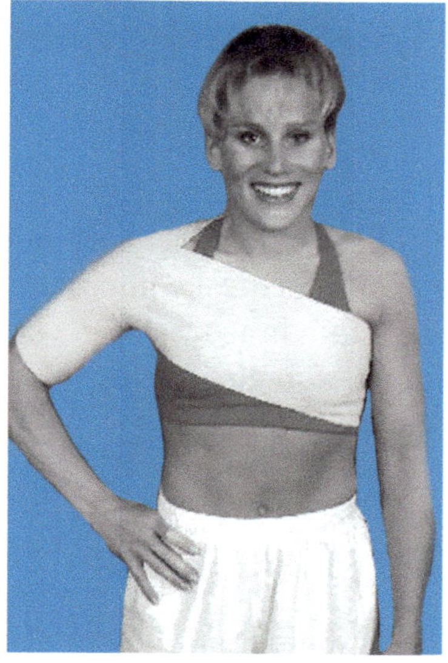

3. Repeat this procedure a second time.

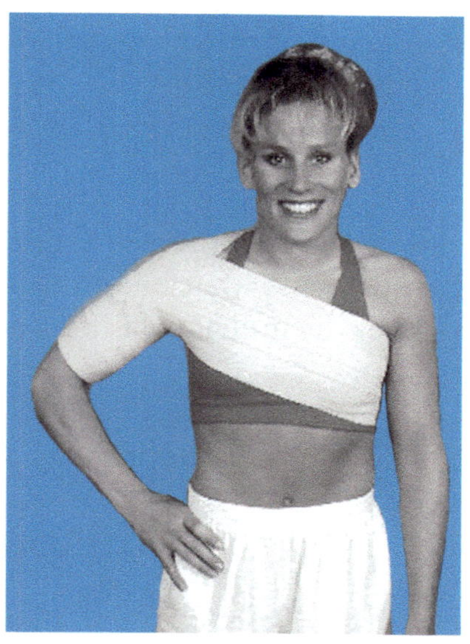

4. Secure the wrap by using a continuous strip of elastic tape in the same pattern as the wrap. Anchor the wrap with 2-in. elastic tape following the same pattern as the wrap.

**Upon completion of the procedure, make sure you check for neatness and gaps, adequate support, along with proper function of the affected area. In certain situations, the individual might be asked to perform function tests to establish appropriate technique application.*

Protective Devices

The use of protective devices is beneficial if they are properly selected, used in the appropriate setting, correctly fitted, properly applied, and used within the rules and guidelines of the specific sport. Consultation with a medical equipment specialist is highly encouraged! In some cases, a prescription from a licensed physician may result in insurance reimbursement. Listed below are various protective devices that are commercially available for use in sports and/or physical activity.

PRO #450 Shoulder Support

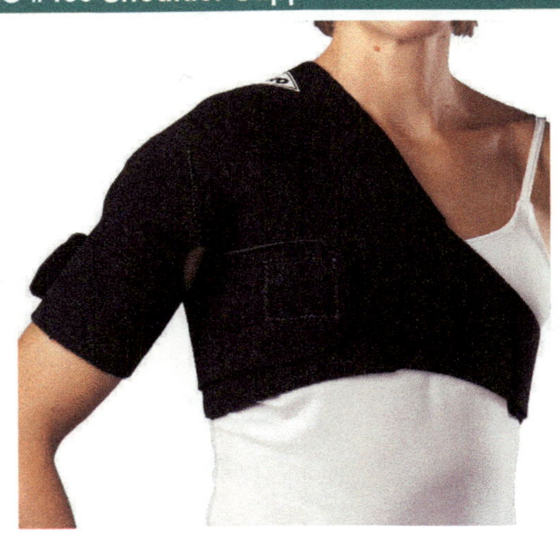

Shoulder Brace

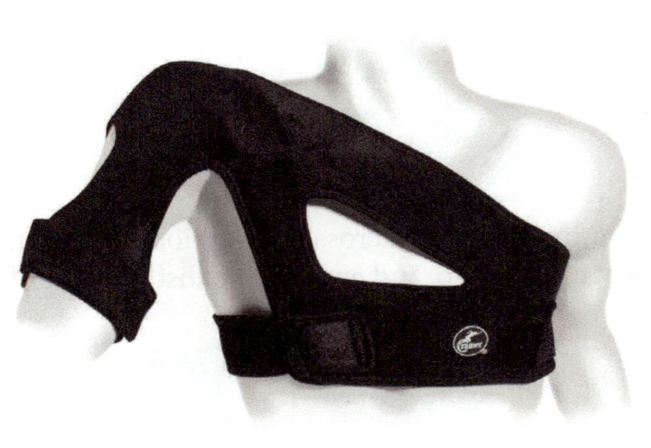

Listed below are various protective devices available to use in sport. Because a variety of protective devices are available, a qualified physician or qualified health care professional and medical equipment specialist can determine whether the individual is best suited for an off-the-shelf or custom brace

AC Joint Pad
Blockers exostosis pad
Glenohumeral joint stailizer brace
Sports compression girdle
Sternum protector

Musculoskeletal Disorders

The following is a list of common musculoskeletal disorders of the shoulder and upper arm. For definitions of these terms, the authors encourage the learner to consult these medical references: *Taber's Medical Dictionary*, *Stedman's Medical Dictionary for the Health Professions and Nursing*, and/or *Signs and Symptoms of Athletic Injuries* (listed in Appendix B).

Shoulder and Upper Arm
Blockers exostosis
Bursitis
Contusion
Dislocation
Nerve injury
Rotator cuff dysfunction
Rotator cuff impingement
Rotator cuff strain
Separation
Sprain
Strain
Subluxation
Synovitis
Tendonitis
Tenosynovitis

Chapter 6

Elbow, Forearm, Wrist, and Hand

EDUCATIONAL OBJECTIVES

Upon completing this chapter, the reader will be able to do the following:

- Identify anatomical structures and landmarks critical for correct taping procedures
- Describe the purpose for the applications of adhesive and elastic tape
- Select the proper supplies and specialty items used for taping
- Explain the steps in preparing the body for taping, wrapping, or protective device
- Describe and demonstrate the purposes, clinical applications, anatomical structures, supplies needed, and pretaping and taping procedures for anatomical areas
- Identify the proper use and application of protective devices for the elbow, forearm, wrist, and hand

Introduction

The ability to use the elbow, forearm, wrist, and hand for active use is important for daily living. Nevertheless, the occurrence of an injury is possible and can be problematic. This chapter will cover terminology, taping techniques, wrapping techniques, protective devices, and musculoskeletal disorders for the elbow, forearm, wrist, and hand to assist with injury care.

Terminology

Flexion. Movement around a transverse axis in an anterior–posterior plane with the angle between the anterior aspects of the displaced parts becoming smaller, as in bending the forearm toward the arm at the elbow joint; the act of drawing a body segment away from a straight line with its proximally conjoined body segment or toward that smallest acute angle of the joint.

Extension. The reverse movement during which the angle between the anterior aspects of the displaced parts is increased, as in moving the forearm away from the upper arm; the act of drawing a body segment toward a straight line position with its proximally conjoined body segment or away from the body joint.

Pronation. Act of rotating the hand or foot internally on its long axis; medial rotation of the forearm, as in turning the palm of the hand downward.

Supination. Act of rotating the hand or foot externally on its long axis; lateral rotation of the forearm, as in turning the palm of the hand upward

Anatomical snuffbox. Space at the base of the thumb created by the extensor pollicis longus and brevis tendons.

Elbow, Forearm, Wrist, and Hand

Taping and Wrapping Techniques and Protective Devices

Developing a thorough knowledge regarding the fundamentals about the application of taping/wrapping procedures is imperative. Review Chapter 1 before applying any technique.

Proper Assessment of Injury

Before applying a preventive technique (tape, wrap, and/or device), a qualified physician should complete a proper injury evaluation. Following the injury evaluation, a qualified health care professional can then recommend proper taping techniques. This ensures that proper taping techniques are applied for support and stabilization. Also, developing a thorough knowledge of taping application fundamentals is imperative.

Purpose and Application of Adhesive and Elastic Tape

The primary purpose for tape application is to provide additional support and stability for the affected body part. Through proper application, taping techniques can be applied to shorten the muscle's angle of pull; to decrease joint range of motion; to secure pads, bandages, and protective devices; and to apply compression to reduce swelling.

Medical Supplies and Specialty Items

Purchasing supplies depends on budget, philosophy of medical staff regarding taping techniques, and occurrence of injury. Review Chapter 1 before applying any technique.

Specific Rules on Taping, Wrapping, and/or Protective Device

If you apply supportive techniques to an individual, you should be aware of specific rules governing tape application in that particular sport or physical activity. Your application must fall within the guidelines established for each sport by appropriate governing bodies.

Special Techniques: Adjunct Taping Procedures

The taping techniques presented are the fundamental procedures. Adjunct techniques will be shown to provide additional support; however, you should still follow the fundamental procedures. Variations can be achieved by adapting these techniques to a particular injury situation. Always give special consideration to

- purpose of the taping procedure
- clinical application
- correct anatomical position
- supply selection
- tape/wrap technique or protective device

Preparation of Body Part for Taping

In preparing the body for tape application, consider these items:

- removal of hair (optional)
- clean the area
- special considerations
- spray adherent (optional)
- skin lubricants
- underwrap or cohesive tape
- proper body positioning

Proper Body Positioning

Before beginning a taping procedure, select a comfortable table height and ask the individual to assume an anatomically correct and comfortable position.

- Neutral Position of Elbow: From the anatomical position, the elbow joint should be held in slight flexion (10 to 15 degrees).
- Neutral Position of Wrist and Hand: This position can vary, so consult specific taping techniques for anatomical structure placement.

When applying a technique, learn to stand at a comfortable and stationary position and place the body part to be taped at your elbow height.

Bones and Ligaments

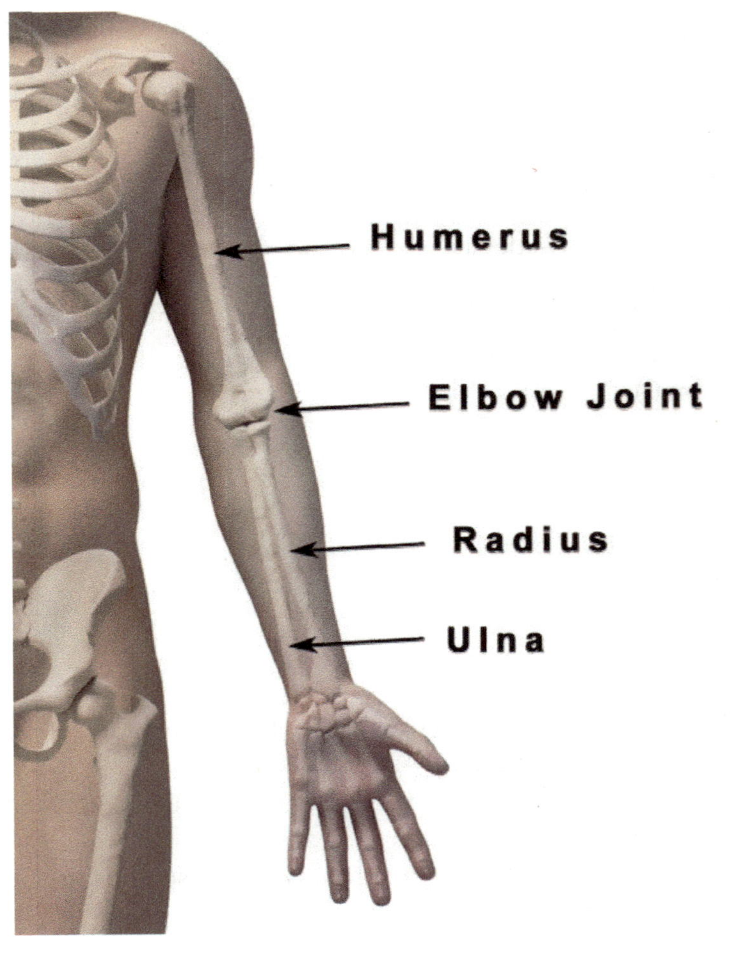

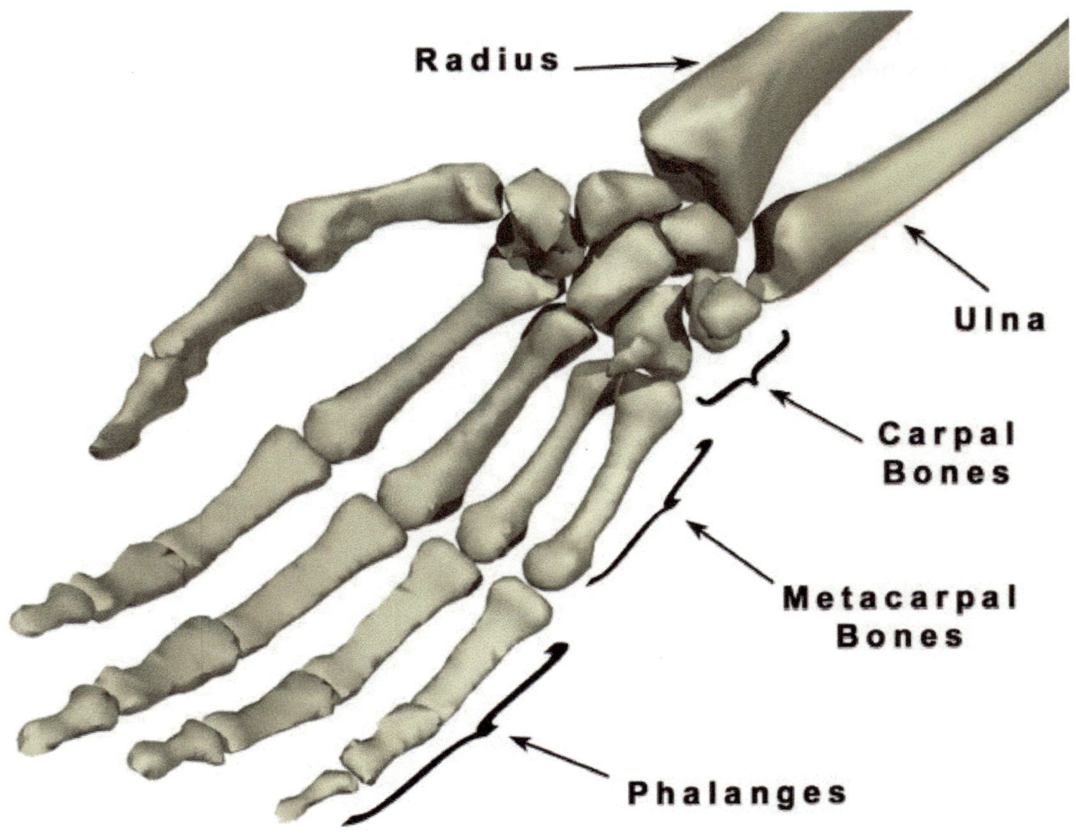

Muscles and Tendons

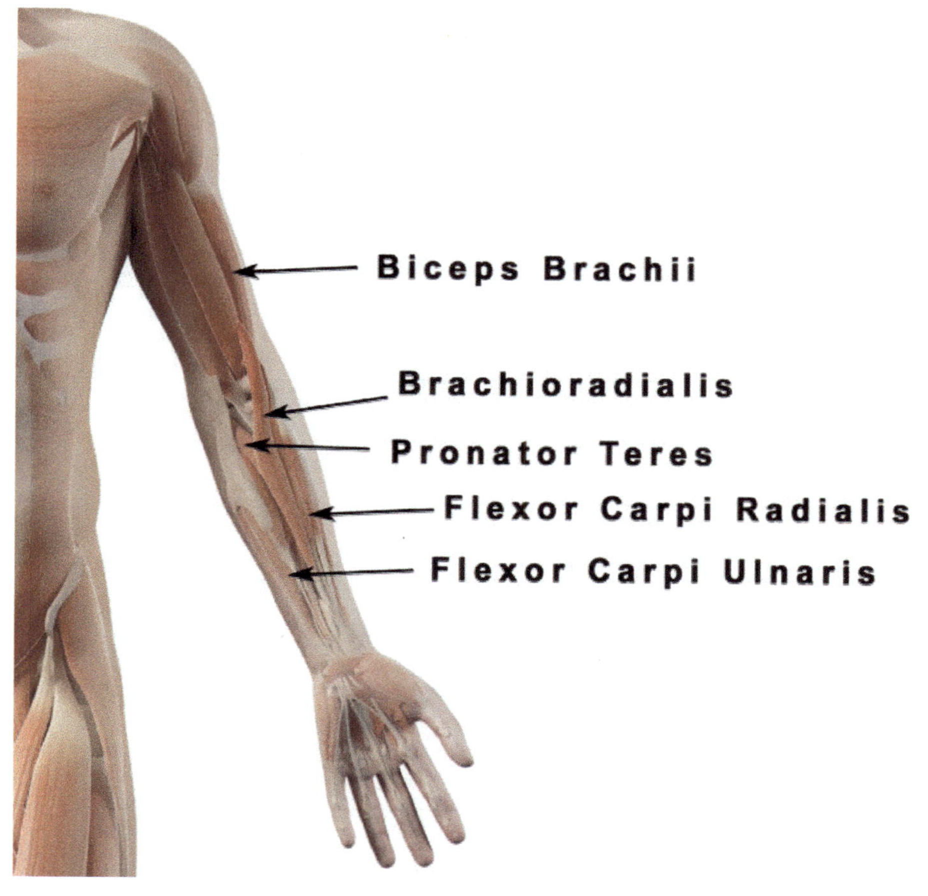

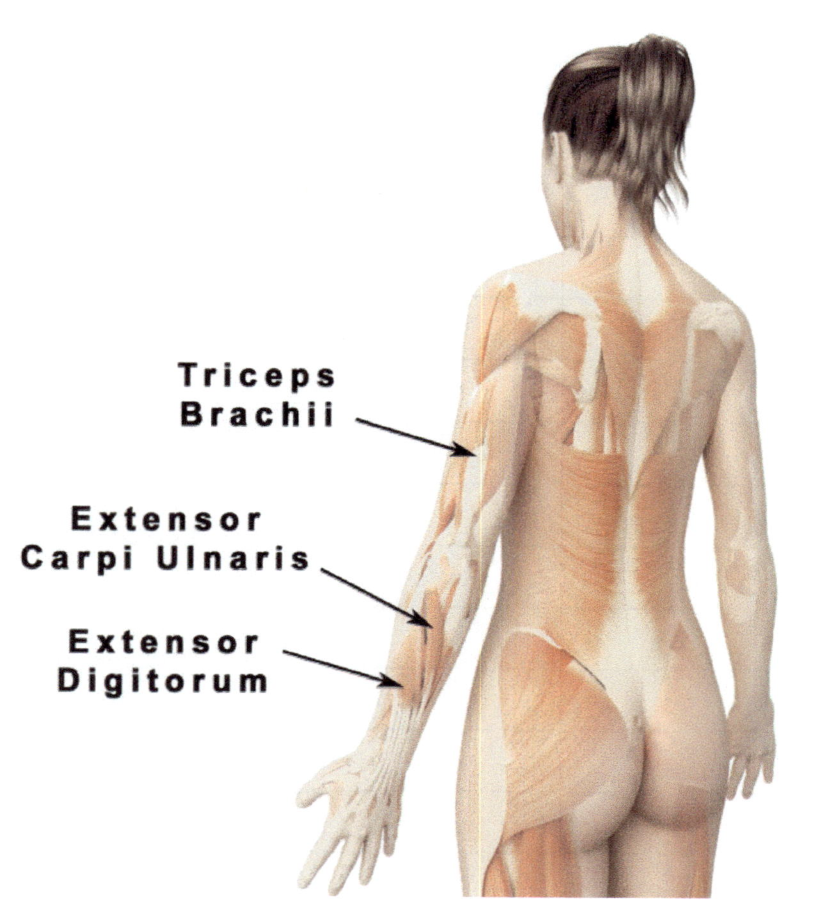

Taping and Wrapping Techniques

The taping techniques presented are the fundamental procedures. A strong knowledge of anatomy, physiology, biomechanics and pathology is essential. Developing a thorough knowledge regarding the fundamentals about the application of taping/wrapping procedures is imperative. Review Section 1–Chapter 1 before applying any technique.

The Kinesio® Taping Method is a therapeutic taping technique not only offering your patient the support they are looking for, but also rehabilitating the affected condition as well. Please consult Chapter 9 for specific application instructions.

NOTES:

ELBOW HYPEREXTENSION

Purpose: To provide support and stability to the elbow joint

Clinical Application: Sprains and contusions

Anatomical Structure: Elbow

Anatomical Position: Forearm supinated and in slight flexion

Supplies: 2-in. elastic tape, 1½-in. adhesive tape

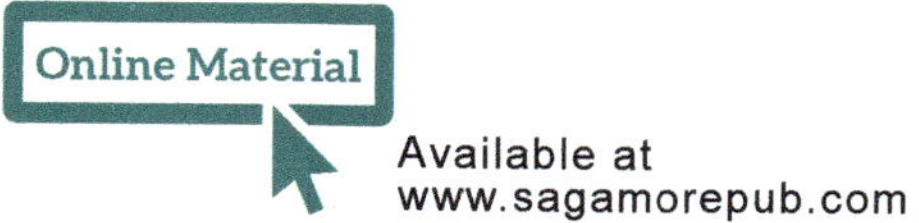

Taping Procedures

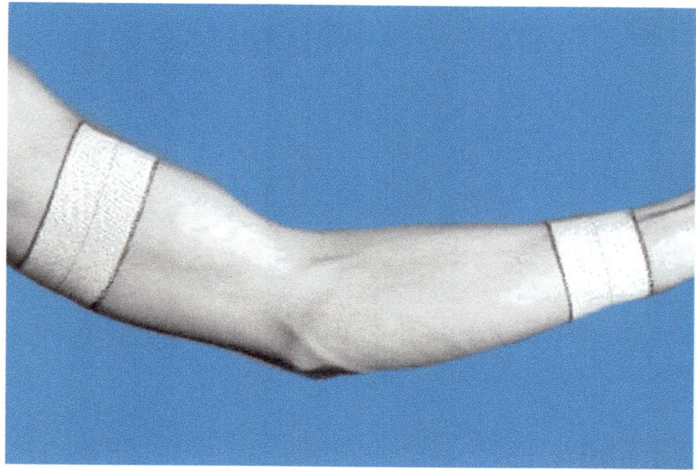

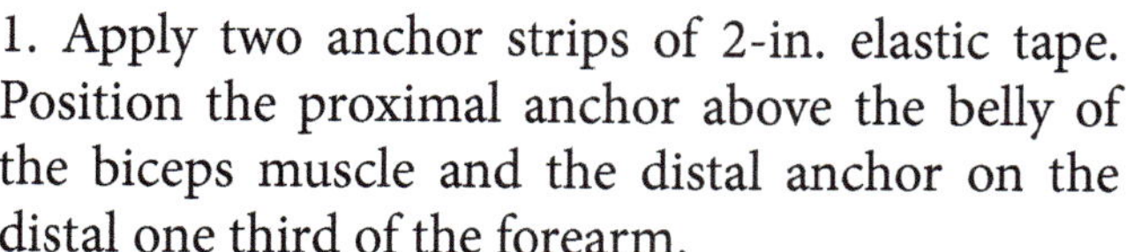

1. Apply two anchor strips of 2-in. elastic tape. Position the proximal anchor above the belly of the biceps muscle and the distal anchor on the distal one third of the forearm.

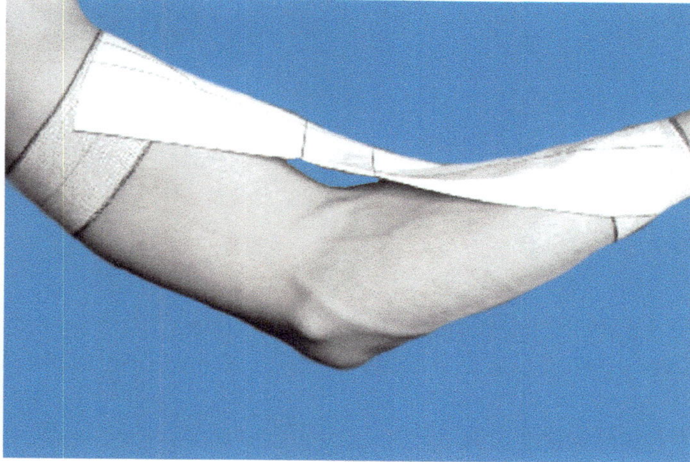

2. Using 1½-in. adhesive tape, construct a five- to seven-strip butterfly. Prior to application, place a strip of tape around the mid-portion of this support pattern. Apply the butterfly pattern from the proximal anchor to the distal anchor. Apply proper tension to ensure that the elbow does not reach full extension.

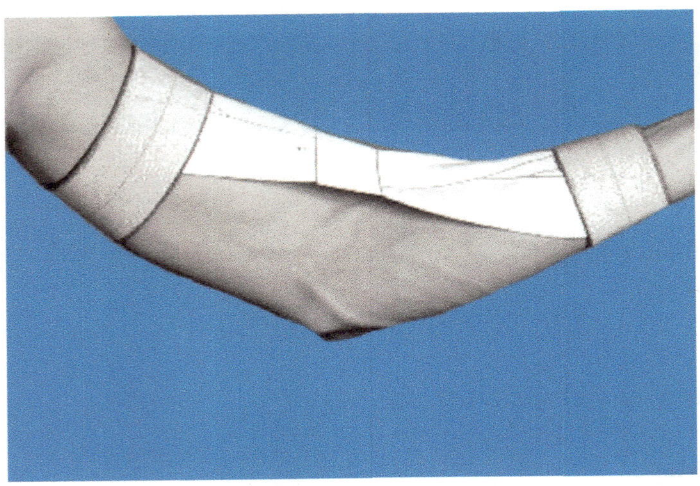

3. Apply a second series of anchor strips using elastic tape.

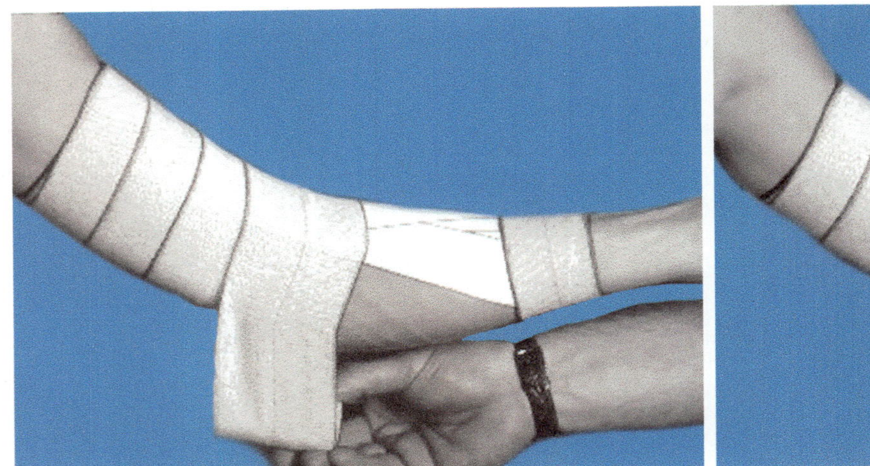

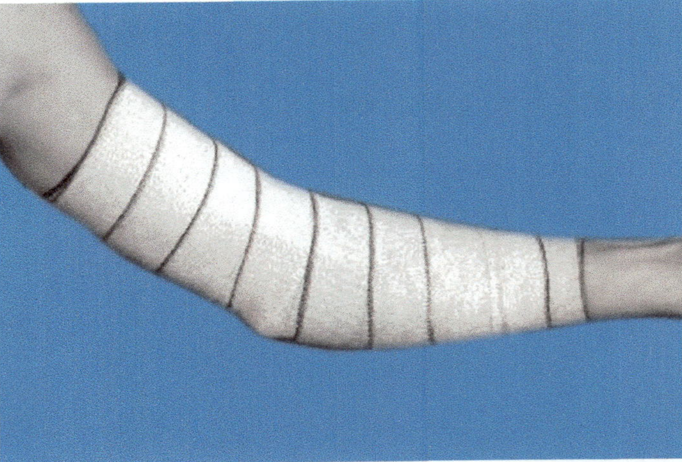

4. Apply a final continuous closure strip with 2-in. elastic tape. Beginning on the distal anchor, spiral the tape, overlapping one half of its width, and end on the proximal anchor.

**Upon completion of the procedure, make sure you check for neatness and gaps, adequate support, along with proper function of the affected area. In certain situations, the individual might be asked to perform function tests to establish appropriate technique application.*

Adjunct Taping Procedures: Elbow Hyperextension

These adjunct taping procedures can be used in conjunction with the basic technique presented.

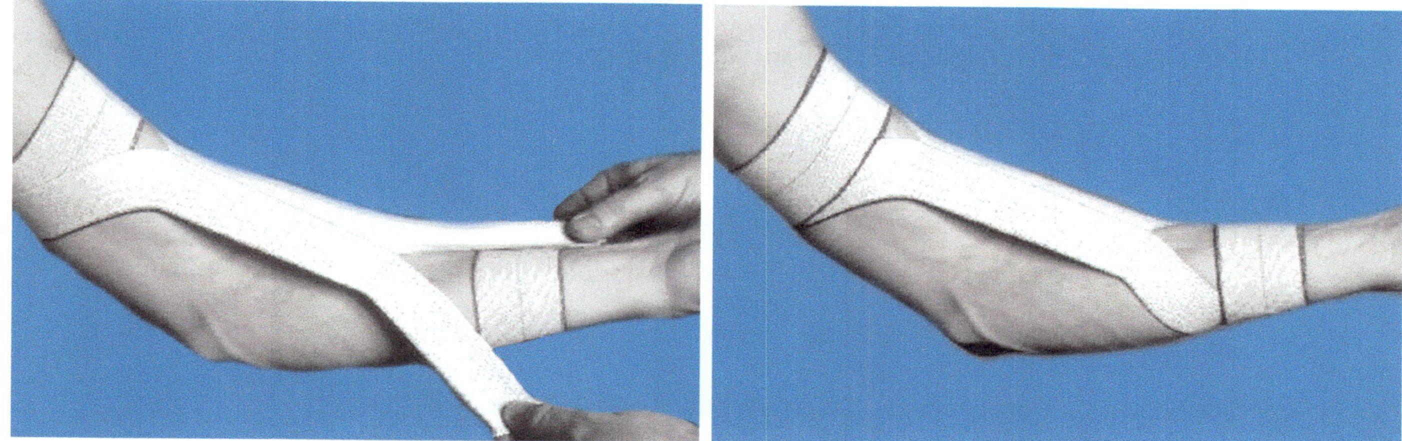

Technique A. This technique aids in preventing the elbow joint from excessive extension. Using 2-in. elastic tape, cut a strip 9 in. to 12 in. in length, split both ends lengthwise approximately 3 in. With the elbow in slight flexion, encircle the proximal anchor with the split ends of the elastic tape. Pull the tape to full tension and encircle the distal anchor with the other split end of the elastic tape. Apply 2-in. elastic tape to secure the anchors.

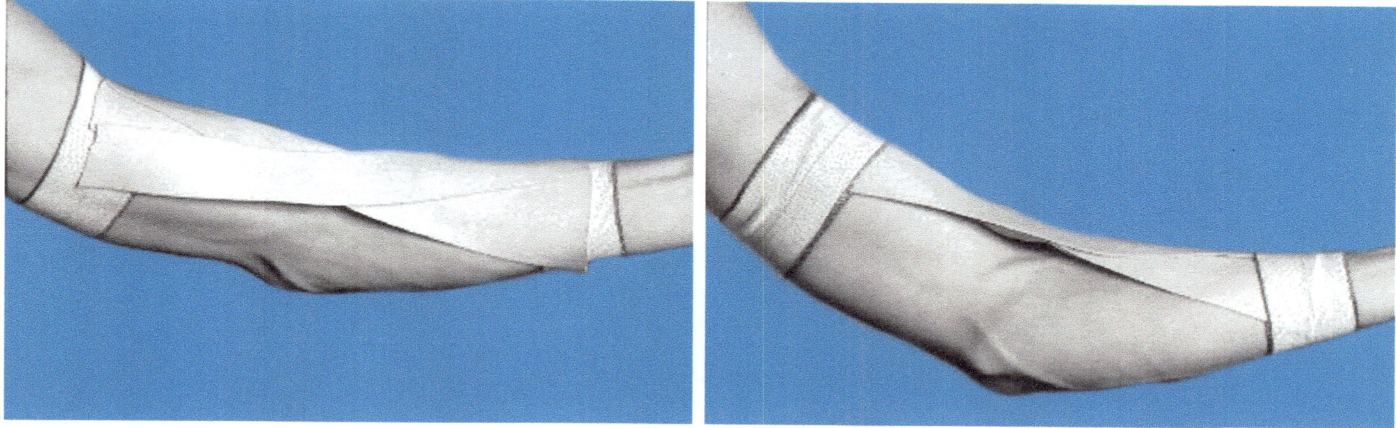

Technique B. Use adhesive felt in place of the adhesive tape butterfly pattern.

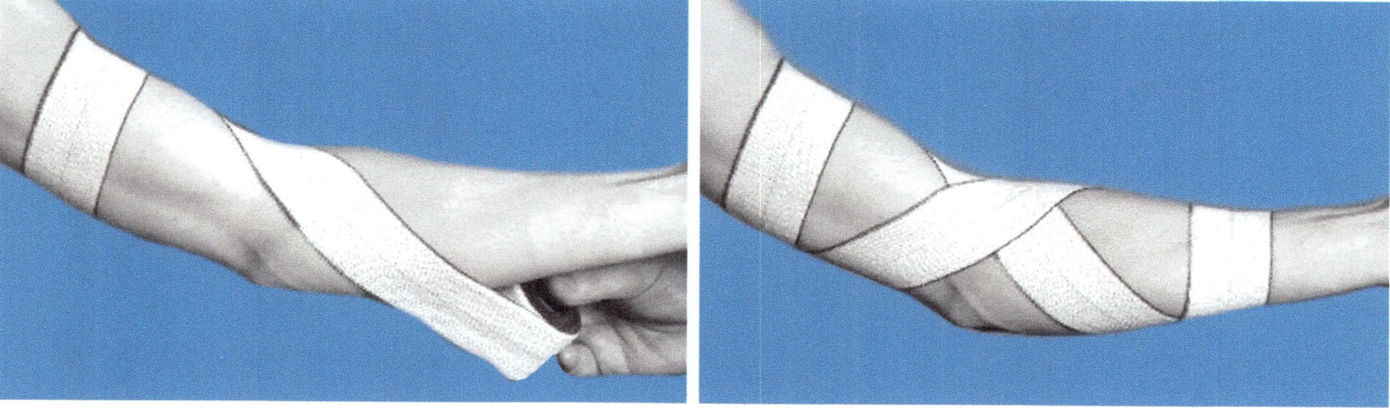

Technique C. Apply a figure of 8 pattern using 2-in. elastic tape. Beginning on the anterior lateral aspect of the upper arm, cross the elbow joint at the medial epicondyle, encircle the forearm, cross the lateral epicondyle, and anchor on the anterior medial aspect of the upper arm. Use caution to avoid circulatory dysfunction.

ELBOW EPICONDYLITIS

Purpose: To help reduce the pain associated with epicondylitis

Clinical Application: Epicondylitis

Anatomical Structure: Elbow

Anatomical Position: Medial epicondylitis: Elbow extended and forearm supinated

Lateral epicondylitis: Elbow extended and forearm pronated

Supplies: 2-in. elastic tape, 1-in. adhesive tape, and ½-in. or ¼-in. felt pad

Pre-taping Procedure: Cut felt to cover affected area.

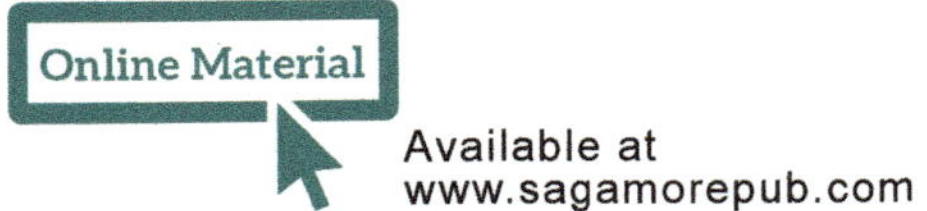

Taping Procedures

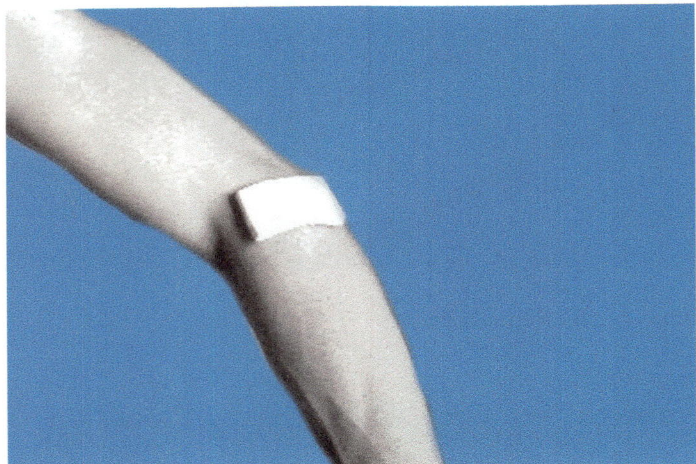

1. Place felt pad over affected area.

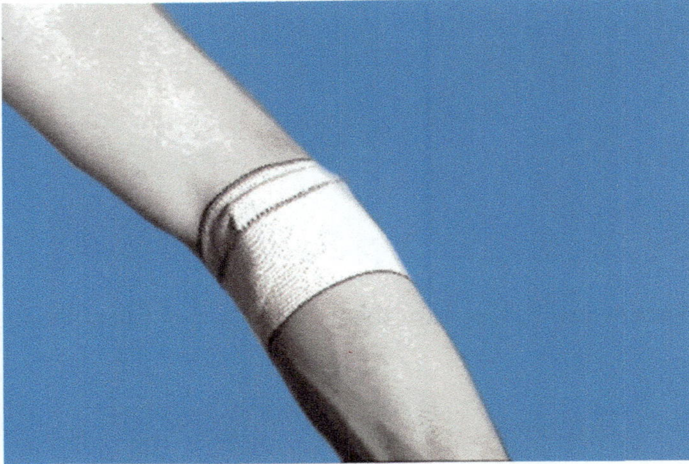

2. Anchor the felt pad using elastic tape. Encircle the forearm two or three times.

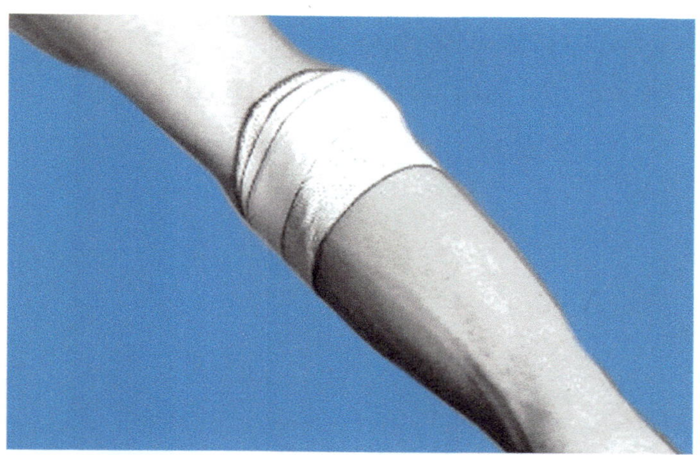

3. Secure the elastic tape ends with two or three support strips of adhesive tape, overlapping the tape by one half of its width.

**Upon completion of the procedure, make sure you check for neatness and gaps, adequate support, along with proper function of the affected area. In certain situations, the individual might be asked to perform function tests to establish appropriate technique application.*

Adjunct Taping Procedures: Elbow Epicondylitis

These adjunct taping procedures can be used in conjunction with the basic technique presented.

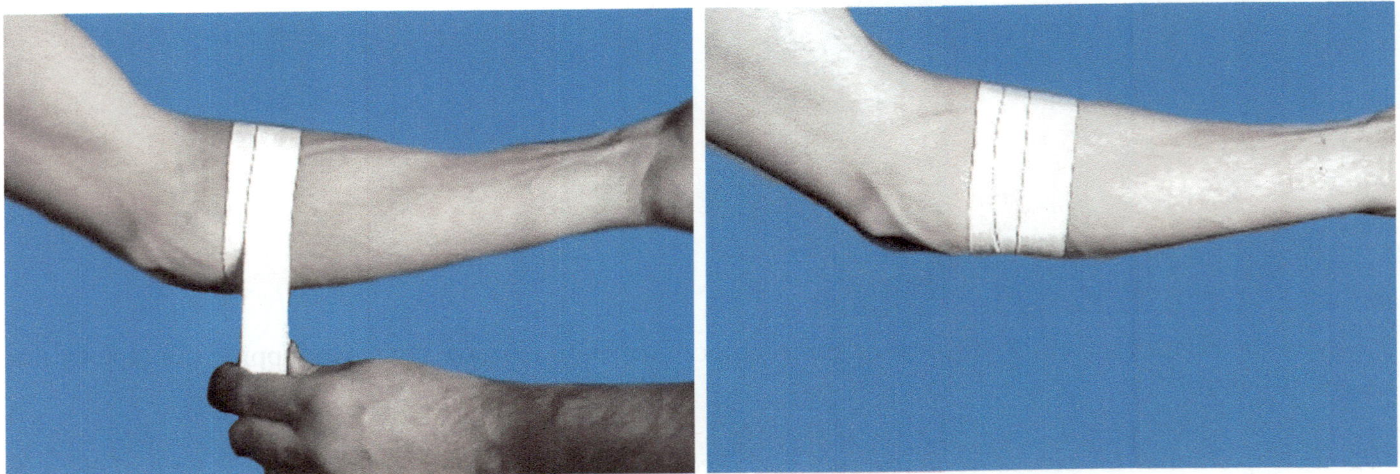

Technique A. Use 1-in. adhesive tape to apply two to three circular strips approximately 2 in. below the condyles of the elbow.

FOREARM SPLINT

Purpose: To help reduce the pain associated with forearm splings

Clinical Application: Forearm Splints

Anatomical Structure: Forearm

Anatomical Position: Elbow joint places in slight flexion (10 to 15 degrees)

Supplies: 1½-in. adhesive tape and 2-in. elastic tape

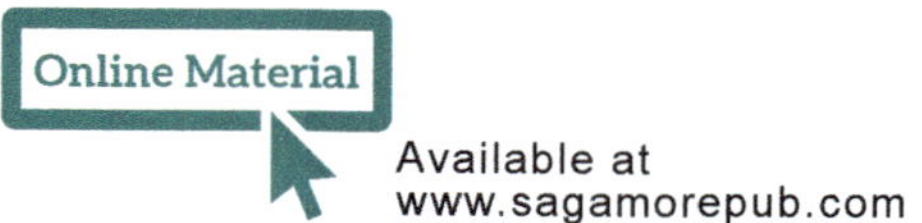

Available at www.sagamorepub.com

Taping Procedures

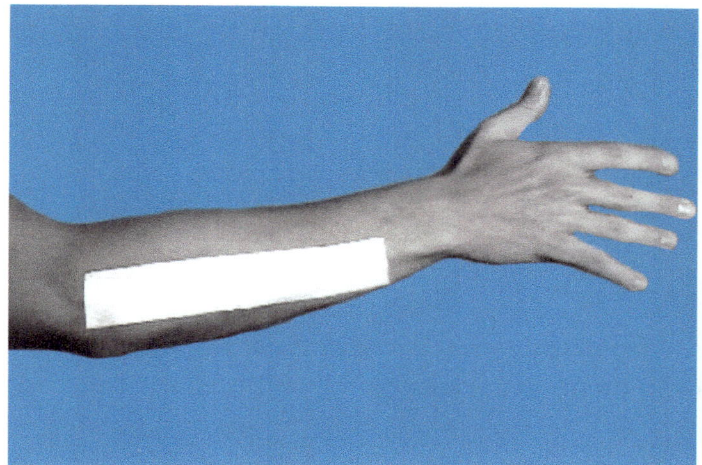

1. Apply anchor strips on the medial and lateral aspects of the forearm using 1½-in. adhesive tape.

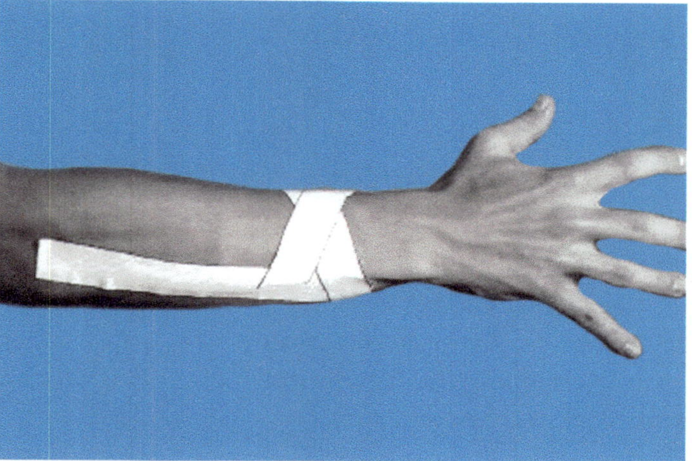

2. Apply a modified X pattern that will cover the affected area. Begin on the distal ends of the anchors and work toward the proximal ends.

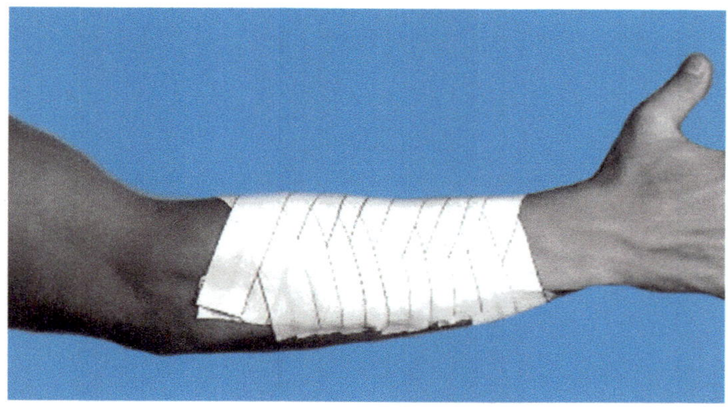

3. Apply three to six sets of X patterns, overlapping the tape by one half of its width.

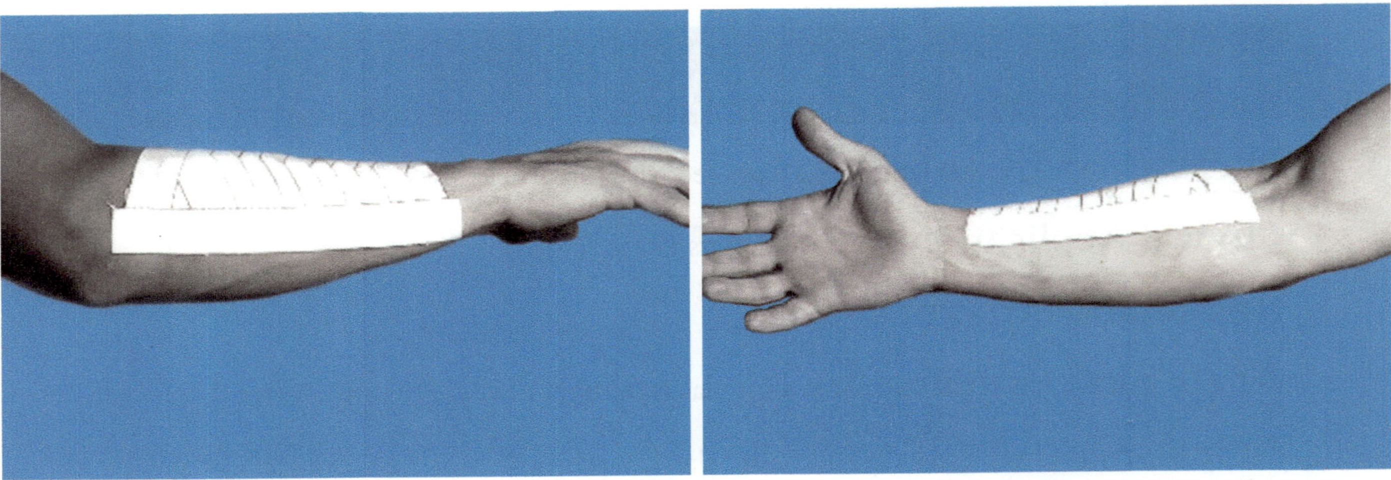

4. Apply a second set of anchors to help hold the technique in place. Do not cover the posterior aspect of the forearm with adhesive tape.

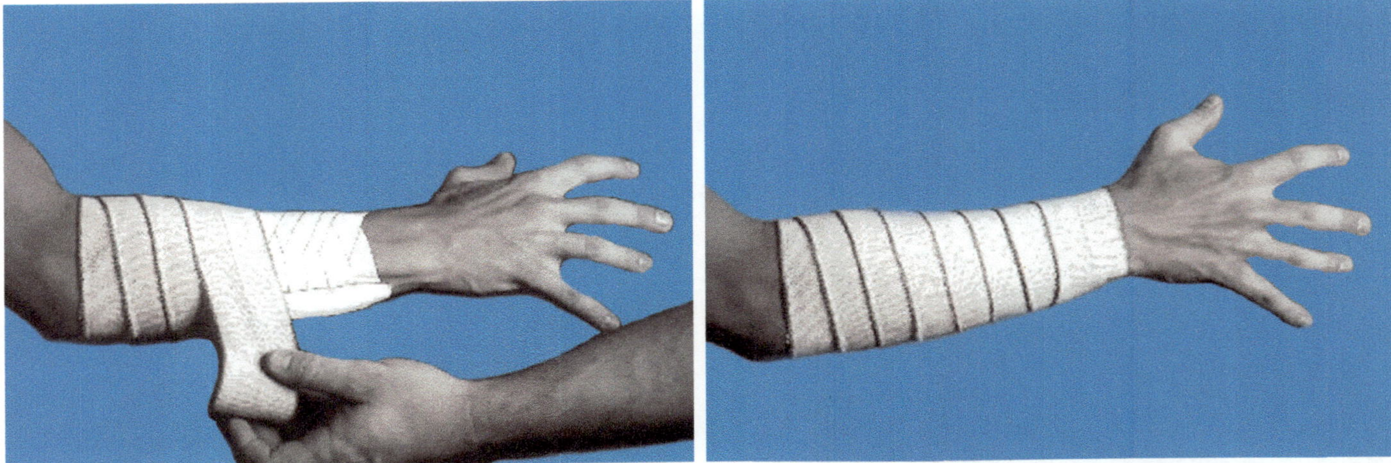

5. Apply a final continuous closure strip with 2-in. elastic tape. Begin on the proximal anchor and spiral the tape, overlapping the tape by one half of its width, and end on the distal anchor. Secure the elastic tape ends with adhesive tape anchors.

**Upon completion of the procedure, make sure you check for neatness and gaps, adequate support, along with proper function of the affected area. In certain situations, the individual might be asked to perform function tests to establish appropriate technique application.*

Adjunct Taping Procedure: Forearm Strain

This adjunct taping procedure can be used in conjunction with the basic technique presented.

Technique A. Using either 2-in. elastic tape or 3-in. cohesive tape, or elastic wrap, apply a compression technique over the forearm area.

WRIST

Purpose: To provide support and stability for the wrist

Clinical Application: Sprains and strains

Anatomical Structure: Dorsal and palmar radiocarpal ligaments

Anatomical Position: Hyperextension: Wrist positioned in slight flexion and fingers spread apart

Hyperflexion: Wrist positioned in slight extension and fingers spread apart

Supplies: 1-in. and 1½-in. adhesive tape and 2-in. elastic tape

Pre-taping Procedure: With the wrist in a supinated position, in slight extension and fingers spread apart

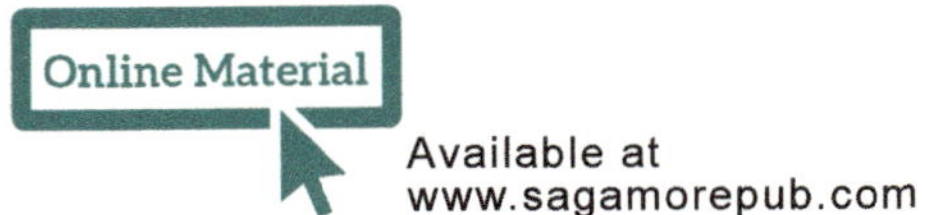

Available at www.sagamorepub.com

Taping Procedures

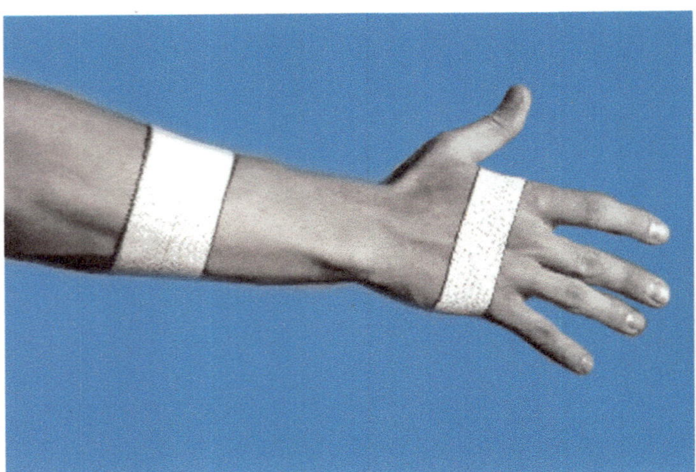

1. Apply two anchor strips of 1-in. and 2-in. elastic tape. Apply the 2-in. anchor around the mid-forearm and the 1-in. anchor around the second through fifth metacarpal heads.

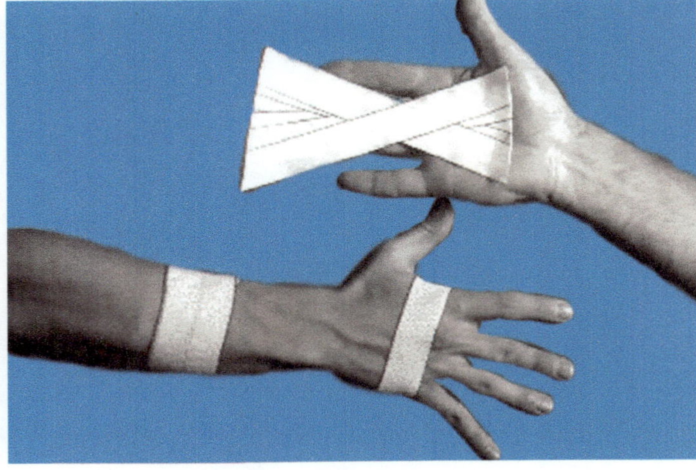

2. Using adhesive tape, construct a five- to seven-strip butterfly pattern that will extend from the proximal anchor to the distal anchor. To prevent hyperflexion, place this butterfly pattern on the dorsal aspect of the hand. To prevent hyperextension, place the butterfly pattern on the palmar aspect of the hand.

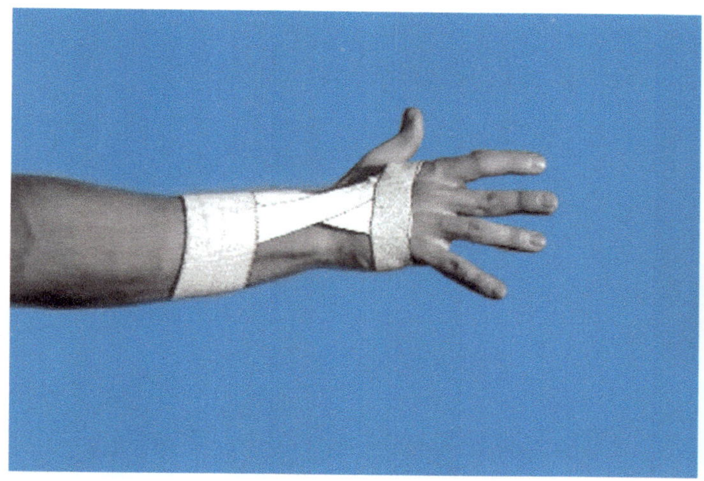

3. Apply a second series of anchor strips.

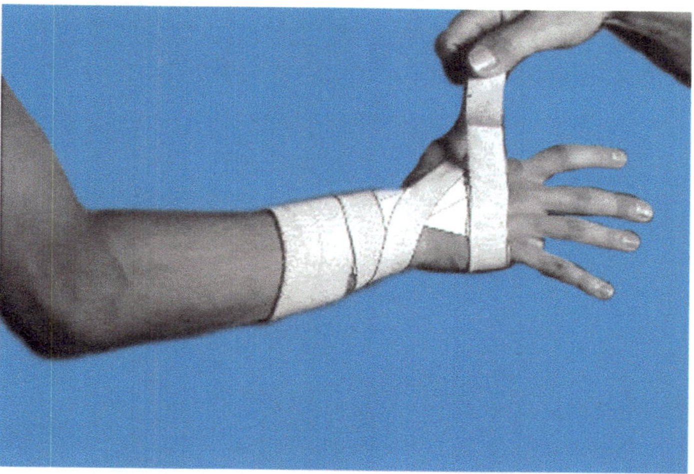

4. Apply a 1-in. strip of elastic tape in a figure of eight pattern. Begin on the dorsal aspect of the forearm, cross diagonally to the second metacarpal, encircle the distal aspect of the second through fifth metacarpals, continue across the palmar aspect to the fifth metacarpal, and cross diagonally to the radial aspect of the wrist and encircle the wrist. Apply two to three figures of eight.

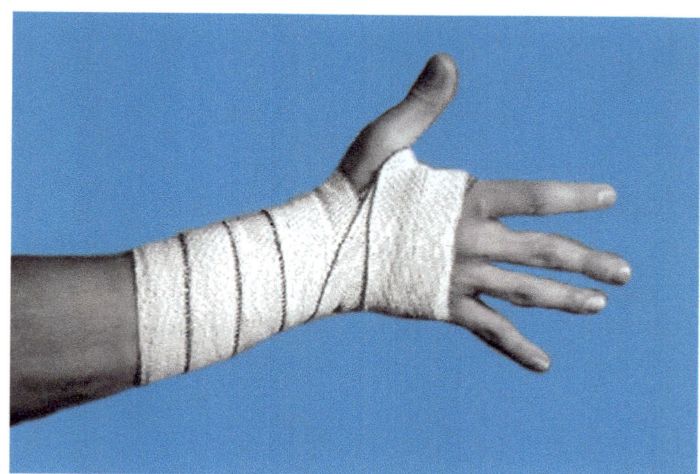

5. Apply a final continuous closure strip with 2-in. elastic tape. Begin on the proximal anchor and spiral the tape, overlapping one half of its width, and end on the distal anchor. Secure the elastic tape ends with anchors of adhesive tape.

**Upon completion of the procedure, make sure you check for neatness and gaps, adequate support, along with proper function of the affected area. In certain situations, the individual might be asked to perform function tests to establish appropriate technique application.*

Adjunct Taping Procedures: Wrist

This adjunct taping procedure can be used in conjunction with the basic technique presented.

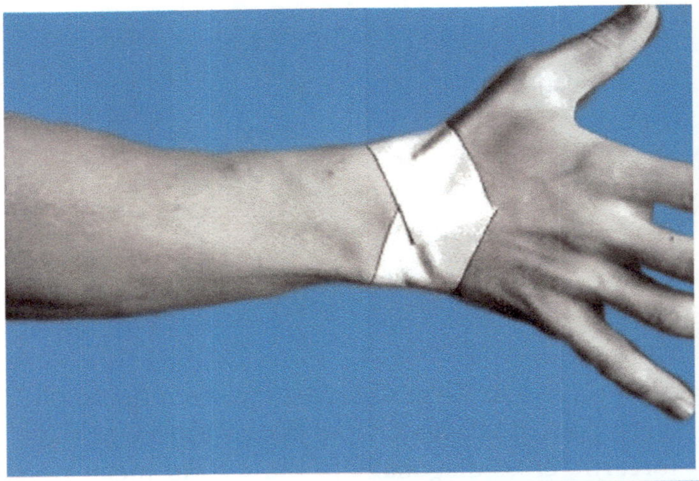

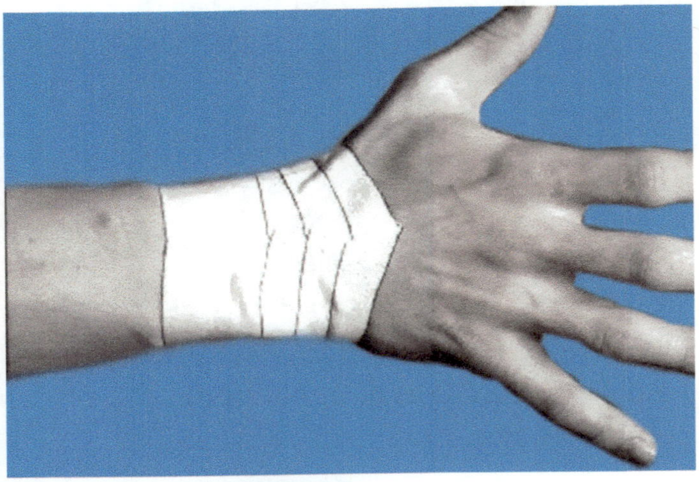

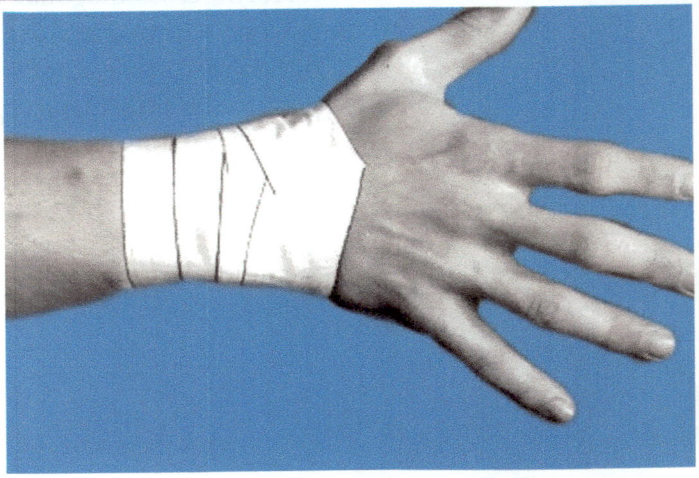

Technique A. In certain sporting activities, tape should not be applied to the palm of the hand. In such situations, apply two layers of four support strips. Begin proximally and work distally. Apply the 1½-in. adhesive tape around the wrist starting at the ulnar styloid process, cross the dorsal aspect of the distal forearm, and encircle the wrist. Overlap the tape by one half of its width each time. Apply the second layer proximally to distally and cover the same area.

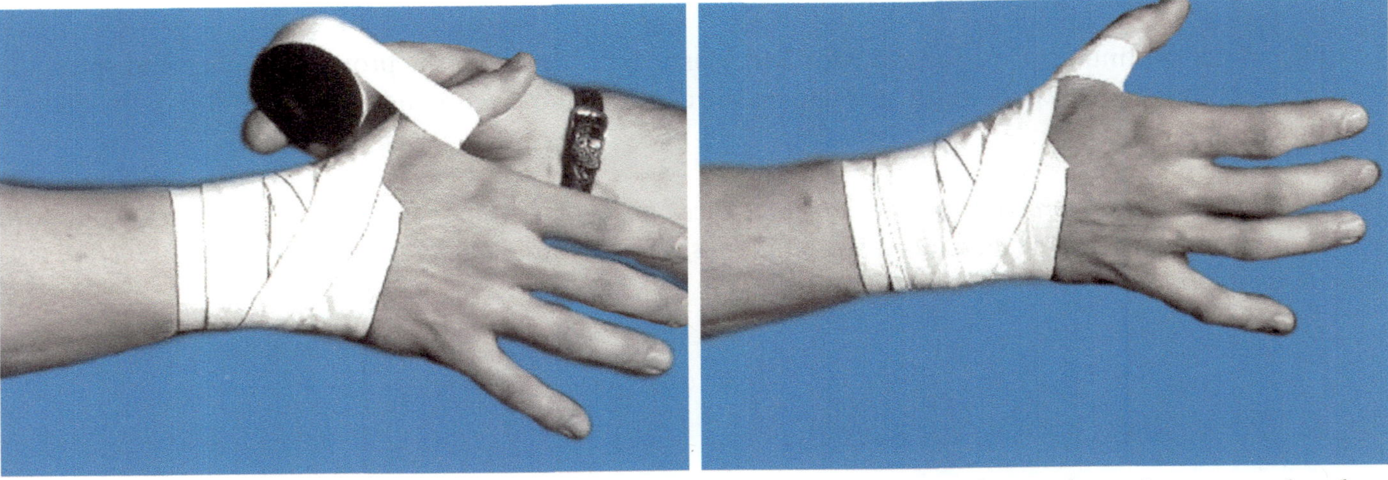

Technique B. In conjunction with Technique A, include a thumb spica taping procedure. Starting at the ulnar styloid process, cross the dorsum of the hand, cover the lateral joint line, encircle the thumb, proceed across the palmar aspect of the hand, and finish at the ulnar styloid process.

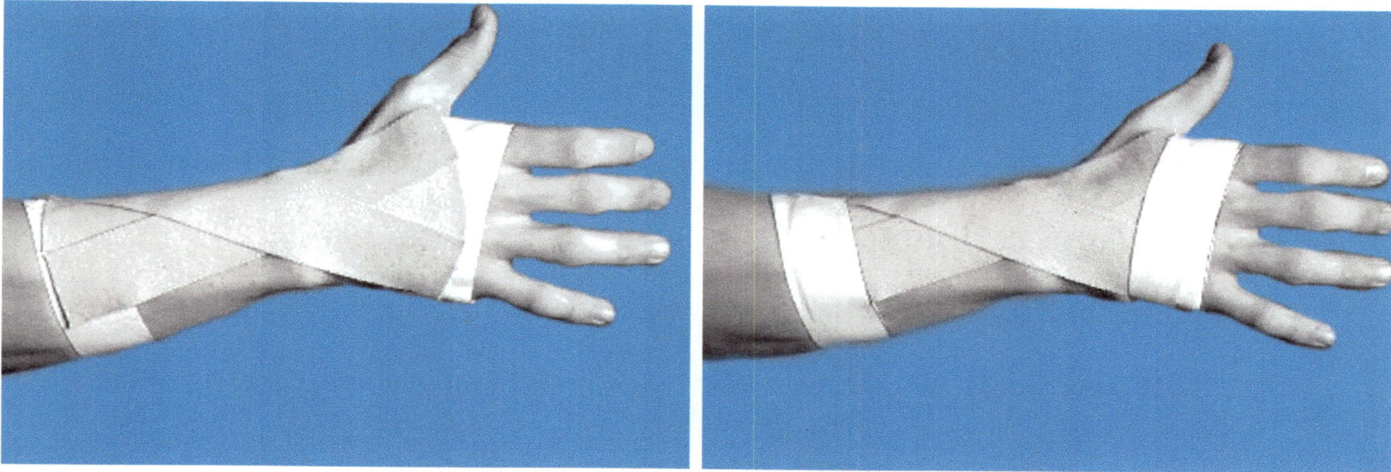

Technique C. Use adhesive felt in place of the adhesive tape butterfly pattern.

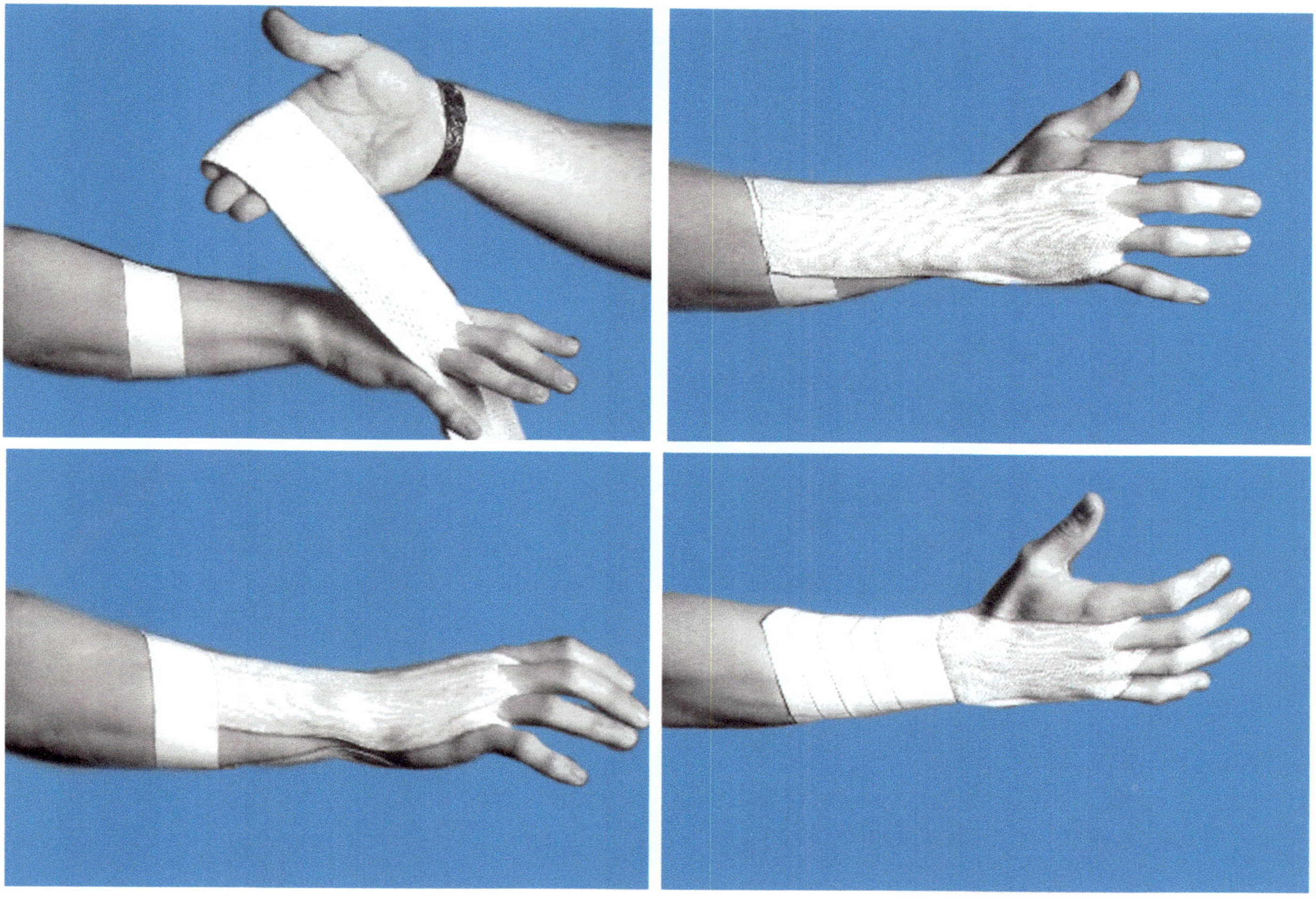

Technique D. Apply an anchor strip of 1½-in. adhesive tape around the mid-forearm. Using 3-in. elastic tape, cut a strip 12 in. to 16 in. in length. In the middle of the tape strip, cut two small holes, approximately 1 in. from each side of the tape. With full tension applied to the tape, place the third and fourth phalanges through the cutouts. Attach the ends of the elastic tape to the mid-forearm anchor. Secure the procedure by applying an anchor of 1½-in. adhesive tape over the tape ends.

THUMB SPICA

Purpose: To provide support and stability for the first metacarpophalangeal (MP) joint of the hand

Clinical Application: Sprain

Anatomical Structure: Thumb and Wrist

Anatomical Position: Hand in palm-down position, with thumb slightly flexed and phalanges abducted

Supplies: 1-in. adhesive tape

Pre-taping Procedure: With the wrist in a supinated position, in slight extension and fingers spread apart

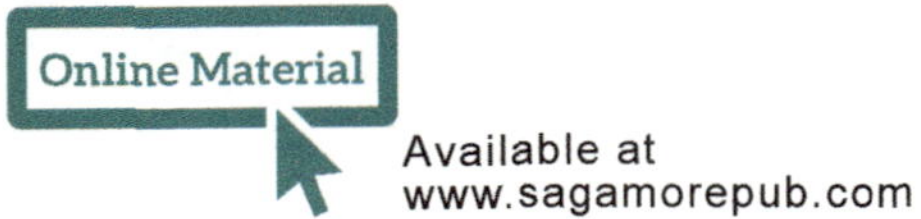

Taping Procedures

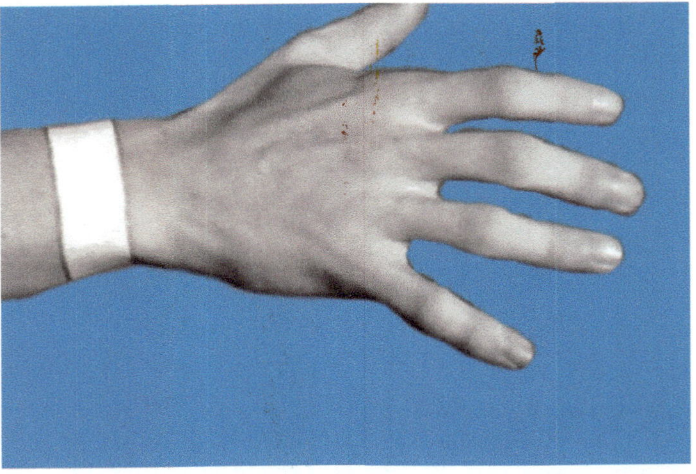

1. Apply an anchor strip of adhesive tape around the wrist. Start at the ulnar styloid process, cross the dorsal aspect of the distal forearm, and encircle the wrist.

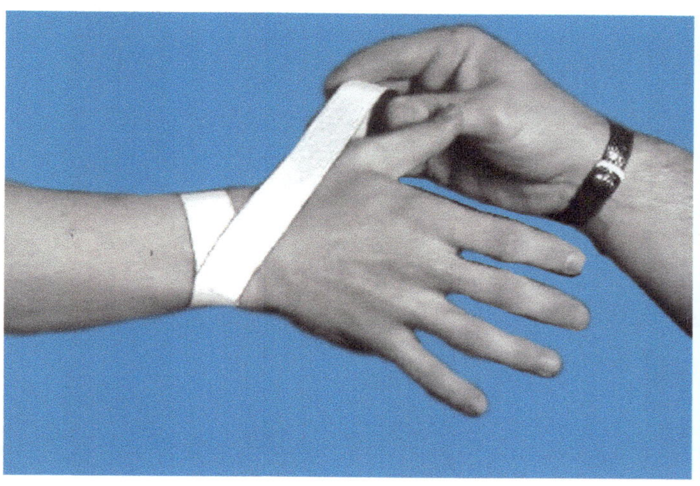

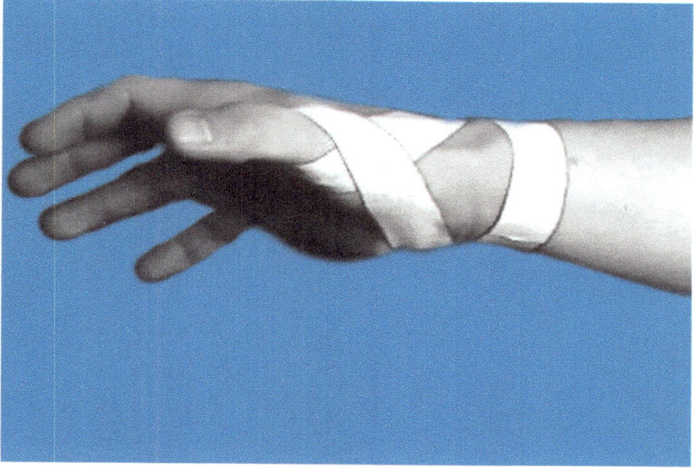

2. Apply the first of three support strips for the first MP joint. Starting at the ulnar styloid process, cross the dorsum of the hand, cover the lateral joint line, encircle the thumb, proceed across the palmar aspect of the hand, and finish at the ulnar condyle.

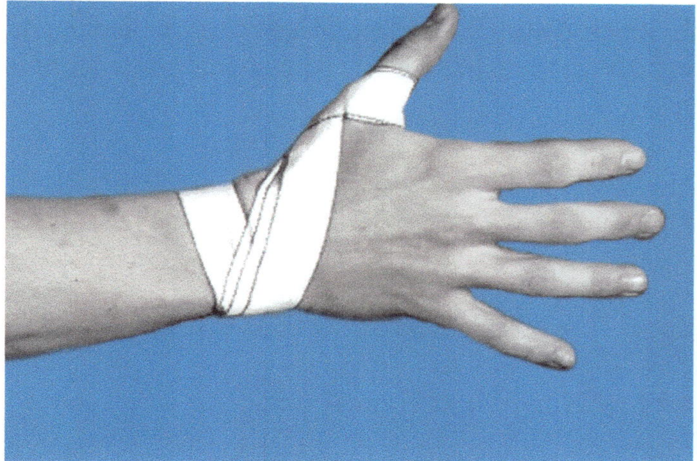

3. This is commonly referred to as a thumb spica. Repeat this procedure.

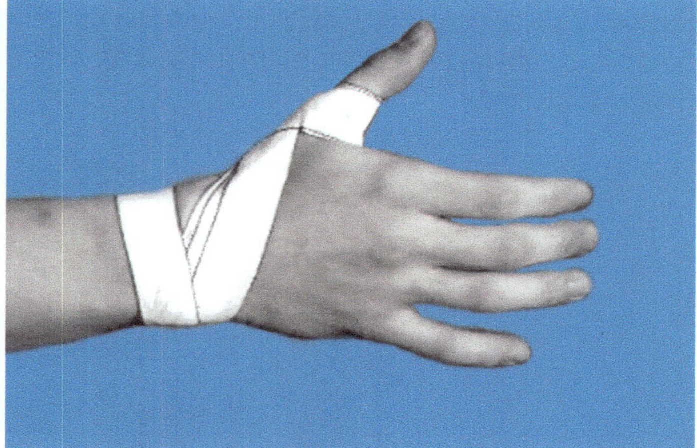

4. To help hold this procedure in place, apply a final anchor strip around the wrist. Check for circulation/skin color at the distal phalanx once you complete the tape procedure.

**Upon completion of the procedure, make sure you check for neatness and gaps, adequate support, along with proper function of the affected area. In certain situations, the individual might be asked to perform function tests to establish appropriate technique application.*

Adjunct Taping Procedures: Thumb Spica

This adjunct taping procedure can be used in conjunction with the basic technique presented.

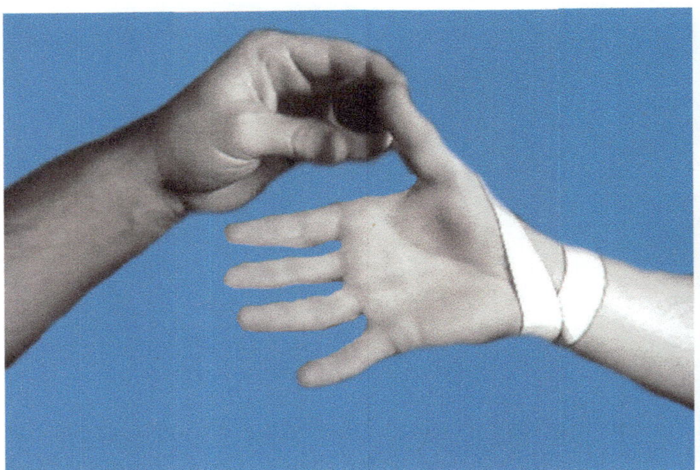

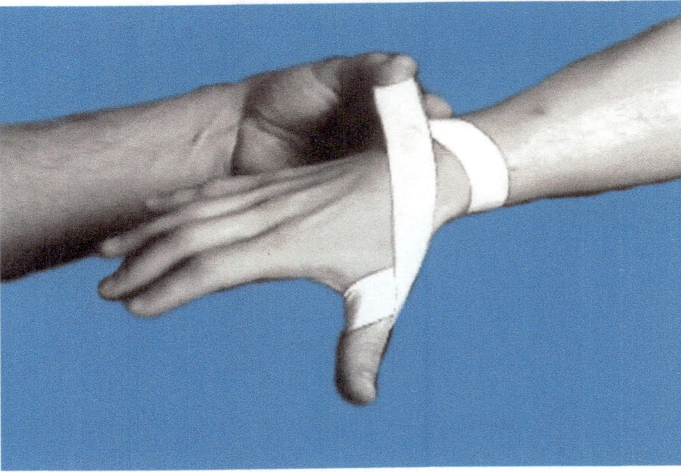

Technique A. In another application of the thumb spica, apply tape in the opposite direction. Apply the first of three support strips for the first MP joint. Starting at the ulnar styloid process, cross the palmar portion of the hand, cover the medial joint line, encircle the thumb, proceed across the dorsum aspect of the hand, and finish at the ulnar styloid process. When you are taping to support the ulnar collateral ligament, this technique may be preferred.

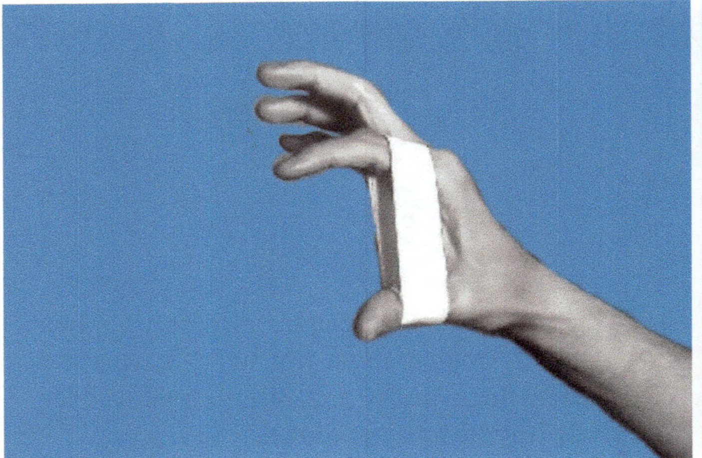

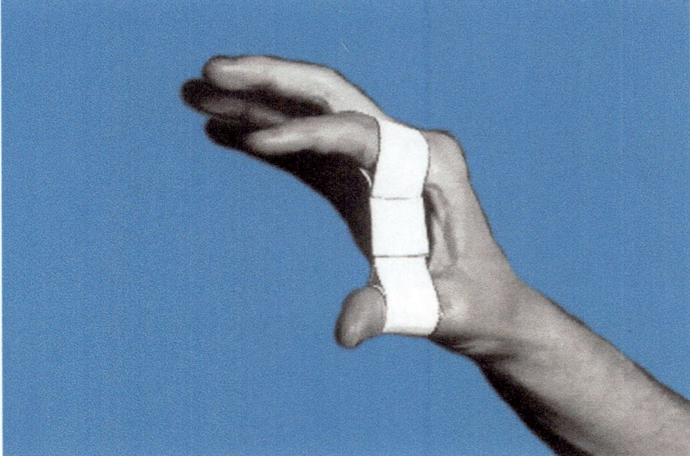

Technique B. Apply thumb c-lock for additional support.

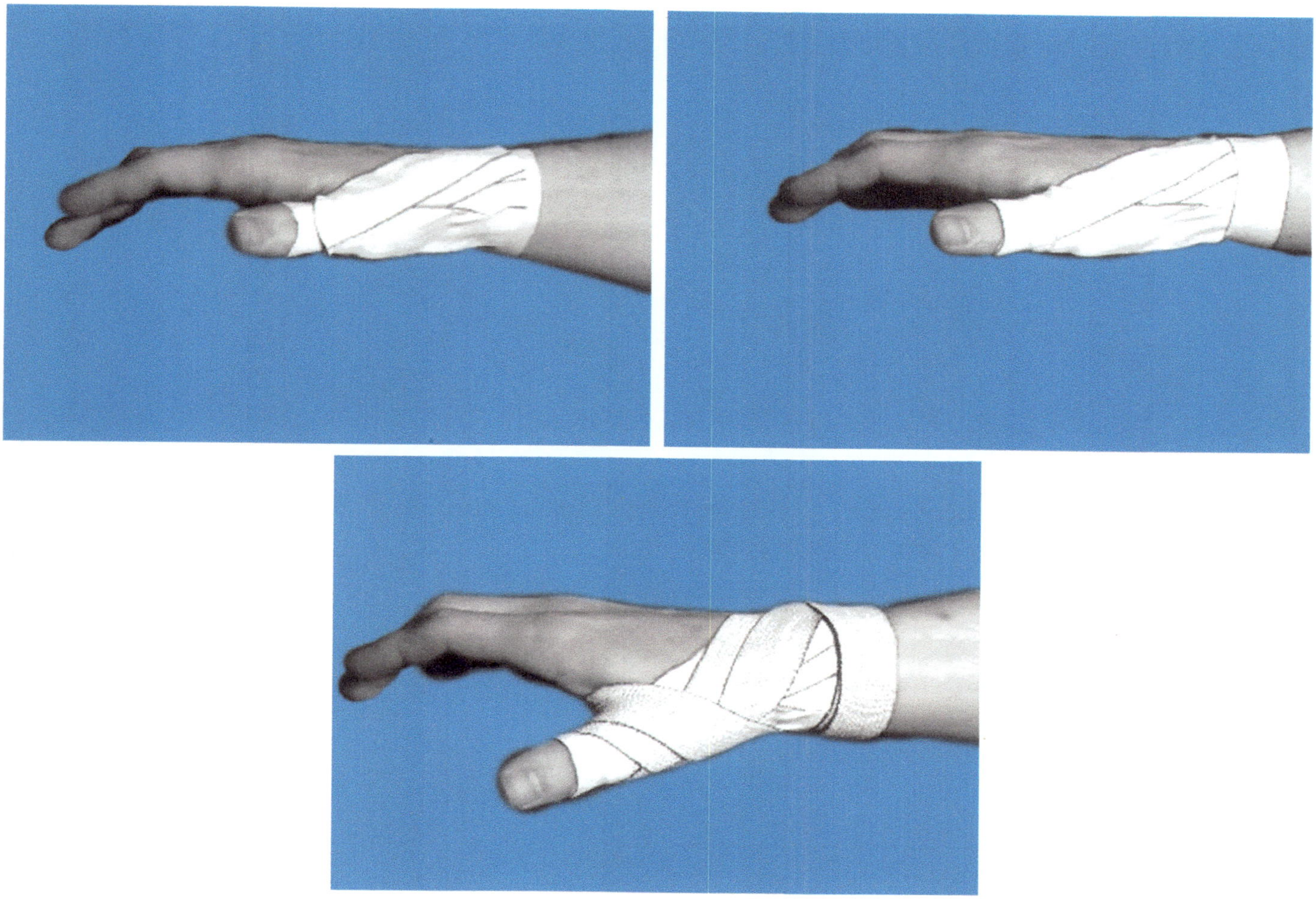

Technique C. For additional support, apply adduction strips. Apply these strips from the dorsal aspect of hand across the thumb and end on palmar surface of the hand. Overlap the tape one half of its width until the first IP joint is covered.

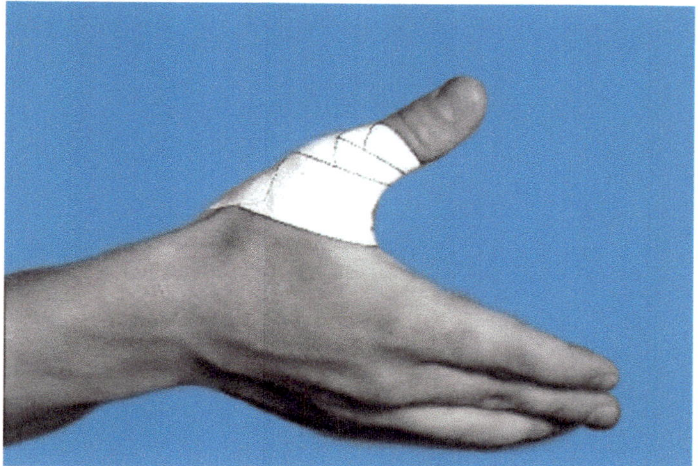

Technique D. Use adhesive tape to form a fan shape (apply four to six strips to provide adequate support). Place the fan-shaped tape from the proximal phalange, cover the affected area, and end on the radial aspect of the wrist. Adhesive felt can be used in place of the adhesive tape. To secure, apply a continuous strip of elastic tape around the thumb and wrist. This joint spica will provide additional support.

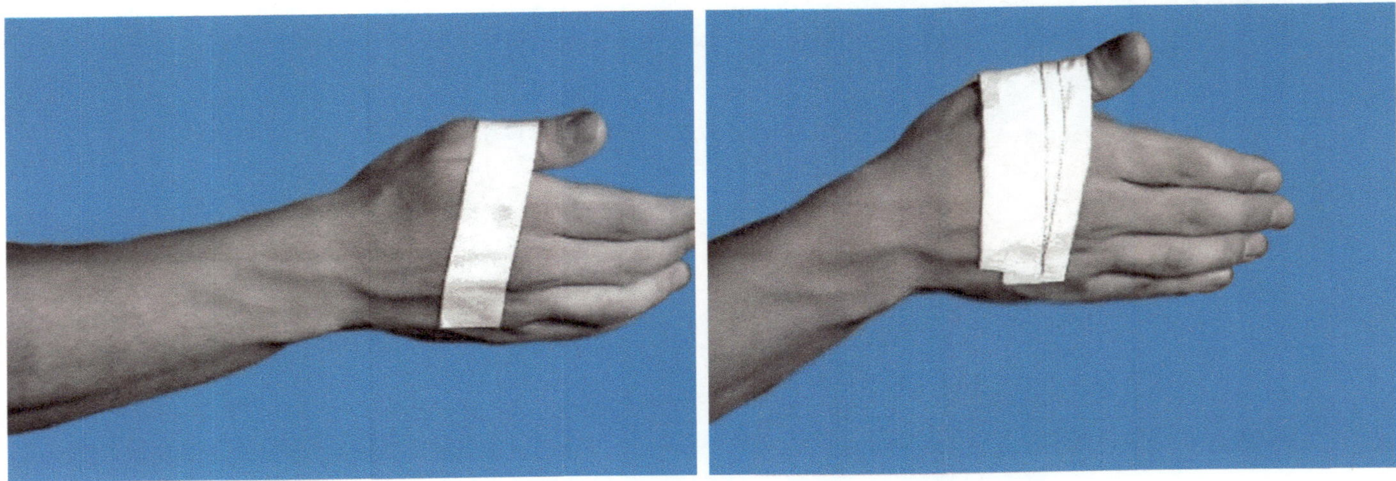

Technique E. Using 1-in. adhesive tape, apply three to four support strips. Begin distally and work proximally. Each strip will resemble a half figure of eight pattern.

FINGER SPLINT

Purpose: To aid in support of the injured interphalangeal (IP) joint

Clinical Application: General conditions procedure used for sprains to the phalanges of the hand

Anatomical Structure: Interphalangeal joint

Anatomical Position: Phalanges placed in extension

Supplies: ½-in. adhesive tape and gauze, felt, or foam rubber

Pre-taping Procedure: Cut the gauze to appropriate size before you begin. Place the phalanges in extension

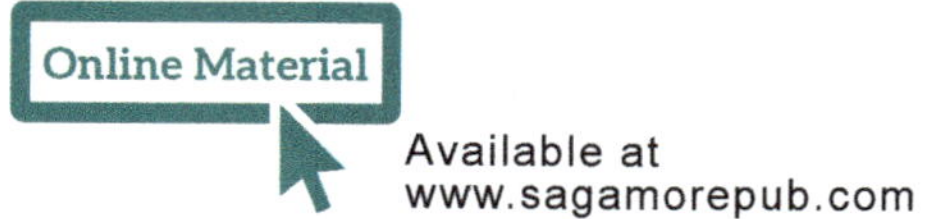

Available at www.sagamorepub.com

Taping Procedures

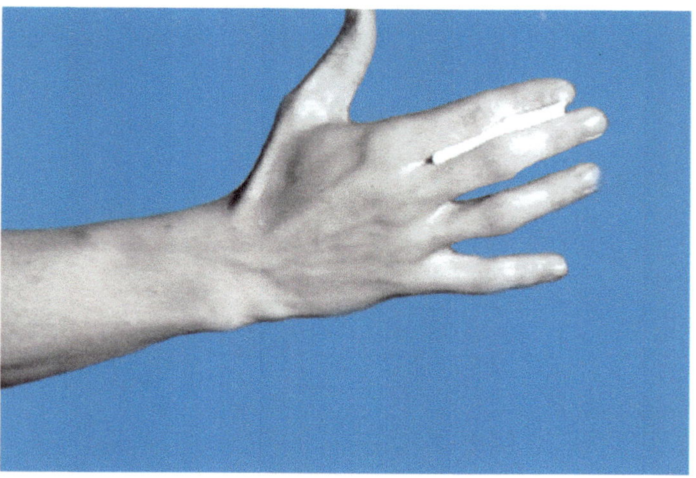

1. Place gauze between affected and adjacent phalanges.

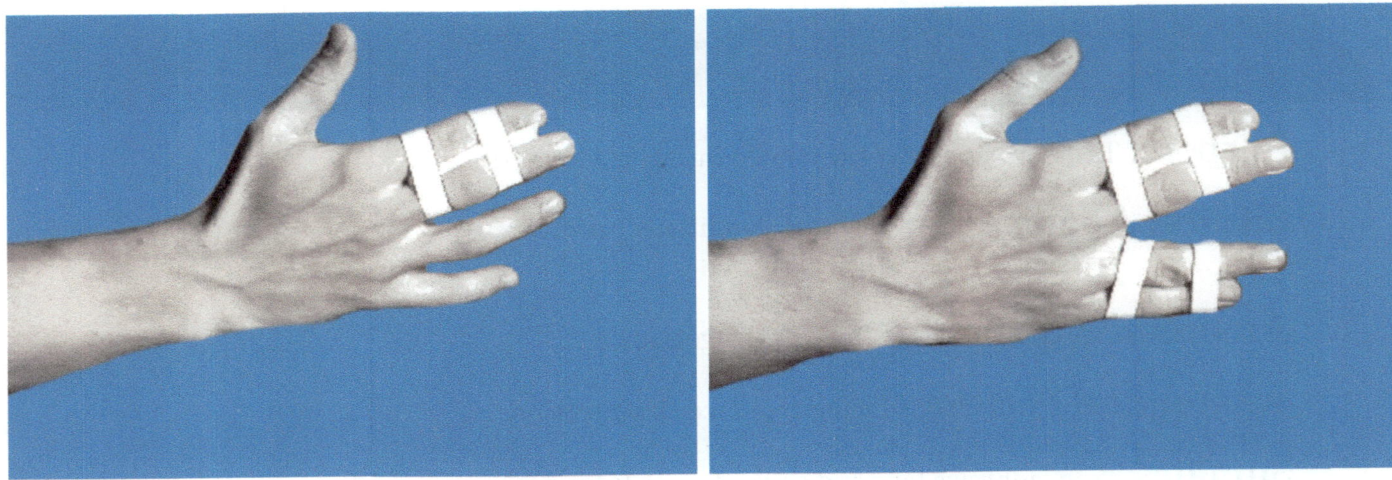

2. Apply ½-in. adhesive tape around the proximal and distal aspects of the affected and adjacent phalanges. This technique is known as buddy taping. In high-risk sports, pair and tape the second and third phalanges and the fourth and fifth phalanges together.

**Upon completion of the procedure, make sure you check for neatness and gaps, adequate support, along with proper function of the affected area. In certain situations, the individual might be asked to perform function tests to establish appropriate technique application.*

COLLATERAL INTERPHALANGEAL JOINT

Purpose: To provide support and stability to the proximal interphalangeal (PIP) joint of the phalanges

Clinical Application: Sprain to PIP joint

Anatomical Structure: Interphalangeal joint

Anatomical Position: With the palmar side of the hand up, phalanges slightly flexed and abducted

Supplies: ½-in. adhesive tape

Pre-taping Procedure: Slightly flex the PIP joint

Taping Procedures

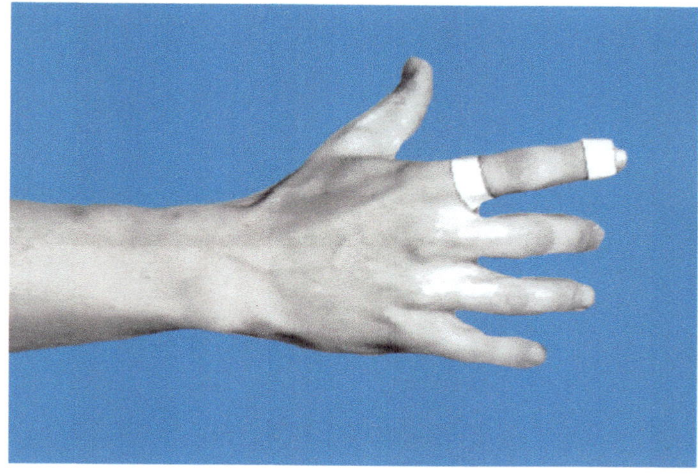

1. Apply anchor strips around proximal and distal aspects of phalanges.

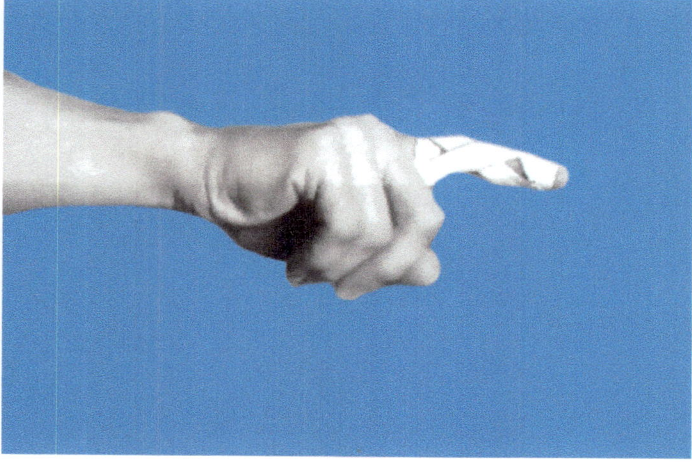

2. Starting on the anterior portion of the proximal anchor, apply the tape, crossing the lateral joint line, going under the finger, and ending on the distal anchor.

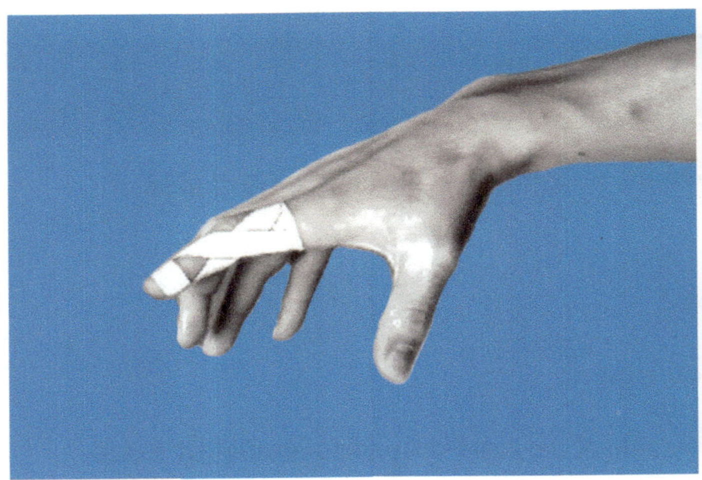

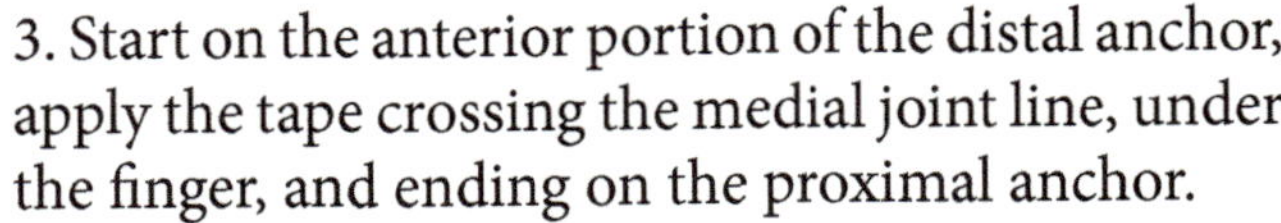

3. Start on the anterior portion of the distal anchor, apply the tape crossing the medial joint line, under the finger, and ending on the proximal anchor.

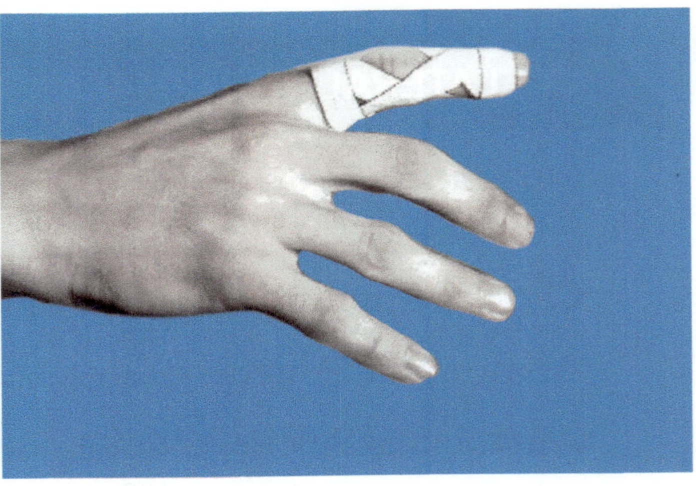

4. To secure this technique, apply a second anchor over the tape ends. For additional support and to allow greater mobility of the affected joint, this technique can be combined with finger splinting.

**Upon completion of the procedure, make sure you check for neatness and gaps, adequate support, along with proper function of the affected area. In certain situations, the individual might be asked to perform function tests to establish appropriate technique application.*

HYPEREXTENSION OF PHALANGES

Purpose: To provide support and stability to the proximal interphalangeal (PIP) joint of the phalanges

Clinical Application: Sprain to PIP joint

Anatomical Structure: Interphalangeal joint

Anatomical Position: With the palmar side of the hand up, phalanges slightly flexed and abducted

Supplies: ½-in. adhesive tape

Pre-taping Procedure: Slightly flex the PIP joint

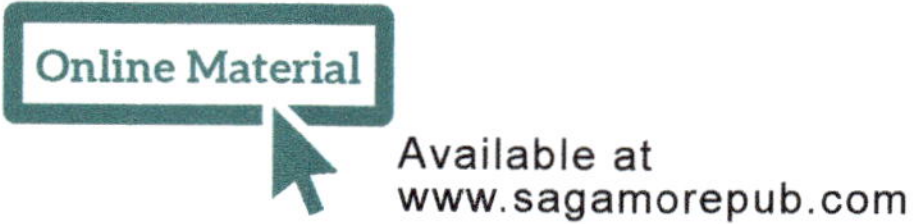

Available at www.sagamorepub.com

Taping Procedures

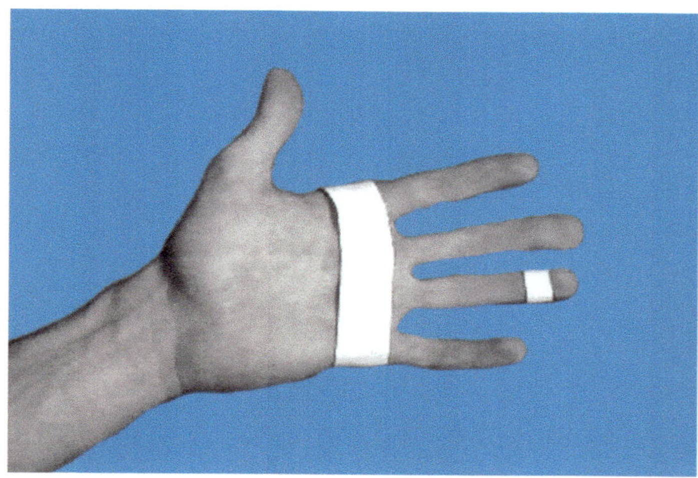

1. Apply an anchor strip around the distal aspect of the second through fifth metacarpals and a second anchor around the distal portion of the affected phalange.

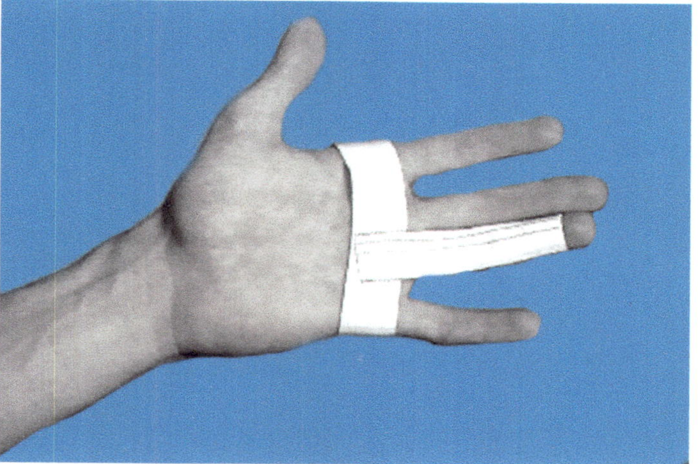

2. Apply two to three stabilizing bars of tape from the proximal anchor to distal anchor on the palmar aspect of the hand.

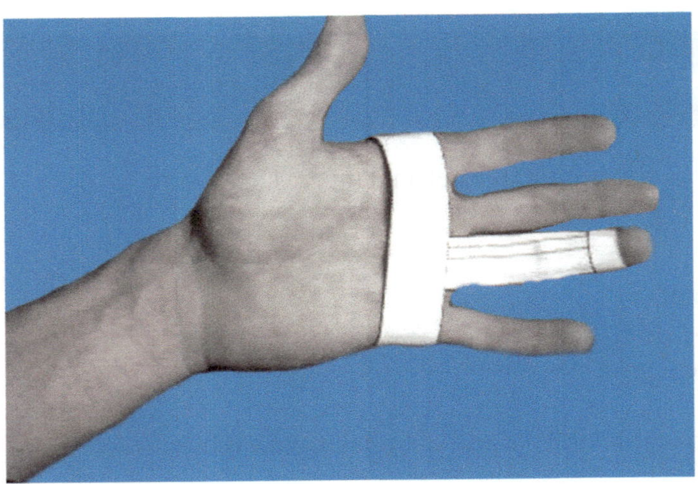

3. To secure this technique, apply a second anchor over the original anchors.

**Upon completion of the procedure, make sure you check for neatness and gaps, adequate support, along with proper function of the affected area. In certain situations, the individual might be asked to perform function tests to establish appropriate technique application.*

Adjunct Taping Procedures: Hyperextension of Phalanges

This adjunct taping procedure can be used in conjunction with the basic technique presented.

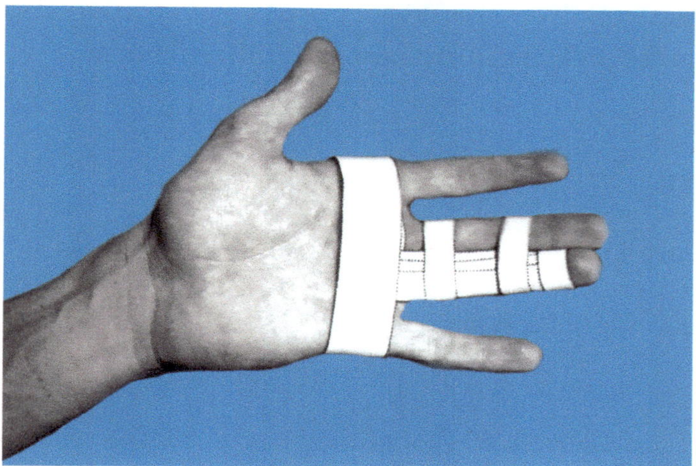

Technique A. For additional support, combine this technique with finger splinting (buddy taping), which will allow greater mobility of the affected joint.

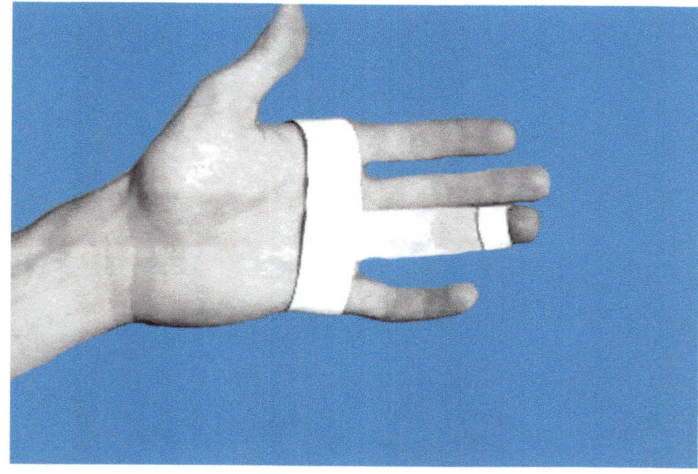

Technique B. Adhesive felt, cut to an appropriate size, can be used as stabilizing bars in place of adhesive tape.

CONTUSION TO HAND

Purpose: To provide support and stability to the proximal interphalangeal (PIP) joint of the phalanges

Clinical Application: Sprain to PIP joint

Anatomical Structure: Interphalangeal joint

Anatomical Position: With the palmar side of the hand up, phalanges slightly flexed and abducted

Supplies: ½-in. adhesive tape

Pre-taping Procedure: Slightly flex the PIP joint

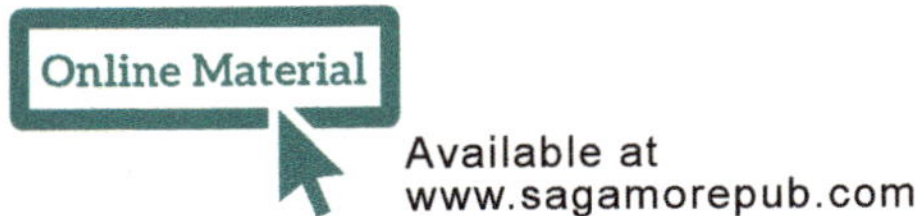

Taping Procedures

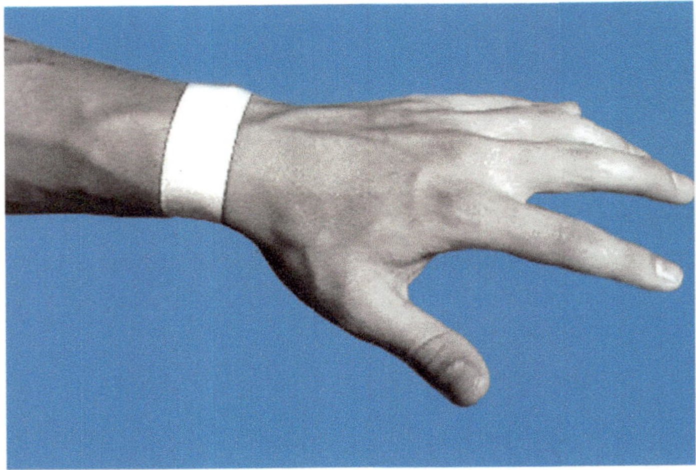

1. Apply an anchor strip of 1-in. adhesive tape around the wrist. Start at the ulnar condyle, cross the dorsal aspect of the distal forearm, and encircle the wrist.

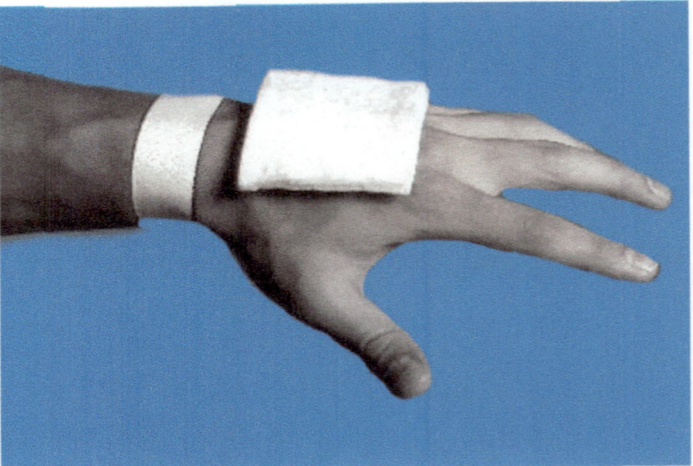

2. Apply the foam pad over the affected area of the hand.

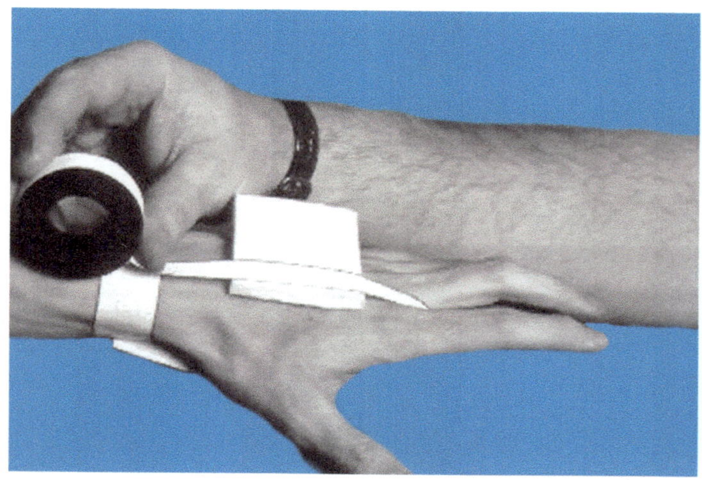

3. Apply strips of ½-in. tape. Start on the palmar aspect of the anchor strip, cross between the phalanges, and end on the dorsal aspect of the anchor strip.

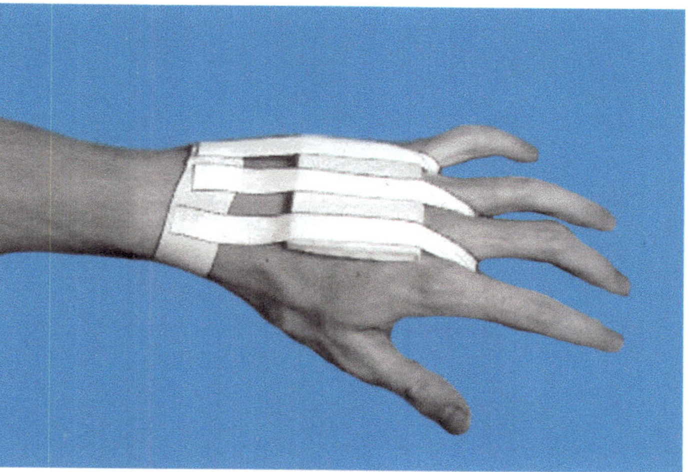

4. Apply three strips, between the second and third, third and fourth, and fourth and fifth phalanges.

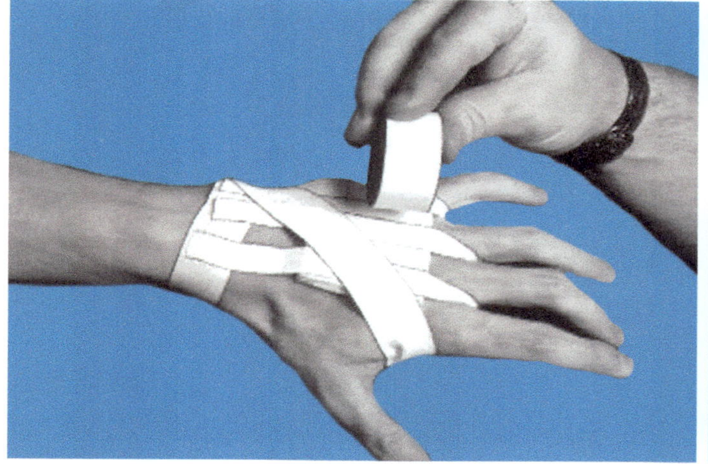

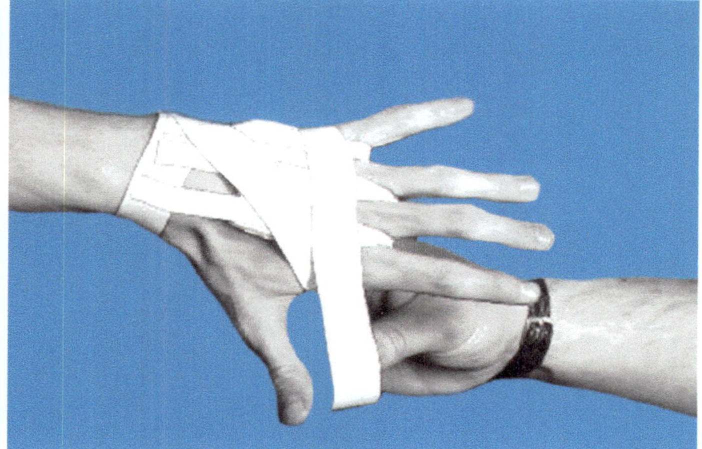

5. Apply a strip of 1-in. adhesive tape in a figure of eight pattern. Begin on the dorsal aspect of the wrist near the ulnar condyle, cross diagonally to the second metacarpal, and encircle the distal aspect of the second through fifth metacarpals. Continue across the palmar aspect to the fifth metacarpal, crossing diagonally to the radial aspect of the wrist and encircling the wrist.

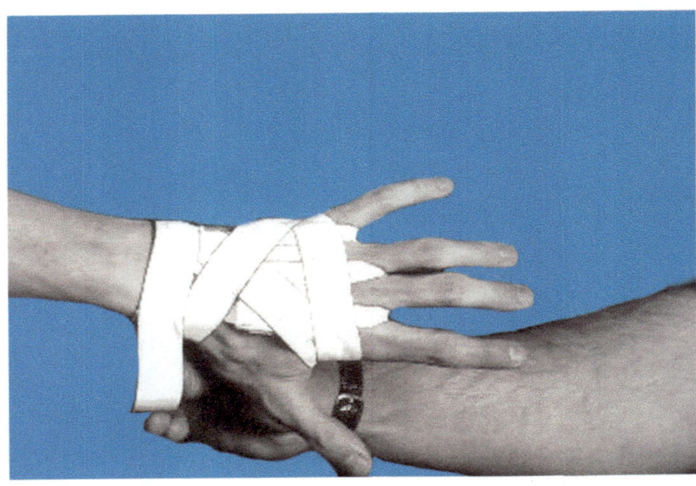

6. Apply two to three figure of eights. Complete this technique by applying a second anchor strip of 1-in. adhesive tape around the wrist.

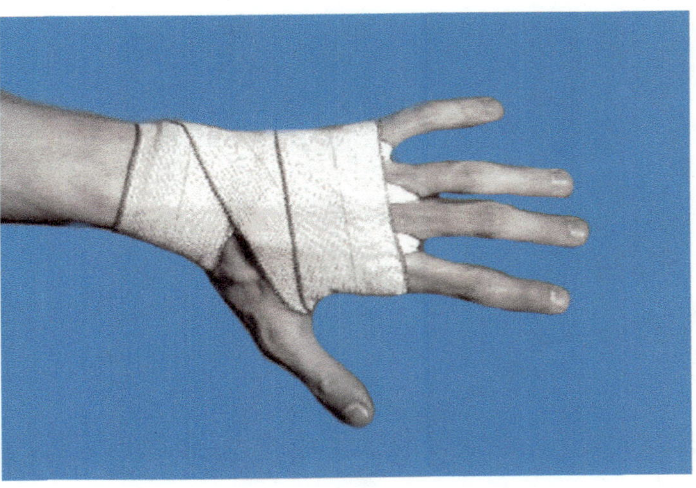

7. Apply a continuous figure of eight strip of 2-in. elastic tape for additional support.

**Upon completion of the procedure, make sure you check for neatness and gaps, adequate support, along with proper function of the affected area. In certain situations, the individual might be asked to perform function tests to establish appropriate technique application.*

Protective Devices

The use of protective devices is beneficial if they are properly selected, used in the appropriate setting, correctly fitted, and follow the guidelines of the specific sport. Consultation with a medical equipment specialist is highly encouraged! In some cases, a prescription from a licensed physician may result in insurance reimbursement. Listed below are various protective devices that are commercially available in use in sport and/or physical activity.

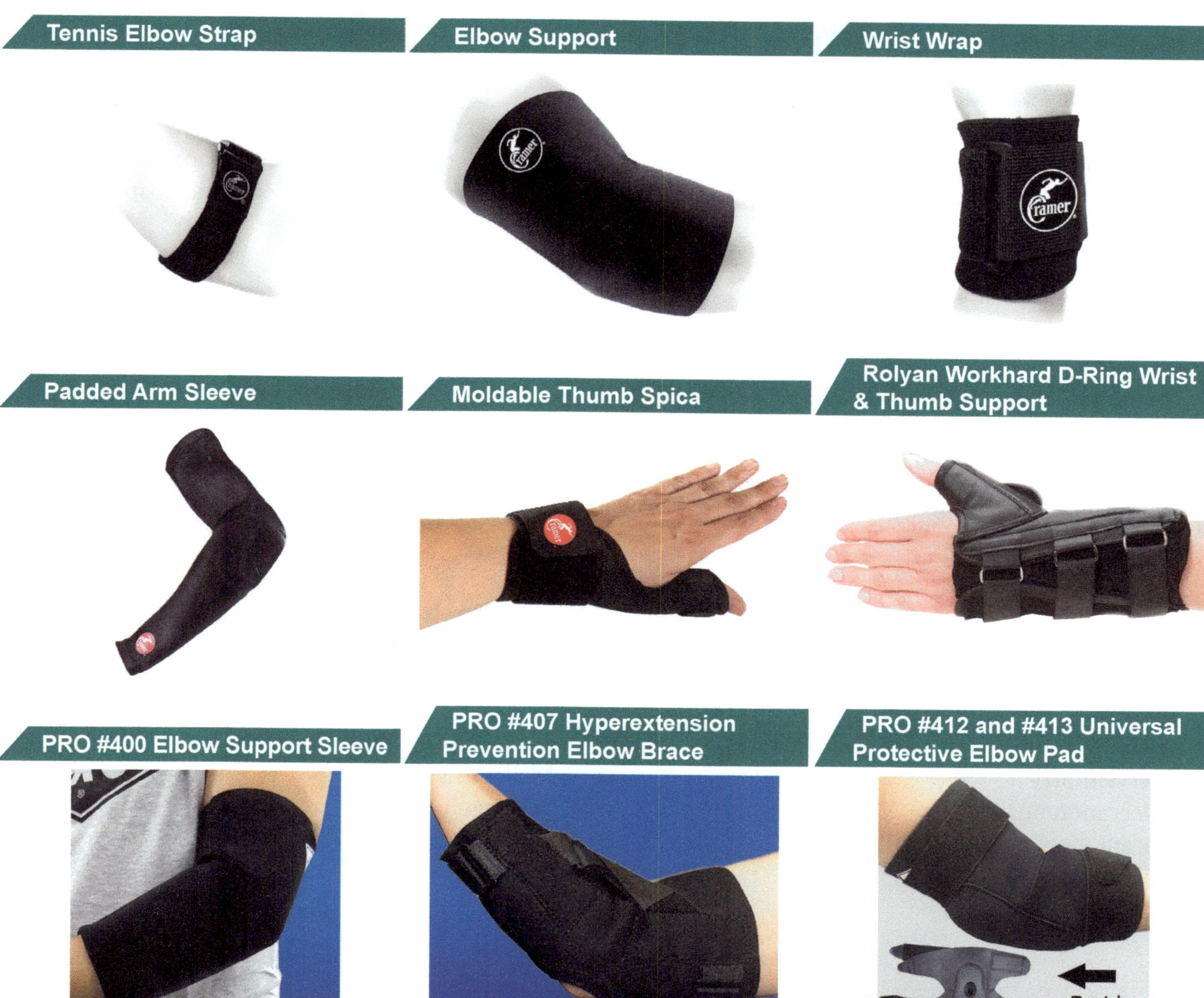

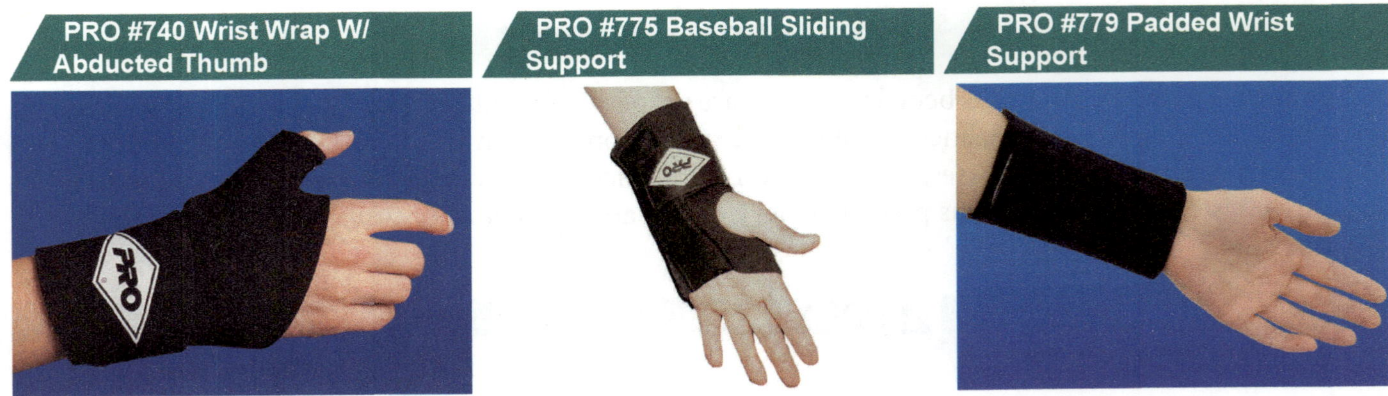

Listed below are various protective devices available to use in sport. Because a variety of protective devices are available, a qualified physician or qualified health care professional and medical equipment specialist can determine whether the individual is best suited for an off-the-shelf or custom brace.

Olecranon pad

Sports compression sleeve

Musculoskeletal Disorders

The following is a list of common musculoskeletal disorders of the elbow, forearm, wrist, and hand. For definitions of these terms, the authors encourage the learner to consult these medical references: *Taber's Medical Dictionary*, *Stedman's Medical Dictionary for the Health Professions and Nursing*, and/or *Signs and Symptoms of Athletic Injuries* (listed in Appendix B).

Elbow, Forearm, Wrist, and Hand
Contusion
Dislocation
Epicondylitis
Forearm splints
Hyperextension
Nerve injury
Olecranon bursitis
Sprain
Tendonopathies of elbow
Ulna nerve contusion
Wrist and hand
Bontonniere deformity
Carpal tunnel syndrome
De Quervain's tenosynovitis
Dislocation
Mallet finger
Subungual hematoma
Sprain
Strain

PART IV
Recommendations for Selected Protective Devices

Chapter 7

Facial, Thorax, Abdomen, and Low Back

EDUCATIONAL OBJECTIVES

Upon completing this chapter, the reader will be able to do the following:

- Identify anatomical structures and landmarks critical for correct taping procedures
- Explain the purpose for a protective device
- Develop skills in the selection of and fit of proper protective devices for specific anatomical structures
- Identify the athletic governing bodies for standards and protection
- Describe and demonstrate the purposes, clinical applications, anatomical structures, supplies needed, and pretaping and taping procedures for the ribs and low back

Introduction and Disclaimer

The procedures in this text are based on current research and recommendations from professionals in sport medicine and related health care professions. The information is intended to supplement, not substitute, recommendations from a qualified physician, qualified health care professional, and medical equipment specialist. Sagamore Publishing LLC and the authors disclaim responsibility for any adverse effect or consequences resulting from the misapplication or injudicious use of the material contained in the text. It is also accepted as judicious that health care professionals, sport industry professionals, and students must work under the guidance of a qualified physician, qualified health care provider, and medical equipment specialist.

Proper Assessment of Injury

Before applying a preventive technique (tape, wrap, and/or device), a qualified physician or qualified health care professional should complete a proper injury evaluation. Following the injury evaluation, a qualified health care professional and a medical equipment specialist can then recommend a proper protective device. This ensures that the proper device is applied for protection, support, stability, and compression. Also, developing a thorough knowledge of protective devices is imperative for health care professionals.

Terminology

Flexion. The act of bending or condition of being bent in contrast to extension; decrease in the angle between the bones forming a joint.

Extension. A movement that pulls apart both ends of any part; the act of drawing a body segment toward a straight line position with its proximally conjoined body segment, or away from the body joint.

Rotation. Process of turning on an axis; movement around a longitudinal axis which passes through a joint as in turning the palm of the hand up or down with the arm abducted.

Protective Devices

The primary purpose for a protective device is to prevent an injury and to protect injured anatomical structures from further aggravation. Through proper application, a protective device can be applied for additional protection, support, stability, and compression. The use of a protective device can be highly beneficial to the particular body part if properly selected. To avoid violating the manufacturer's specifications, follow suggested guidelines for proper selection, application, and maintenance. A protective device is a commercial product that is well designed and provides manufacturing liability and proper application instructions. The protective device is worn for protection, support, stability, or compression of an anatomical body part. To ensure safety and product effectiveness, the protective device should have product liability coverage from the manufacturer and instructions for proper application. There are sport-specific regulations, rules, and warnings concerning proper athletic equipment. Sport-specific equipment is worn as a standard uniform for participation in order to address the individual's safety. Standards of protection have improved through the combined efforts of athletic governing bodies, the American Society for Testing and Materials (ASTM), the National Operating Committee on Standards for Athletic Equipment (NOCSAE), and the Hockey Equipment Certification Council (HECC).

Medical Device Authorization

As required, a qualified physician or qualified health care professional must prescribe a custom brace. Upon their recommendations, an individual can work with a qualified health care professional and medical equipment specialist for a recommended custom brace. In some cases, a prescription from a licensed physician may result in insurance reimbursement. Figure 7.1 is an example of a "Medical Device Authorization Form."

MEDCO SPORTS MEDICINE

PRESCRIPTION DRUG & MEDICAL DEVICE AUTHORIZATION FORM

If purchasing prescription pharmaceuticals, please complete sections A & B
If purchasing an Automated External Defibrillator (AED) unit or other medical device, please complete sections A & C

Dear Valued Customer,

In order to ship you prescription pharmaceuticals and/or medical devices, we must have authorization from a licensed physician or other authorized prescriber. This individual needs to fill out the form below and fax a copy of this page and a photocopy of their license to 800-222-1934.

If your School/Facility does not have a licensed physician or other authorized prescriber, but is licensed to purchase prescription pharmaceuticals and/or medical devices, please fax a copy of the license and this form for identification to 800-222-1934.

A) Name of School/Facility: ______________________

Attention: ______________________ Customer #: ______________________

Address: ______________________

City & State: ______________________ Zip: ______________________

Phone: ______________________ Fax: ______________________

E-Mail: ______________________

B) I hereby authorize the internally designated representatives named below to order prescription products for this School/Facility. (please print)

1. ______________________ 2. ______________________

Type of authorization: ❑ Unlimited ❑ Limited (please attach list of products)

Physician/Authorized Prescriber Signature: ______________________

Physician/Authorized Prescriber Name (please print): ______________________

State License Number: ______________________
(please include photocopy of license)

C) I hereby acknowledge that I am aware that medical devices are intended for use by a physician or a person certified or trained to use such device.

Name (please print): ______________________

Title: ______________________

State License/Certification Number: ______________________

Signature: ______________________ Date: ______________________

Rx Pharmaceuticals

Call 1-800-55MEDCO www.medco-athletics.com Fax 1-800-222-1934 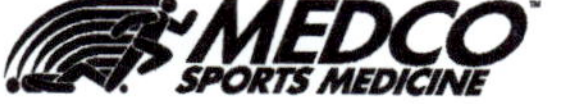 137

Figure 7.1 Medical Device Authorization Form

Protective Devices

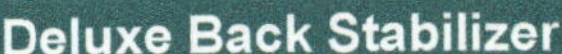

Back Support

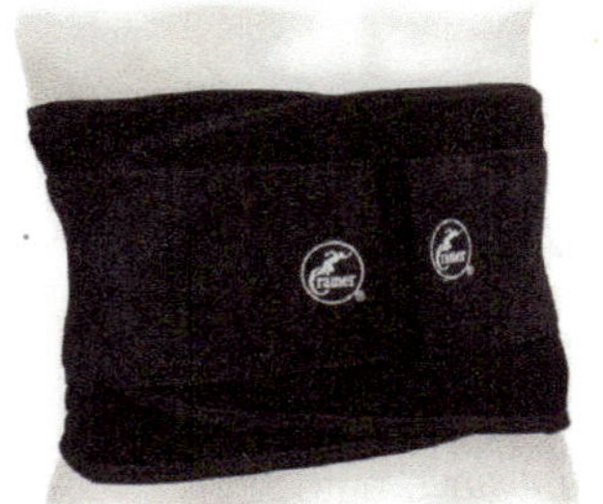

Deluxe Back Stabilizer

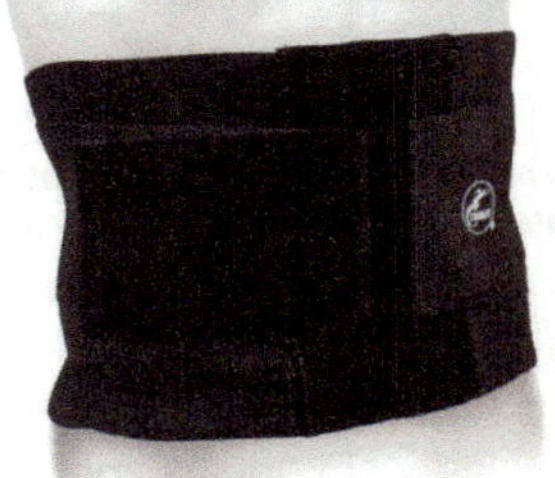

Mouthpiece

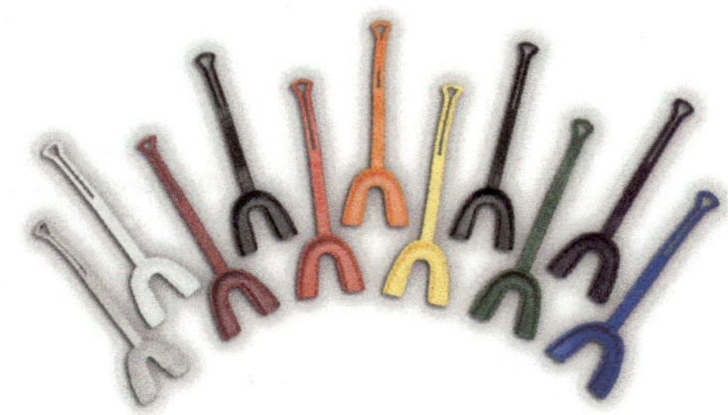

Rolyan Universal Rib Support

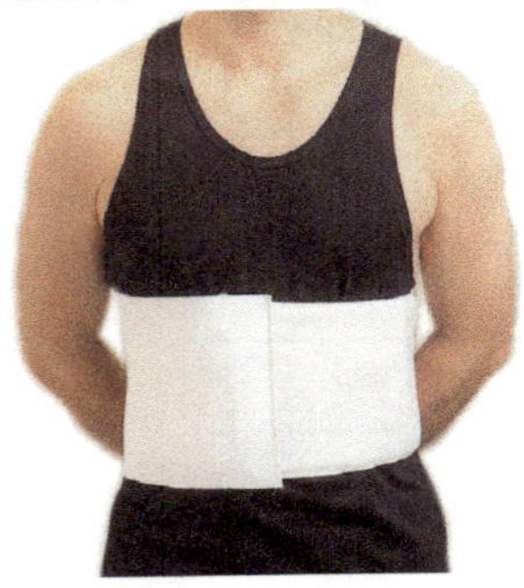

PRO #200 Low Back Support Belt

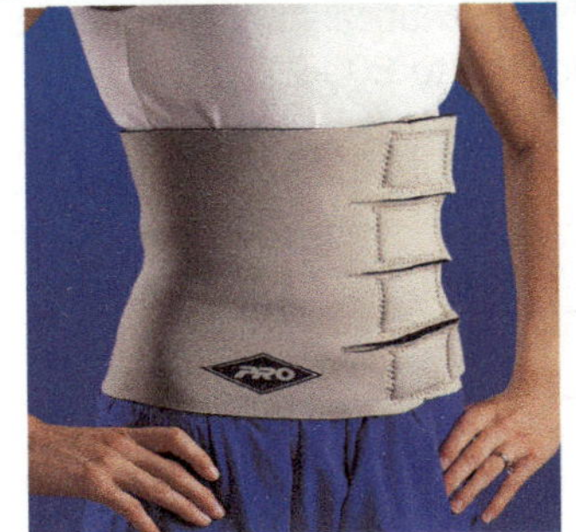

PRO #240 Lightweight Industrial Back Support

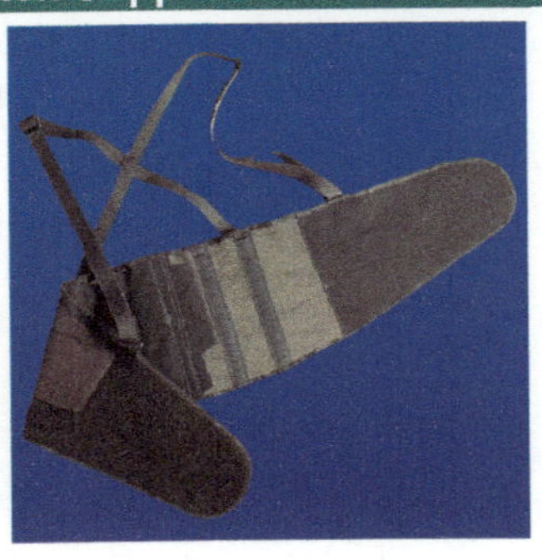

PRO #250 Lumbar –Sacral Back Support Belt

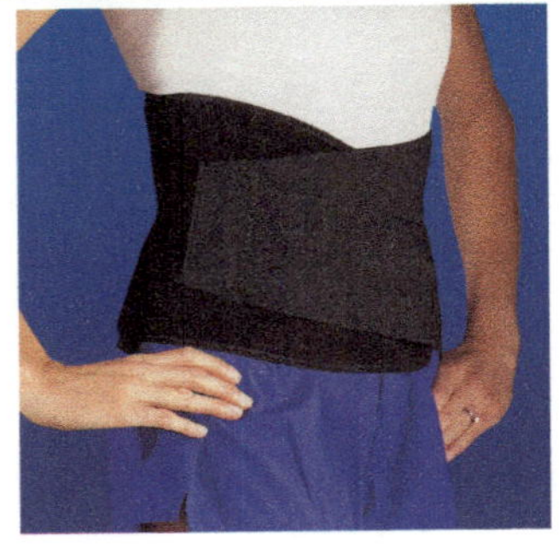

PRO #280 Lumbar Back Support

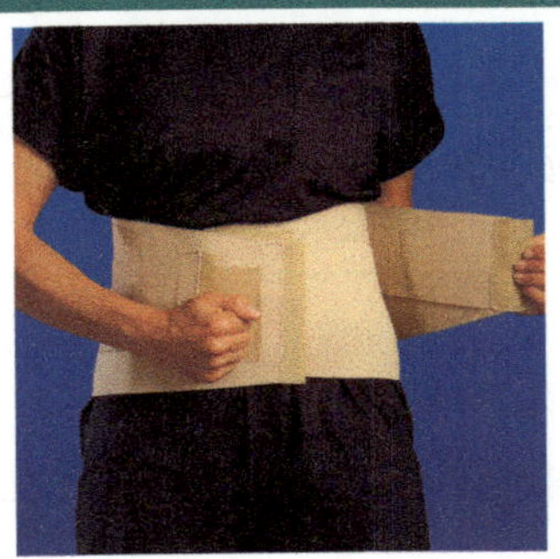

Fastbreak Shirt Front

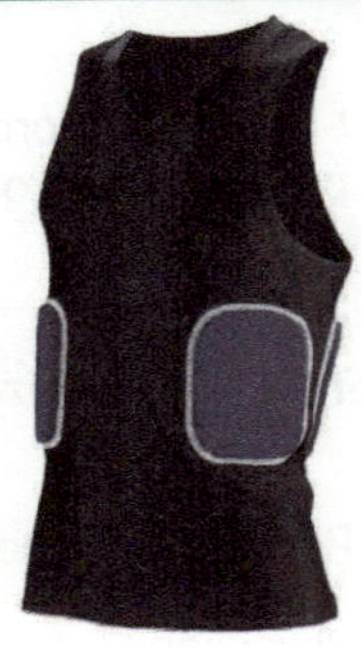

Cramer Black Front

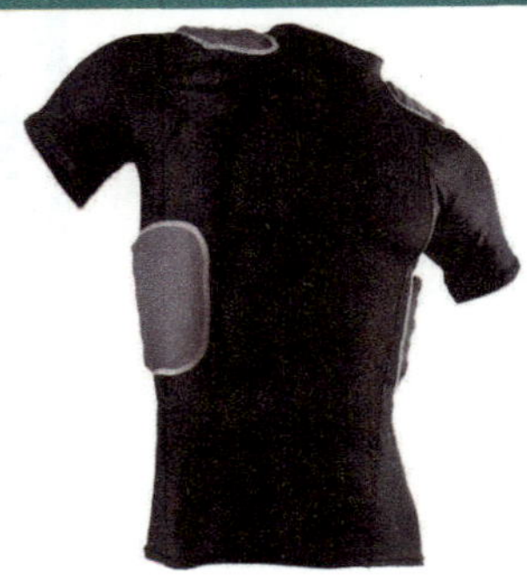

Women Fastbreak Short Front

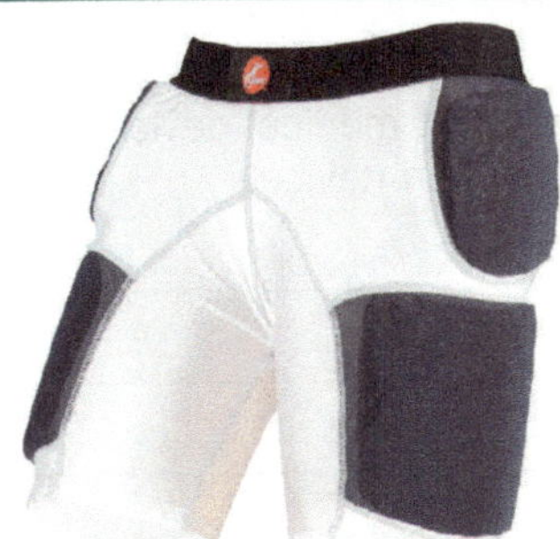

Men Fastbreak Short Front

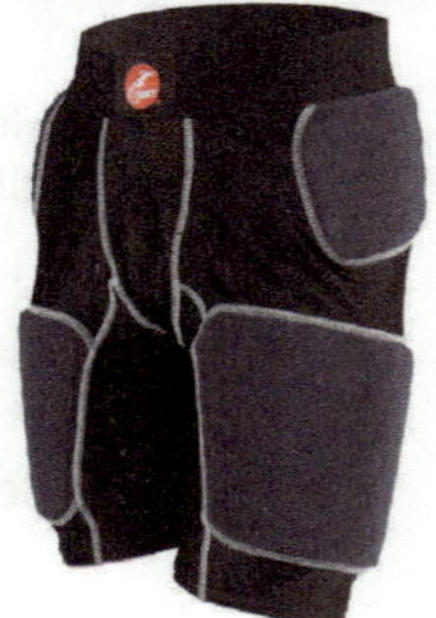

Listed below are various protective devices available to use in sport. Because a variety of protective devices are available, a qualified physician or qualified health care professional and medical equipment specialist can determine whether the individual is best suited for an off-the-shelf or custom brace.

Ear plugs
Hip pointer brace/guard
Nose guard
Sports compression girdle
Throat protector that attaches for face mask

Bones and Ligaments

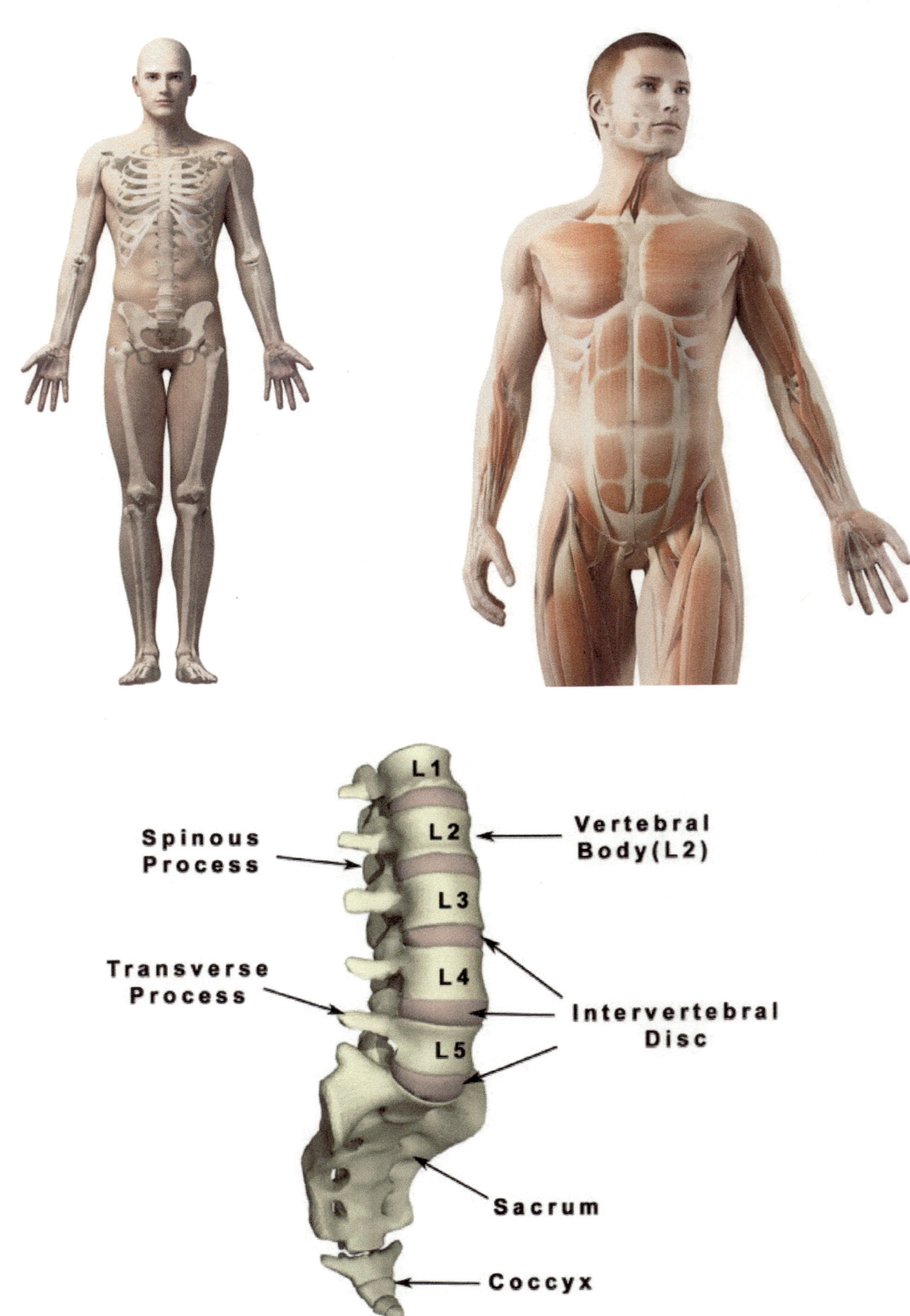

Muscles and Tendons

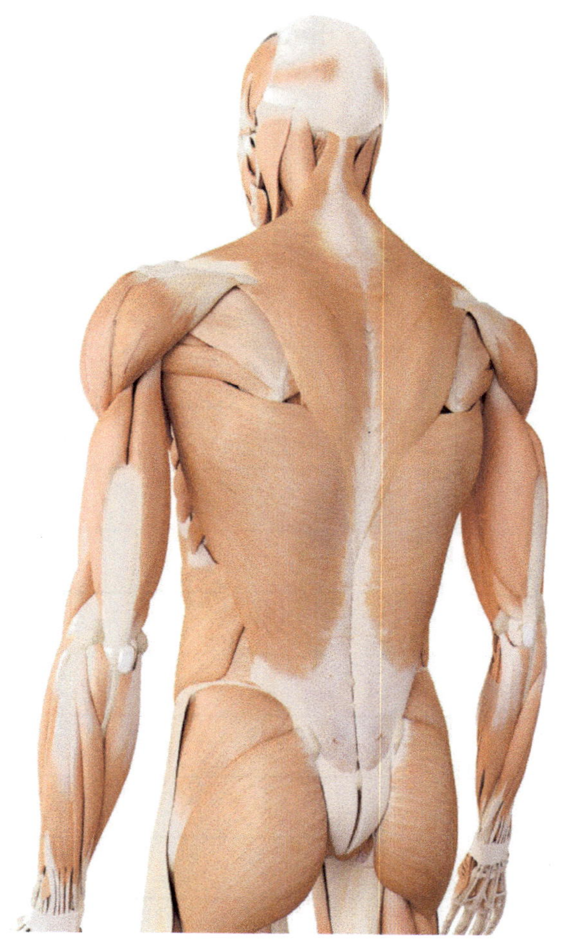

Taping Techniques

The taping techniques presented are the fundamental procedures. A strong knowledge of anatomy, physiology, and biomechanics is essential. Developing a thorough knowledge regarding the fundamentals about the application of taping/wrapping procedures is imperative. Review Chapter 1 before applying any technique.

NOTES:

RIB

Purpose: To provide support and compression to the ribs

Clinical Application: Contusion and strains

Anatomical Structure: Thoracic cavity

Anatomical Position: Standing upright, the arm of the affected side abducted

Supplies: 1½-in. adhesive tape, 4-in. or 6-in. extra long elastic wrap, and gauze pad or large Band-Aid, and 2-in. or 3-in. elastic tape

Pre-taping Procedure

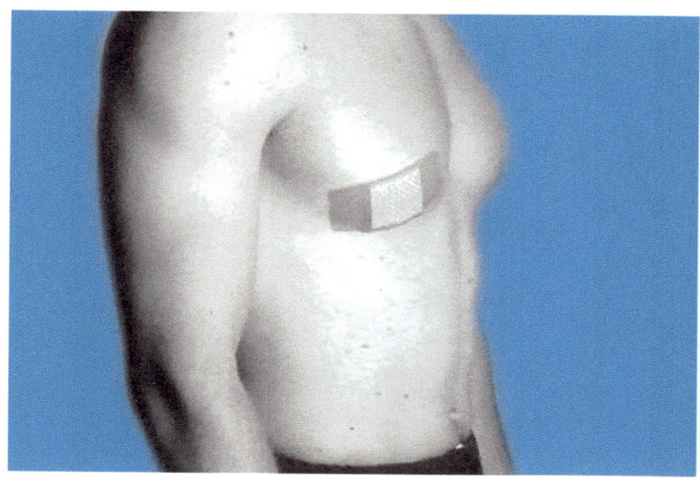

Cover the nipple with either gauze pad or Band-Aid.

Taping Procedure

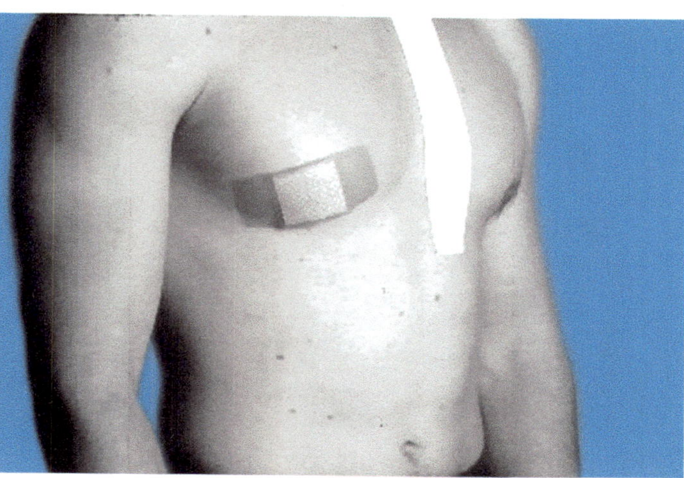

1. On the uninjured side, apply two vertical anchor strips near the anterior and posterior midline of the body. Advise the individual to inhale and expand thorax cavity.

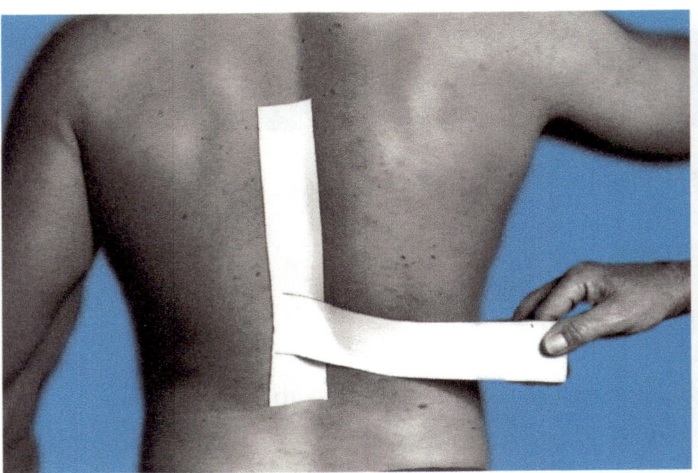

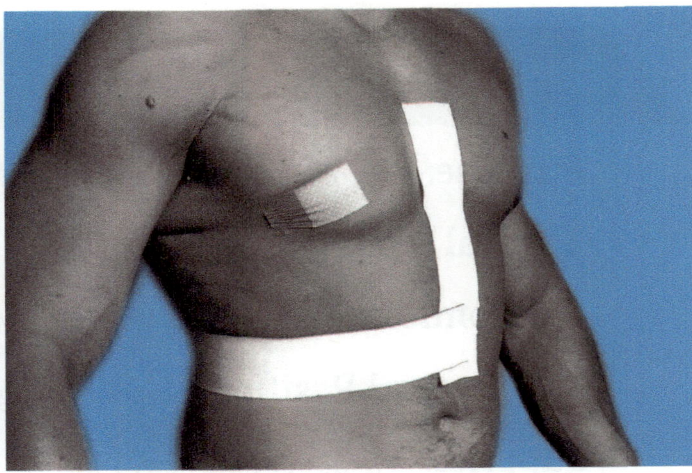

2. Begin with a strip of adhesive tape on the distal aspect of the posterior anchor, follow the contour of the ribs, and end on the distal aspect of the anterior anchor. When applying the tape, have the person inhale.

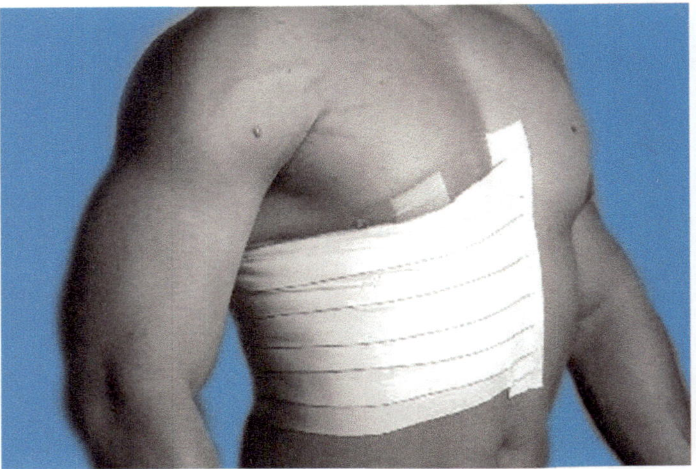

3. Repeat Step 2, applying six to eight strips of adhesive tape. Overlap the tape by one half of its width. Begin interiorly and work superiorly.

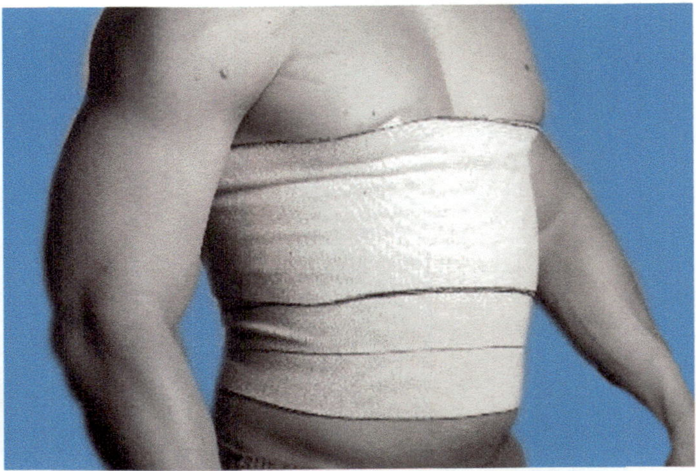

4. Apply a 4-in. or 6-in. extra long elastic wrap over the top. With the person's chest expanded, apply the wrap in a circular manner around the torso, beginning inferiorly and working superiorly.

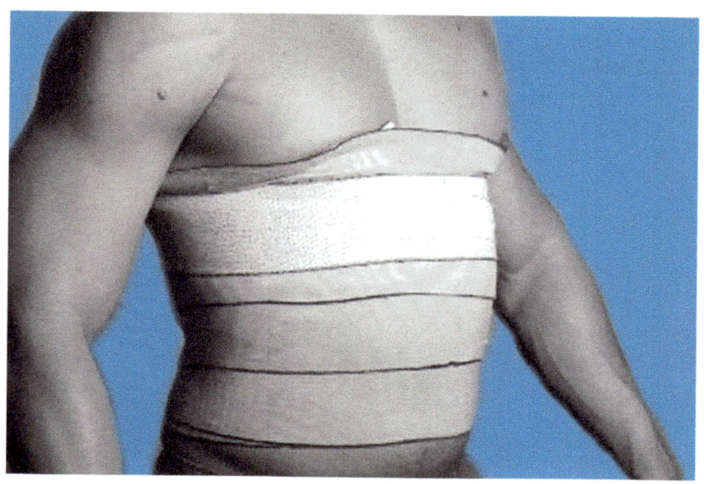

5. Secure the wrap with a continuous strip of elastic tape. Anchor the elastic tape with adhesive tape.

**Upon completion of the procedure, make sure you check for neatness and gaps, adequate support, along with proper function of the affected area. In certain situations, the individual might be asked to perform function tests to establish appropriate technique application.*

Adjunct Taping Procedures: Rib

These adjunct taping procedures can be used in conjunction with the basic technique presented.

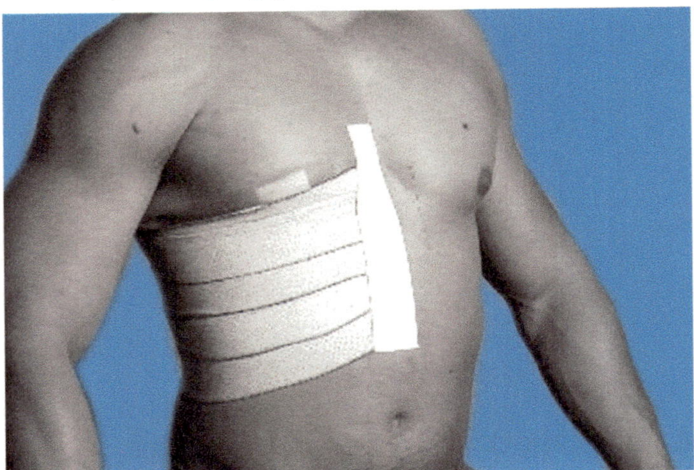

Technique A. Use 3-in. elastic tape in place of the adhesive tape.

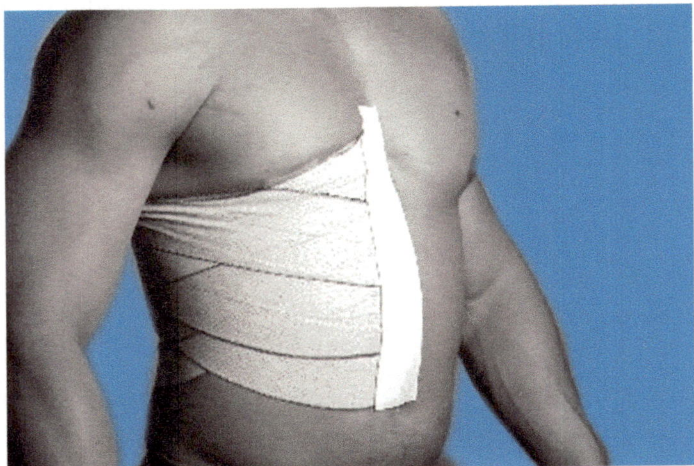

Technique B: The "X" Pattern Technique. Apply the X pattern technique. Begin at the distal aspect of one anchor, cross the affected area, and end on the opposite anchor. Apply the second strip in the same pattern beginning from the opposite anchor. Repeat step 2, three to five times, overlapping the tape by one half of its width.

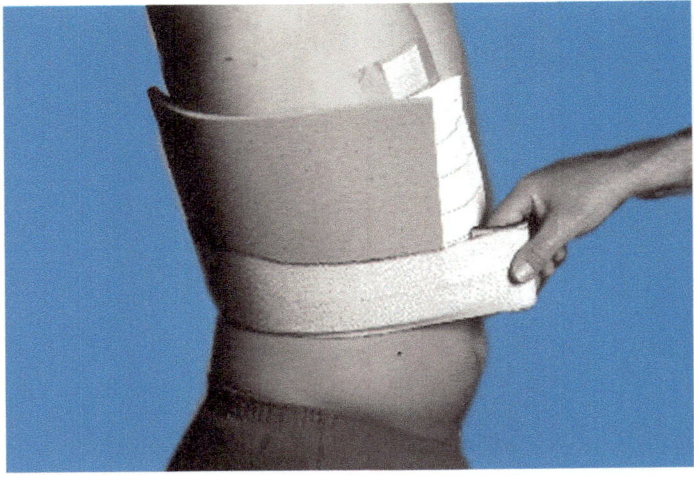

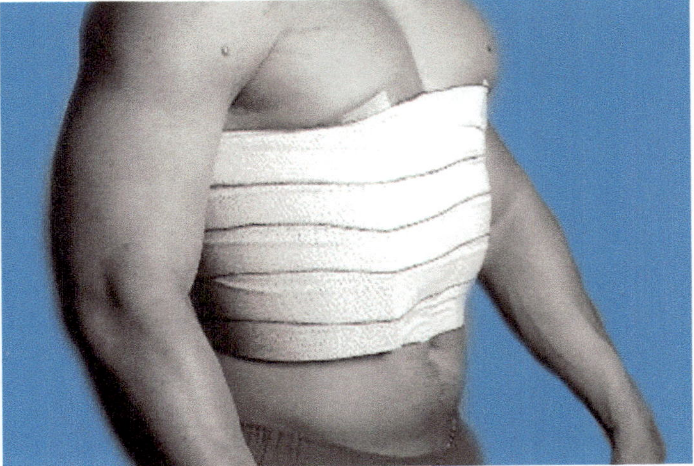

Technique C. Use foam rubber to pad the affected area for additional protection and then secure with elastic tape or elastic wrap.

LOW BACK

Purpose: To provide support to the low back

Clinical Application: Sprains, strains, and contusions

Anatomical Structure: Low back (lumbar and sacral)

Anatomical Position: Standing position, knees and waist slightly flexed

Supplies: 1½-in. or 2-in. adhesive tape and 6-in. extra long elastic wrap

Taping Procedure

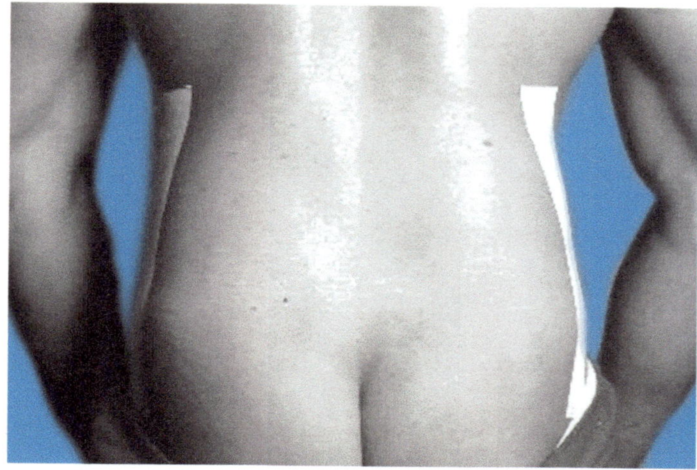

1. Apply two vertical anchor strips, approximately 4 in. to 6 in. in length, over the lateral sides of the torso.

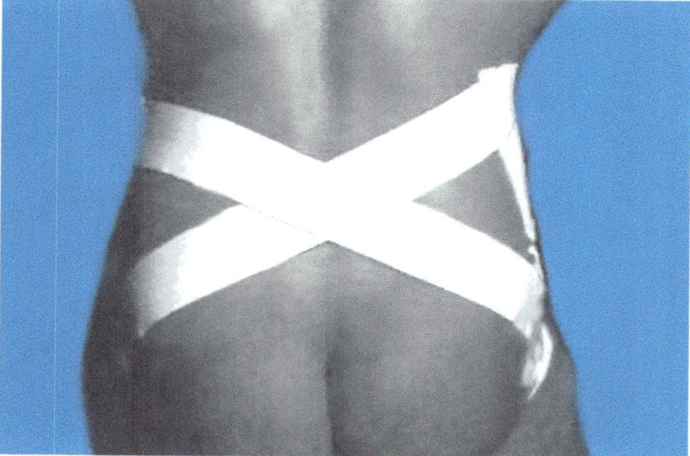

2. Apply the X pattern technique. Begin at the distal aspect of one anchor, cross the affected area, and end on the opposite anchor. Apply the second strip in the same pattern beginning from the opposite anchor.

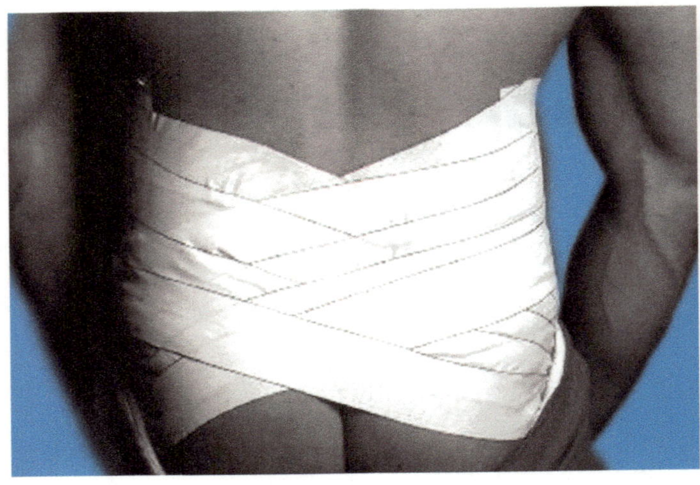

3. Repeat Step 2, seven to nine times, overlapping the tape by one half of its width.

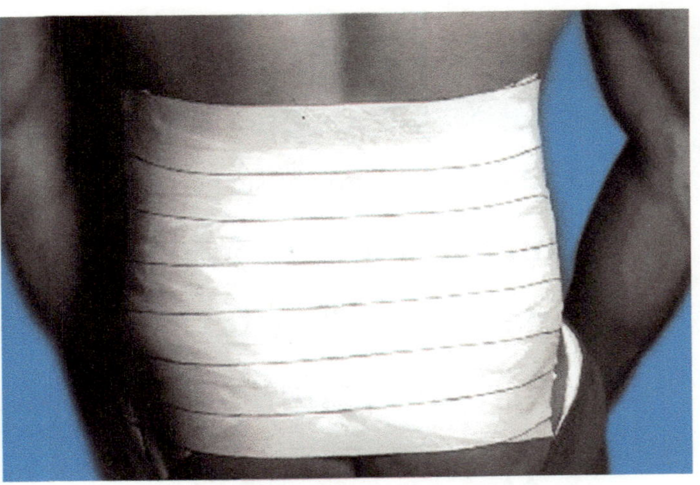

4. Apply parallel strips, working inferior to superior, until the affected area is covered. Overlap each strip by one half of its width. Place a final anchor over each original anchor to help hold the tape in place.

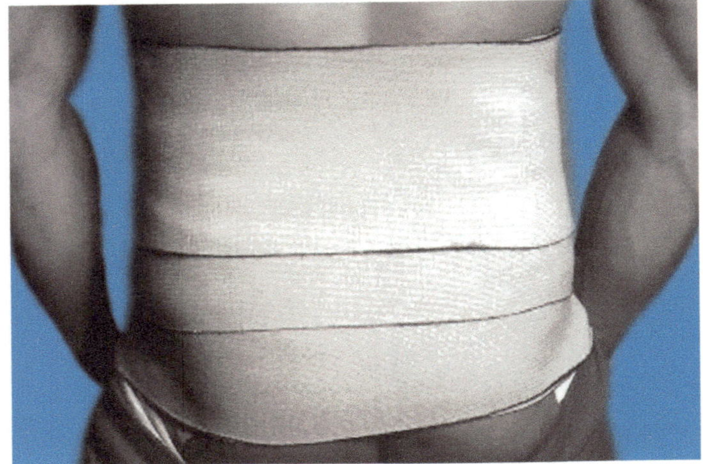

5. Have the individual exhale to expand the abdominal cavity. In a circular fashion, apply the elastic wrap around the waist. Secure the wrap with a strip of adhesive tape.

**Upon completion of the procedure, make sure you check for neatness and gaps, adequate support, along with proper function of the affected area. In certain situations, the individual might be asked to perform function tests to establish appropriate technique application.*

Musculoskeletal Disorders

The following is a list of common musculoskeletal disorders of the facial, thorax, abdomen, and low back. For definitions of these terms, the authors encourage the learner to consult these medical references: *Taber's Medical Dictionary*, *Stedman's Medical Dictionary for the Health Professions and Nursing*, and/or *Signs and Symptoms of Athletic Injuries* (listed in Appendix B).

Facial, Thorax, Abdomen, and Low Back
Contusion
Sprain
Strain

Chapter 8

BSN Medical

EDUCATIONAL OBJECTIVES

Upon completing this chapter, the reader will be able to do the following:

- Explain the purpose for selecting and using the BSN Medial Products for compression and support
- Describe the benefits and advantages of compression support garment for the physically active patient
- Identify the proper use and application of protective devices for the ankle, lower leg, knee, elbow, thumb, and wrist/hand

Compression Supports

There are many benefits and advantages to compressive support garments for the orthopedic patient and more specifically the athlete. Compressive supports can be highly beneficial for the particular body part if it is properly selected, applied and worn. Compression supports can be worn to protect an injured body part, to protect from future injury, and provide proprioception. The use of compression supports around anatomical joints and larger muscular areas has shown to have beneficial results in improving circulation and reducing pain, not only during athletic performance but during recovery.

Compression support garments provide compression through various knitting or neoprene materials to the joint or muscle to help minimize/reduce swelling via decongestion and improve lymphatic flow through muscle stimulation (proprioception) which leads to rapid healing. Compression supports are unobtrusive and do not restrict movement.

BSN medical

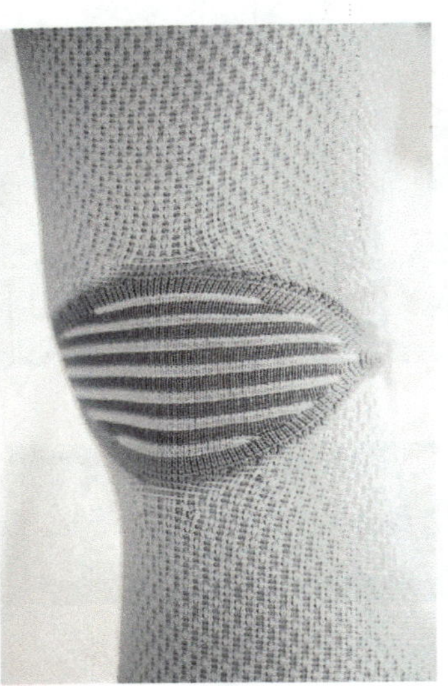

BSN medical's new 3D knit PowerMotion supports series is manufactured using an advanced knitting structure that provides support and compression for weak or injured joints and muscles. This material helps promote the healing process by decreasing pain intensity and improved pain complaints as well as positive experiences with wearing comfort.

Each 3D knit support features a unique design for optimal fit and breathable, light weight material for comfortable wear. 3D knit supports are made of polymide and elastane to create a lightweight, breathable and moisture-wicking material alternative to neoprene.

The knitted structure of each compression support provides specific gradient pressure around the affected area by providing a seamless interwoven layer support. Each support has pressure-free cuffs for secure fit with no constriction. Specially designed motion comfort zones in each compression support allows for improved comfort in areas of the joint. The combination of these components provides gradient pressure and support individualized to the specific body part.

Actimove GenuMotion / 3D Knee Support - Specially designed 3D knit support for the knee provides excellent compression and stabilization for weak or injured knees while providing flexibility.

Indications: Bursitis, Chondromalacia Patella, Contusions, Strains, Osgood-Schlatter Disease, Patellar Instability, Tendinitis

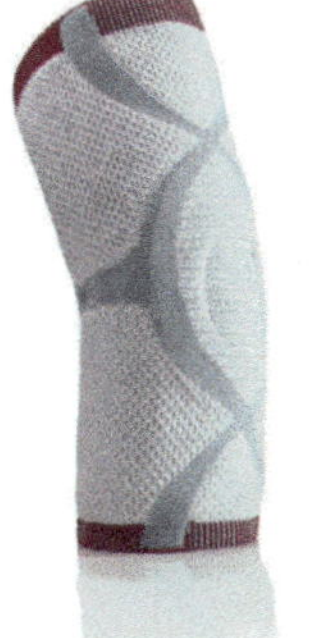

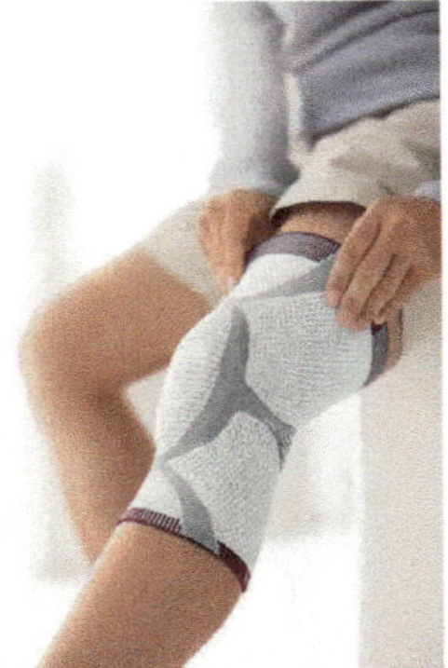

- Premium knit design provides compression, stabilization and support
- Lightweight and breathable
- Motion comfort zone at the popliteal area for more comfortable wear
- Silicone insert surrounds the patella and helps reduce swelling
- Gradient compression around knee to speed healing
- Measurement for sizing: Measure circumference of thigh 5 ½" above center patella and circumference of calf 4 3/3" below center patella.

Actimove TaloMotion / 3D Ankle Support – Specially designed 3D knit ankle support provides excellent compression and stabilization for weak or injured ankles while providing flexibility.

Indications: Sprains and Strains, Contusion, Tendinitis, Arthritis, Postoperative use

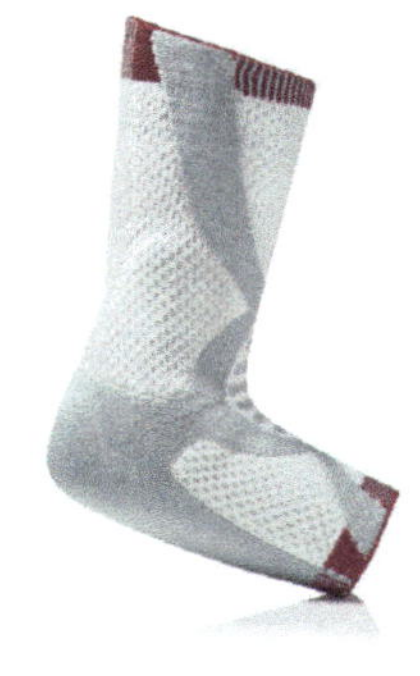

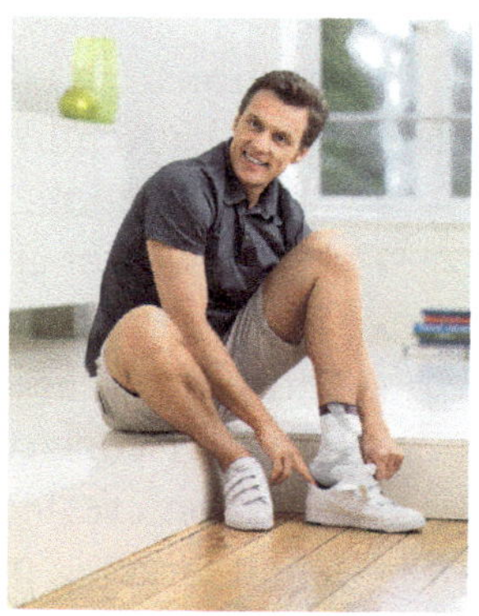

- Premium knit design provides compression, stabilization and support
- Lightweight and breathable
- Motion comfort zone at the dorsum of ankle area for more comfortable wear
- Two viscoelastic pressure pads on both sides of the malleoli create a massage effect for the reduction of swelling of the ankle
- Gradient compression around the ankle and foot to speed healing
- Measurement for sizing: Measure circumference of ankle just above malleoli

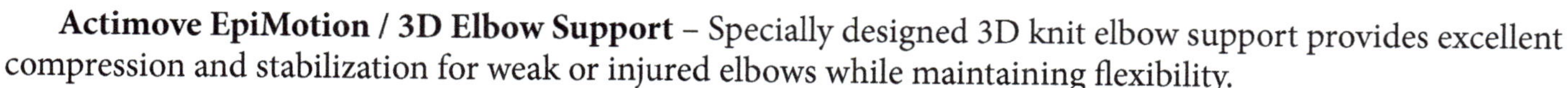

Actimove EpiMotion / 3D Elbow Support – Specially designed 3D knit elbow support provides excellent compression and stabilization for weak or injured elbows while maintaining flexibility.

Indications: Epicondylitis (Tennis or Golfer's elbow), Arthritis, Postoperative use

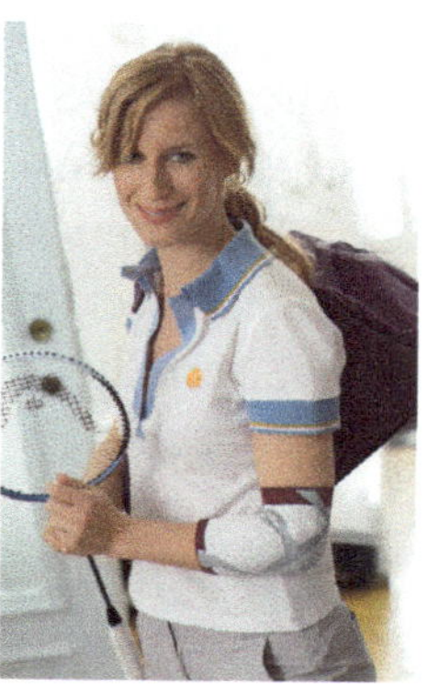

- Premium knit design provides compression, stabilization, and support
- Lightweight and breathable
- Motion comfort zone at the elbow crease for more comfortable wear
- Anatomic inserts pressure pads on both sides of the epicondyles create a massage effect and target pressure on epicondylar tendons for the reduction of swelling and targeted pain relief
- Gradient compression around the elbow and forearm to speed healing
- Measurement for sizing: Measure circumference of forearm 4 ¾" below the center of elbow

Actimove ManuMotion – Specially designed 3D knit wrist support provides excellent compression and support for weak or injured wrists while maintaining functionality.

Indications: Sprains, Strains, Carpal Tunnel Syndrome, Arthritis pain, post-operative use

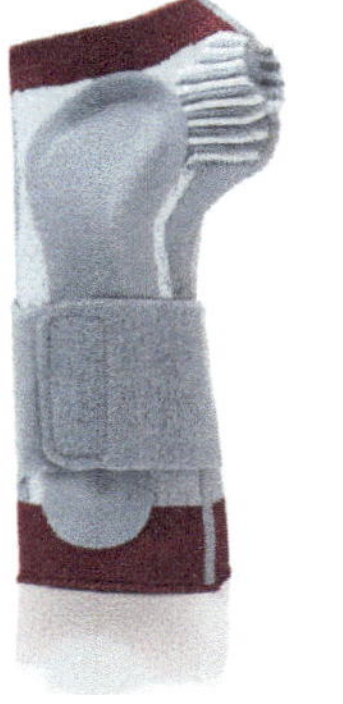

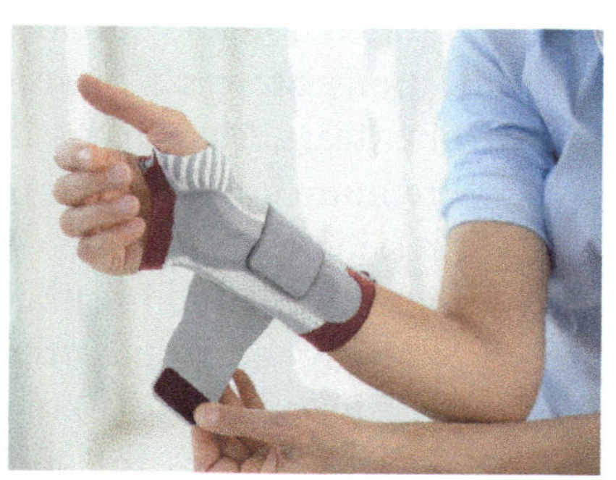

- Premium knit design provides compression, stabilization and support
- Lightweight and breathable
- Moldable aluminum stay on palmer surface for support
- Gradient compression around the wrist and forearm to speed healing
- Adjustable strap for improved comfort
- Measurement for sizing: Measure circumference of the wrist

Actimove AchilloMotion / 3D Achilles Tendon Support – Specially designed 3D knit Achilles tendon support provides excellent compression and support for weak or injured Achilles tendons while maintaining flexibility.

Indications: Achilles tendonitis, Achillobursitis, Degenerative changes in the Achilles tendon postoperative use

- Premium knit design provides compression and support
- Lightweight and breathable
- Motion comfort zone at the dorsum of ankle for more comfortable wear
- Two viscoelastic pressure pads on both sides of the Achilles tendon create a massage effect for the reduction of swelling and targeted pain relief.
- Gradient compression around the ankle, Achilles and foot to speed healing
- Optional heel wedges for additional relief to the Achilles tendon
- Measurement for sizing: Measure circumference of ankle just above malleoli

Actimove PowerMotion Thigh / 3D Thigh Support – Specially designed 3D knit thigh support provides excellent compression and support for sore or injured thigh muscles.

Indications: Strains, Contusions, Minor muscle fiber tears, Myositis ossificans

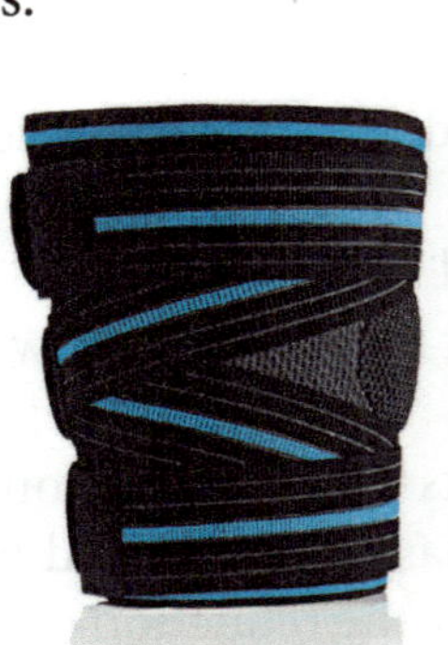

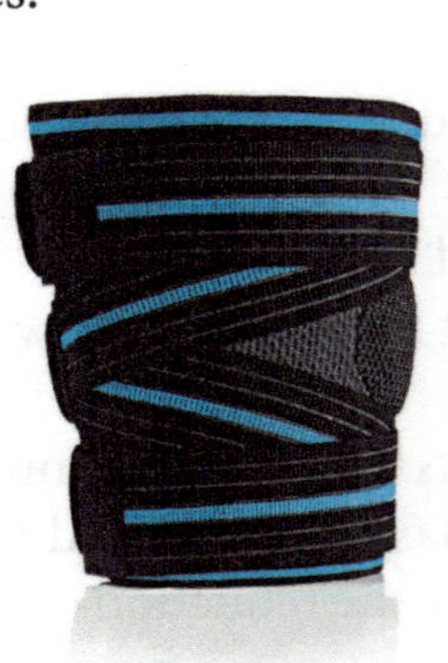

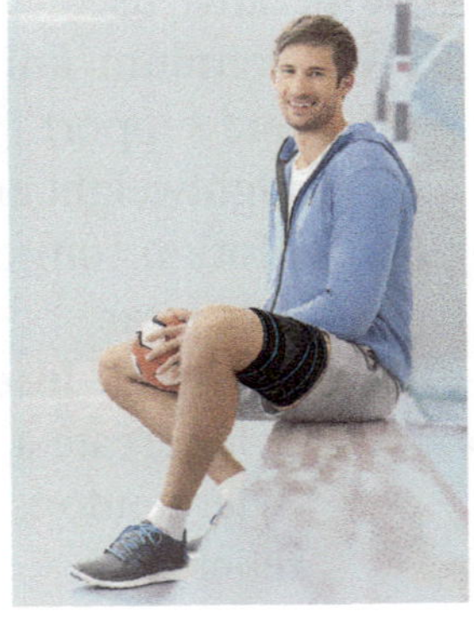

- Premium knit design provides compression and support
- Lightweight and breathable
- Specially designed pressure relief zone for affected area of muscle
- Y-shaped straps for additional adjustable compression around thigh
- Straps uniquely place to surround painful area avoiding direct pressure on injury while providing improved support promoting pain reduction
- Gradient compression around thigh
- Measurement for sizing: Measure circumference around mid-thigh

Actimove PowerMotion Calf / 3D Calf Support – Specially designed 3D knit thigh support provides excellent compression and support for sore or injured calf muscles.

Indications: Strains, Contusions, Minor muscle fiber tears, Myositis ossificans

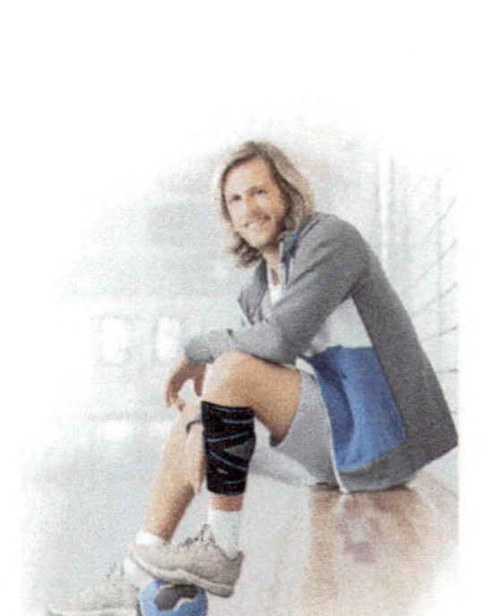

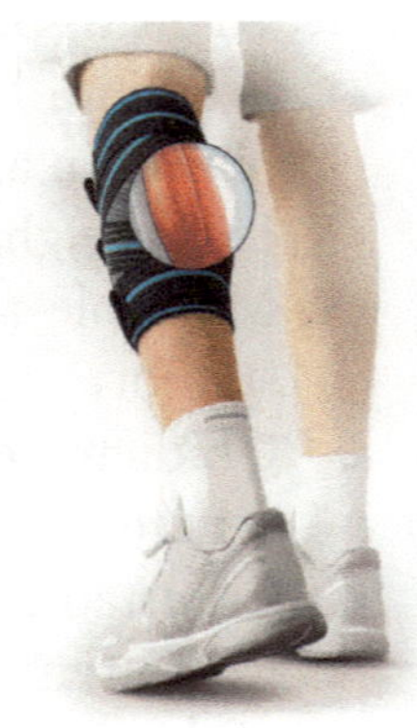

- Premium knit design provides compression and support
- Lightweight and breathable
- Specially designed pressure relief zone for affected area of muscle
- Y-shaped straps for additional adjustable compression on calf area
    - Straps uniquely place to surround painful area avoiding direct pressure on injury while providing improved support promoting pain reduction
- Gradient compression around calf
- Measurement for sizing: Measure circumference around mid-thigh

Actimove® Rhizo Forte Thumb Brace

The thumb and its joints differentiate it from the fingers. It allows a wide range of motion - flexion and extension, adduction and abduction. Combined these movements achieve a opposition and is an important motion for the hand. This makes the thumb unique in its functionality, allowing humans to hold even small objects securely.

Injuries and conditions affecting the thumb can cause loss of motion, instability and pain:

Ulnar Collateral Ligament injuries are encountered frequently in sports with a high risk of falling, such as skiing, biking, soccer, basketball, rugby and inline-skating. This injury is also known as skier's thumb or Gamekeeper's thumb. The main goal of managing UCL injuries is to restore the full functionality of the thumb. Treatment and management is based on the grade and severity of the injury. Partial tears can be managed by immobilization only. Complete tears are usually treated with surgery. Post-operative treatment includes immobilization for up to six weeks to protect the surgical site. After the immobilization period, targeted functional hand training is used to regain range of motion and strength of the thumb.

Osteoarthritis (OA) of the thumb affects the CMC joint and is caused by wear to the cartilage of the joint, resulting in inflammation and pain. It is a chronic disorder and the main treatment goal is to manage symptoms and retain quality of life for the patient. Acute pain management and inflammation reduction is obtained through medication and is supported by using immobilization braces or supports to rest the CMC joint. Surgery may be required when the symptoms and loss or level of activity has become significant and the patient no longer responds to other therapies. Most surgical options remove some or all of the arthritic bone and use different techniques to stabilize the joint. The surgical procedures are followed by an extended immobilization period with splints, casts or braces. After the immobilization period, targeted functional hand training is used to regain range of motion and strength of the thumb.

The Actimove® Rhizo Forte with its unique design and functionality provides reliable support for the injured area, along with high patient comfort. Actimove® Rhizo Forte is a thumb orthosis for the management of painful conditions and irritations of the thumb joints associated with chronic or acute indications. The brace immobilizes the carpometacarpal (CMC) and the first metacarpophalangeal (MCP 1) joints and places the thumb in a functional position. Material composition includes primarily thermoplastic polyurethane, a core out of aluminum alloy and straps made out of polyamide with a latex free formulation.

It is easy to clean and machine washable. The special construction effectively restricts thumb adduction, while leaving the four fingers and the wrist to move freely. The adaptable aluminum core makes it easy to optimally fit the immobilizer to the individual hand shape of the patient. With its fasteners/closures, the brace can be easily secured with one hand. The low profile design and smooth edges contribute to maximum patient comfort. The product is dirt and water resistant and can be dried easily.

Indications:

- Thumb osteoarthritis (OA)
- Ulnar ligament injury (UCL) of the MCP1 joint (e.g. Skier's thumb or Gamekeeper's thumb)
- Rheumatoid arthritis (RA) of the thumb
- Instability of the CMC joint
- After surgical and nonsurgical treatment
- Soft tissue injuries (sprains)
- Traumatic Thumb CMC dislocation
- Ligament instabilities
- Post-operative immobilization

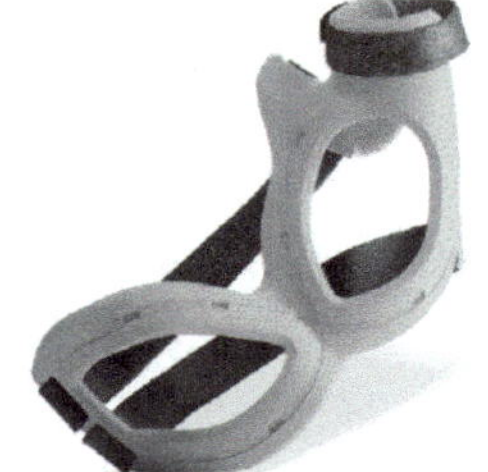

Contraindications:

- Impaired lymph flow or circulatory disorders of the hand and fingers. Fracture of the wrist and hand.

Design Details:

- Its special construction effectively restricts thumb adduction, while leaving the four fingers and the wrist to move freely
- Its adaptable aluminium core makes it easy to optimally fit the immobilizer to the individual hand shape
- With its fasteners/closures, the brace can be easily secured with one hand
- The selected materials and the low profile design with smooth edges contribute to maximum comfort
- The product is dirt and water resistant and can be dried easily

Actimove® Rhizo Forte is an anatomically pre-shaped orthosis.

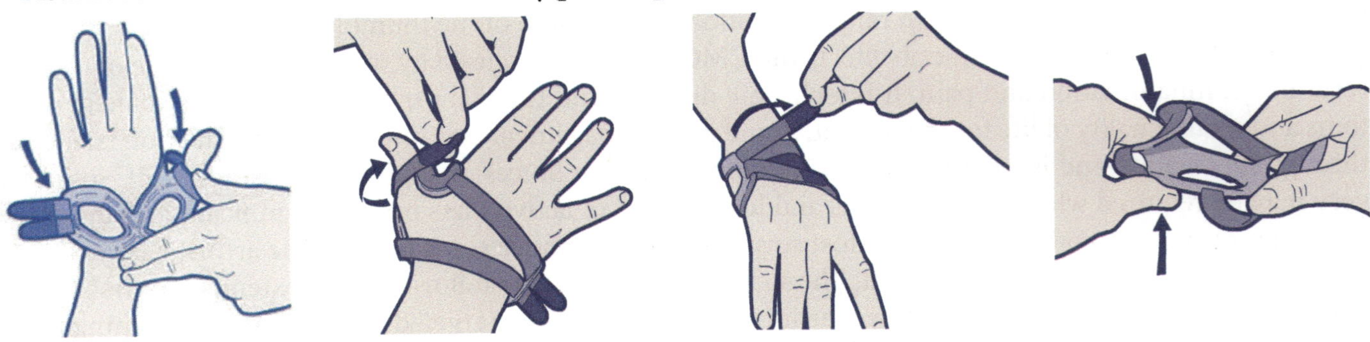

Biomechanical Study - *Stabilization effectiveness and functionality of different thumb CMC OA braces.*

- Hamann, N., et al., Stabilization effectiveness and functionality of different thumb orthoses in female patients with first carpometacarpal joint osteoarthritis, Clin. Biomech. (2014)

Conclusion

Stabilization seems to be at the expense of functionality. MEDI afforded best stabilization at lowest functionality, while PUSH provided best functionality at lowest stabilization. Best compromise of stability and functionality could be reached with BSN.

Method

- 18 females with diagnosed OA of the thumb
- 4 orthoses with different design included
- Stabilization examined by measurement of range of motion at CMC and MCP joints
- Hand functionality was examined by Sollerman test results
- All orthoses significantly restricted the range of motion of the thumb compared to the range of motion without external support
- Braces with high rates in functionality offer lower stability
- Braces with high stability impact strongly the functionality
- **Actimove® Rhizo Forte offers the best compromise between stability and functionality**

Results of the post-market observational study with the novel orthosis for the treatment of osteoarthritis (OA) of the thumb

Conclusions:

The results of this observational study with 10 patients demonstrate that the use of Tricodur® Rhizo Forte thumb orthosis was beneficial in a total of 9 patients with OA of the thumb under conditions of daily practice in an orthopedic specialist practice (1 premature withdrawal due to pain). Pain reduction was reported from all patients. Moreover, ease of use, fit and suitability for everyday use was evaluated as good to very good by the patients and the treating physician. Therefore, the Tricodur® Rhizo Forte thumb orthosis has demonstrated its ability for conservative treatment of the OA of the thumb and may add important value to the existing therapy options.

Delta-Cast soft

Delta Cast Soft is fiberglass free and was designed to provide functional support to fractures and soft tissue injuries. Its semi-rigidity allows for more flexibility and mobility, thus helping to reduce immobilization-related problems such as atrophy or joint stiffness. As a result, the overall healing process tends to shorten.

Earlier patient mobility as cast will allow a limited range of motion
Improved circulation, faster healing, shorter rehabilitation period
Helps to avoid or minimize muscle atrophy and other immobilization-related issues
Lightweight, breathable material offers high wearing comfort
Smooth surface for a snag-free finish
Soft edges for higher patient satisfaction
Available in a wide range of attractive colors and patterns

Delta-Dry Softliner Stockinette

BSN Medical Delta-Dry™ Water Resistant Synthetic Stockinette is used as the first layer in the casting process to cover the skin. The Stockinette when used in conjunction with Synthetic Casting Tape is water resistant. This allows patients to shower, swim, and wash with less disruption in lifestyle for patients. An open knit fiber material allows water to quickly drain from the cast. The Quick Dry Stockinette helps to minimize cast odor and promotes routine hygiene. The stockinette conforms to body contours and is latex free for use on patients with latex allergies. The unique padding of the Delta-Dry™ helps to reduce skin issues like macerations, itching, and odor by providing a soft, comfortable cushion on the skin.

- Unique patented technology outperforms other water resistant orthopaedic products
- Allows patients to shower, swim, bathe and wash hands
- Reduces odor under the cast
- Excellent conformability to body contours
- Better long term water resistance
- Provides comfortable, fast-drying casts
- Leaves the skin healthy under the cast
- Simple and quick application
- Latex Free

Chapter 9
Kinesio Taping® Method

EDUCATIONAL OBJECTIVES

Upon completing this chapter, the reader will be able to do the following:

- Explain the purpose for selecting and using the Kinesio Taping Method
- Identify contraindications and precautions for the Kinesio Taping Method
- Demonstrate the purposes and taping procedures for the following body areas: FanCut™, foot, knee, back, neck, shoulder, and wrist

Introduction

The Kinesio Taping Method is a definitive rehabilitative taping technique that is designed to facilitate the body's natural healing process while providing support and stability to muscles and joints without restricting the body's range of motion, as well as providing extended soft tissue manipulation to prolong the benefits of manual therapy administered within the clinical setting. Latex-free and wearable for days at a time, Kinesio® **Tex Tape is safe for populations ranging from pediatric to geriatric and successfully treats a variety of orthopedic, neuromuscular, neurological, and other medical conditions. The** Kinesio Taping Method is a therapeutic taping technique that not only offers patients support but also rehabilitates the affected condition. By targeting different receptors within the somatosensory system, Kinesio Tex Tape alleviates pain and facilitates lymphatic drainage by microscopically lifting the skin. This lifting effect forms convolutions in the skin, thus increasing interstitial space and decreasing inflammation of the affected areas. Based upon years of clinical use, Kinesio Tex Tape is specifically applied to the patient based upon their needs after evaluation. The findings of the clinical evaluation or assessment dictate the specifics of the Kinesio Taping application and other possible treatments or modalities. With the use of single I Strips or modifications in the shape of an X, Y, or other specialized shape, and with the direction and amount of stretch placed on the tape at the time of application, Kinesio Tex Tape can be applied in hundreds of ways and has the ability to reeducate the neuromuscular system, reduce pain and inflammation, enhance performance, prevent injury and promote good circulation and healing, and assist in returning the body to homeostasis.

The Kinesio® Benefit

Evaluation and assessment are key in the treatment of any clinical condition. To achieve the desired results from a Kinesio Taping application, as well as from any other treatment, a full assessment of your patient is necessary. In some cases, the treatment of a condition may require treatment of other underlying conditions as well. This assessment should include manual muscle testing, range of motion testing, gait assessment, and any other orthopedic special tests that you deem necessary within your scope of practice. The information gained from these assessments will allow for the proper treatment protocol to be laid out. The Kinesio Taping can be a valuable addition to this protocol. It has been proven to have positive physiological effects on the skin, lymphatic, and circulatory systems, fascia, muscles, ligaments, tendons, and joints. It can be used in conjunction with a multitude of other treatments and modalities within your clinic, is effective during the rehabilitative and chronic phases of an injury, and can be used for preventative measures.

Education

Education is a key element of the Kinesio Taping Method and its continued success in the world of therapeutic taping. Along with Certified Kinesio Taping Practitioners® (CKTPs®) and Certified Kinesio Taping Instructors (CKTIs) around the world, Dr. Kase is dedicated to advancing the art and science of the method through education, clinical practice, and research. It is vital that a consistent standard of practice is maintained, and allied health professionals wishing to learn more about the Kinesio Taping Method are encouraged to participate in seminars and courses. After completing the certification program, practitioners join a select group of medical professionals who are able to properly use the Kinesio Taping Method within their realm of practice.

For more in-depth information on Kinesio Taping, contact the Kinesio Taping Association International (KTAI):

3901 Georgia Street NE, Building F
Albuquerque, NM 87110
Toll Free: (855) 488-TAPE
Phone: (505) 797-7818
www.KinesioTaping.com

Kinesio Taping

- Reeducate the neuromuscular system
- Reduce pain
- Optimize performance
- Prevent injury
- Promote improved circulation and healing

Contraindications: Do not apply Kinesio Tex Tape

- Over active malignancy site
- Over active cellulitis or skin infection
- Over open wounds, fragile or healing skin
- Over deep vein thrombosis (clots)
- If patient has had a previous skin reaction to this product

Precautions (consult with a specialist before considering applying Kinesio Taping):

- Diabetes
- Kidney disease
- Lymphoedema
- Respiratory conditions
- Congestive heart failure
- CAD or bruits in the carotid artery
- Pregnancy

Kinesio Taping Don'ts

- Do not blow-dry tape
- Do not attach to nape of hair, through axilla or groin
- Do not "pull" patient into position using Kinesio® Tex Tape
- Do not touch adhesive side of tape
- Do not tape over broken skin

NOTES: ______________________________

Kinesio Precut Methods

FAN CUT APPLICATION INSTRUCTIONS

The Kinesio Strip is applied using a fan cut. The crisscross pattern of the technique is applied over the area of the edema and is adjusted as needed in subsequent applications. If the lymph duct nearest to the edema is nonexistent or dysfunctional, then redirect the lymphatic fluid toward a viable duct using the anastomosis present in the lymphatic system.

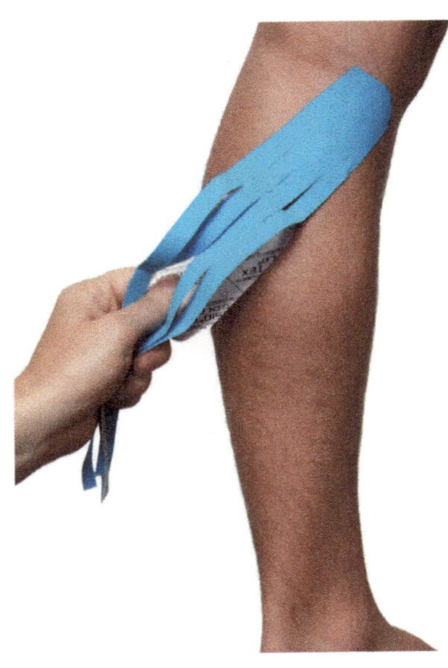

1. Place anchor of fan cut slightly above the lymph node to which lymph drainage is being directed. Have the patient move into a stretch position if appropriate for area to be treated. In example shown, the knee is in extension and the ankle in dorsiflexion.

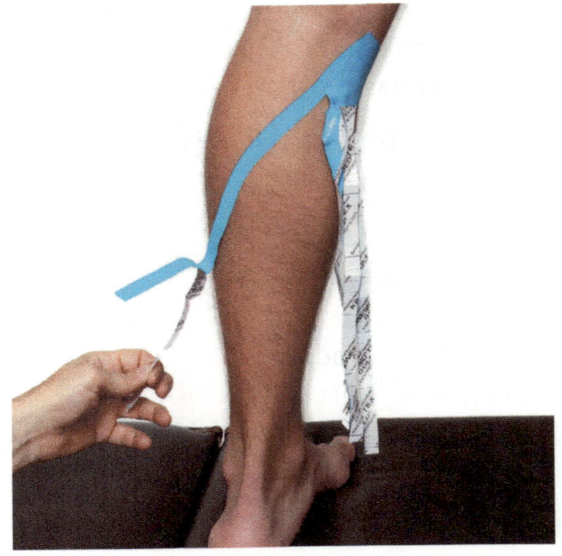

2. Apply the tails of the fan with 0% to 20% of available tension over area of edema.

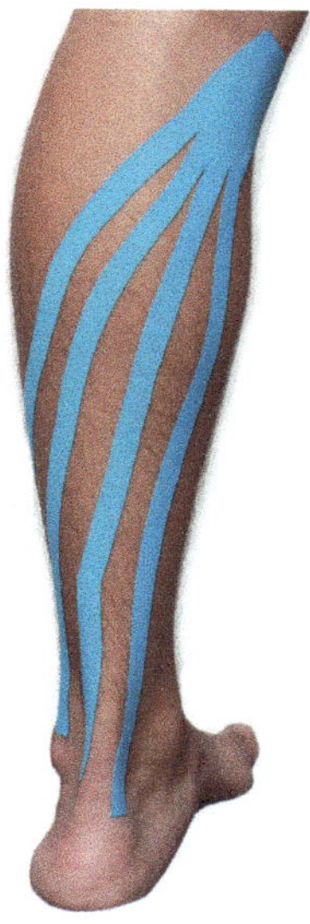

3. The placement of the lymphatic strips is directed over the area of edema. The photo shows drainage from the area of the calf to the posterior medial aspect of the knee, location of the lymph node. After the first fan cut application, pat or gently rub to activate adhesive prior to any further patient movement.

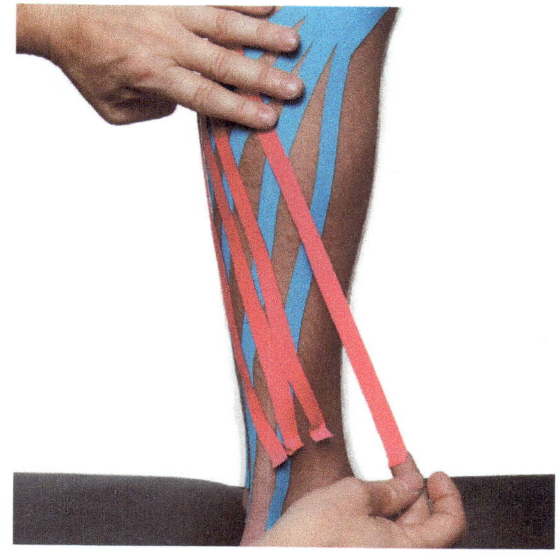

4. The second fan is placed in such a position as to create a crisscross pattern over the area of edema. Fan tails are applied using 0% to 20% of available tension.

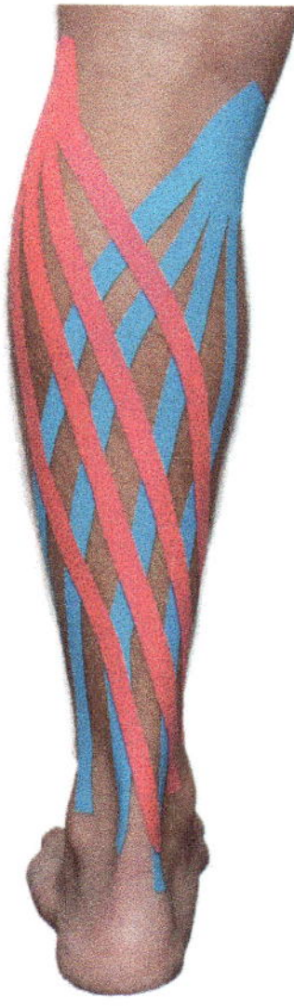

5. Following the application of the second fan strip, gently pat to initiate adhesive prior to any further patient movement. Rubbing will cause the fan strips to roll or curl, limiting wear time and effectiveness. The use of a tape adherent, beeswax, and a noncompressive tape placed on the ends may lengthen wear time.

PRECUT FOOT INSTRUCTIONS

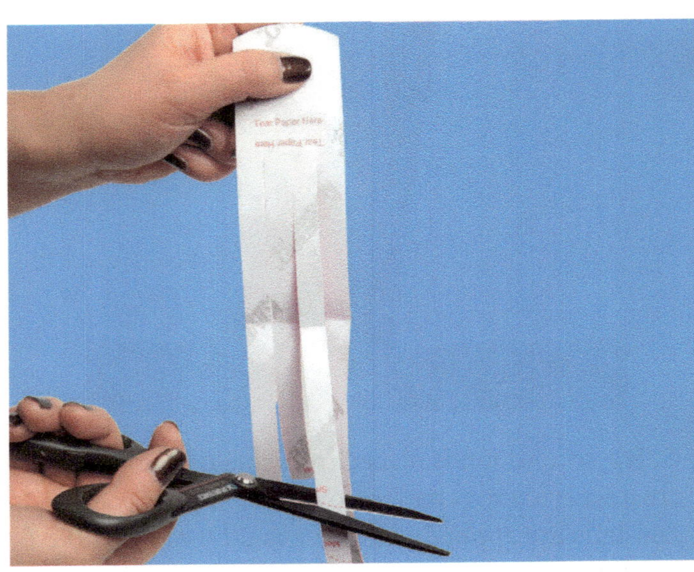

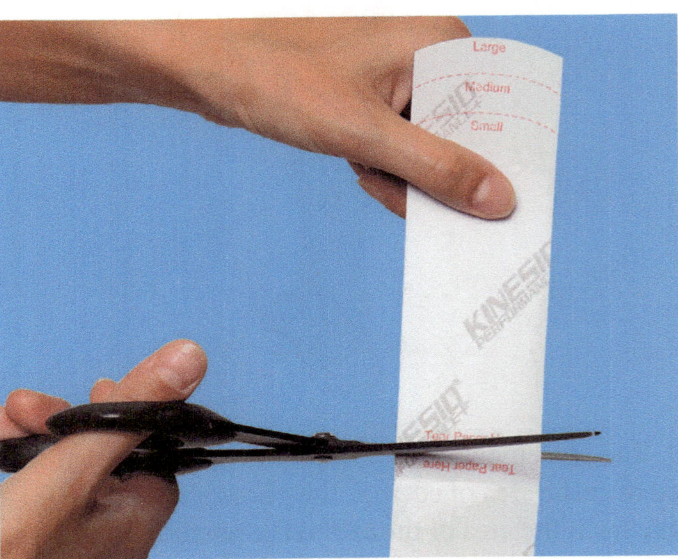

1. Take the pink tape strip and cut it to the small size using the guide on the tape backing. After cutting the strip to small, cut each tape tail in half, creating four tape tails. Take the blue tape strip and cut it in half where the tape backing indicates "tear paper here."

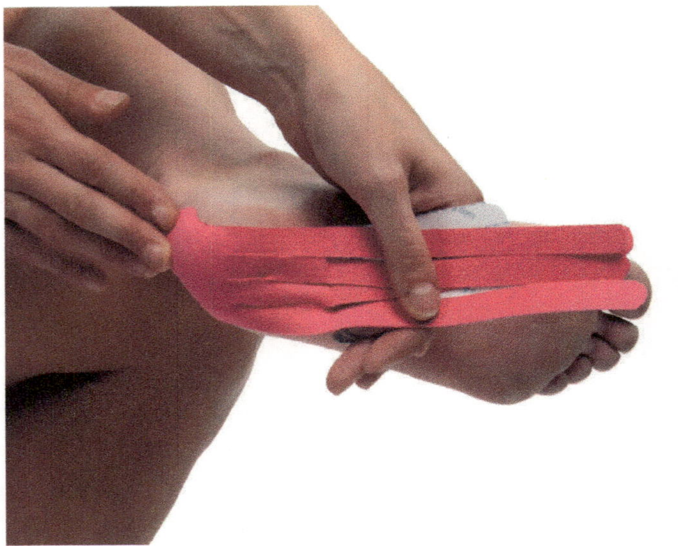

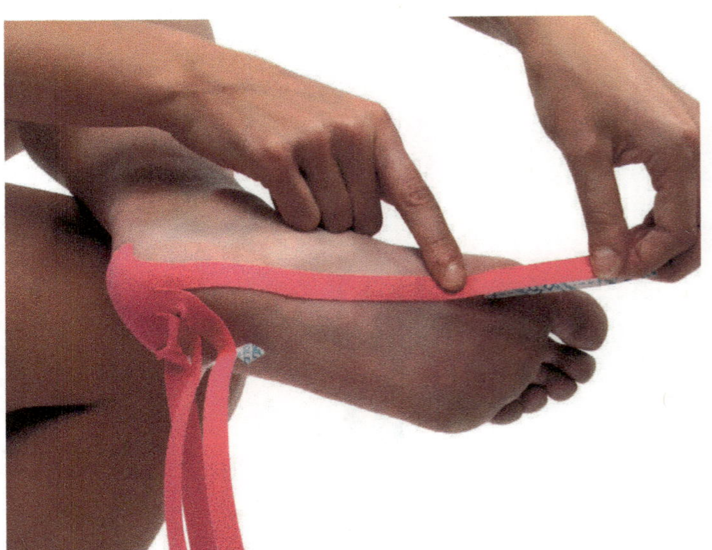

2. Take the pink tape strip and tear the paper backing where indicated on the backing paper. Remove the small section of the paper backing and apply the base of the tape strip to the back of the heel. Once applied in the correct place, the tape should be rubbed to activate the adhesive. For easier application, cut the paper backing where each tape tail begins. Only cut the paper; do not cut the tape itself.

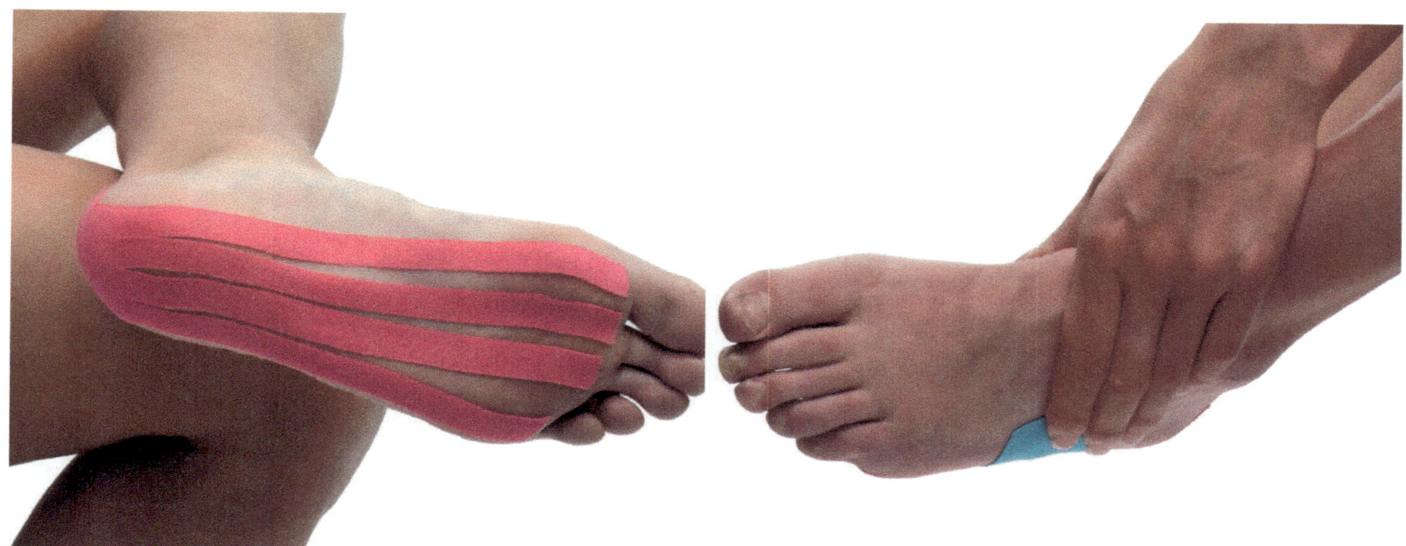

3. Using an outside tape tail, begin removing the paper backing as you apply the tape tail without stretching the tape. Repeat this process for the remaining tails so that the tape tails are spread evenly across the bottom of the foot. *Rub each tape tail to activate the adhesive.*

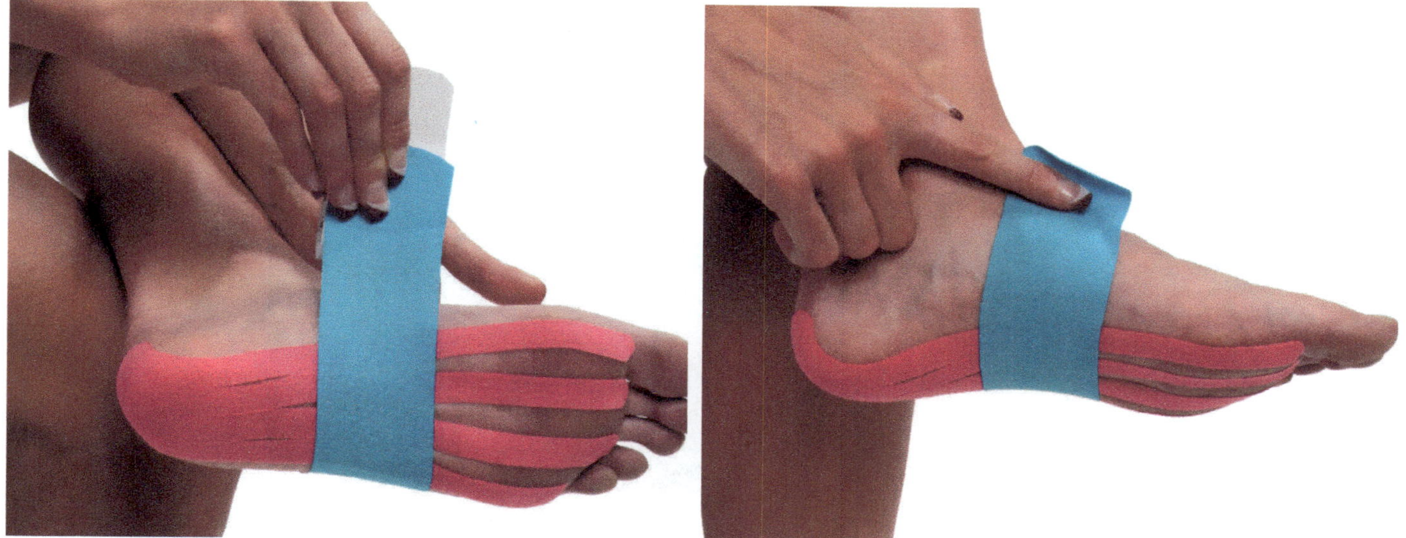

4. Take the blue tape strip and tear the paper backing approximately 1 in. from the end. Place the base of the blue tape strip on the outside of the foot near the center of the outside arch. Begin removing the paper backing and apply the tape strip across the bottom of the foot and pulling up on the arch with moderate tension on the tape. After the tape strip is applied to the arch, continue removing the paper backing while applying the strip to the top of the foot. The end of the tape strip should be applied without stretch. *Rub the tape to activate the adhesive.*

PRECUT KNEE INSTRUCTIONS

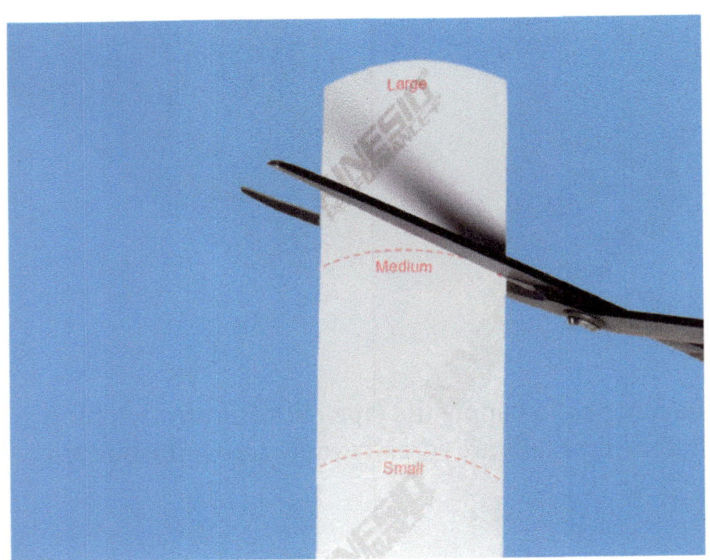

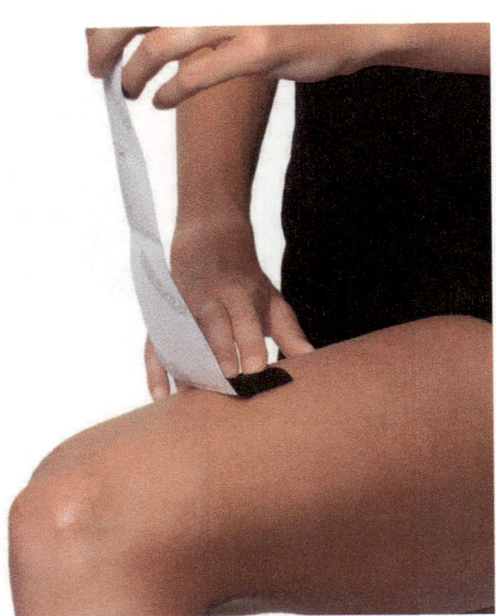

1. Take the black I strip. If required, use the guide on the tape backing to cut the strip to the correct length. Using the tear line, remove the small section of the backing paper from the base of the strip. With your knee bent to 90 degrees, place the base of the tape strip mid-thigh approximately 4 in. to 5 in. above the knee joint.

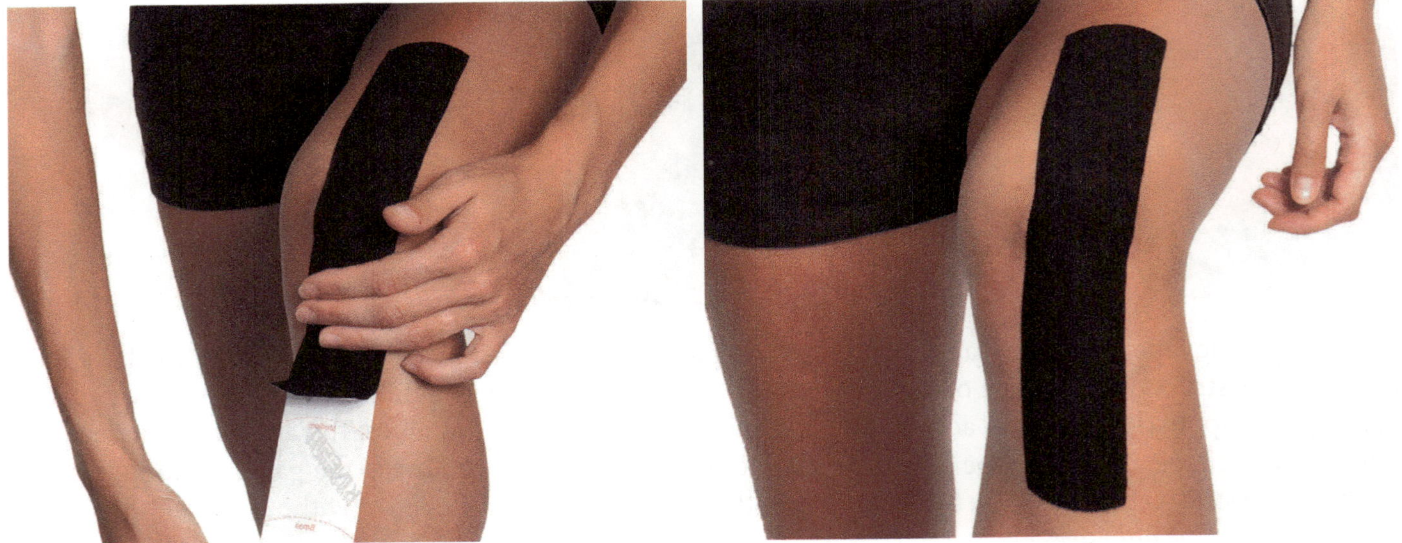

2. Without stretching the tape, begin removing the paper backing while applying the tape strip over the center of the knee joint and ending approximately 2 in. to 3 in. below the joint. *Once applied in the correct place, rub the tape to activate the adhesive.*

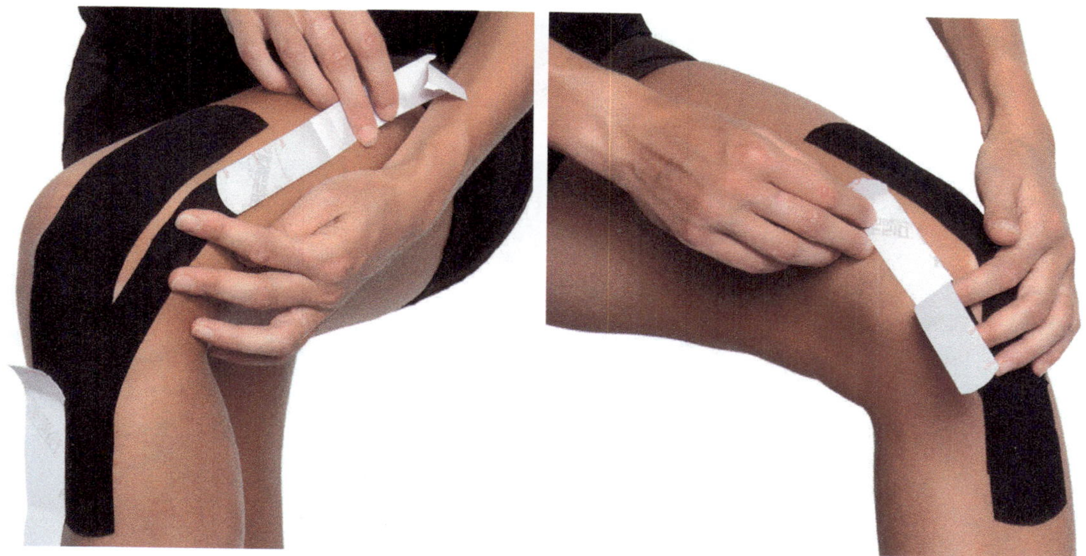

3. Take the black Y tape strip and, if required, use the guide on the tape backing to cut the tape strip to the correct length. Using the tear line, remove the paper backing and apply the base of the tape strip 2 in. to 3 in. below the knee cap. Without stretching the tape, apply each tape tail around each side of the knee joint. *Rub the tape to activate the adhesive.*

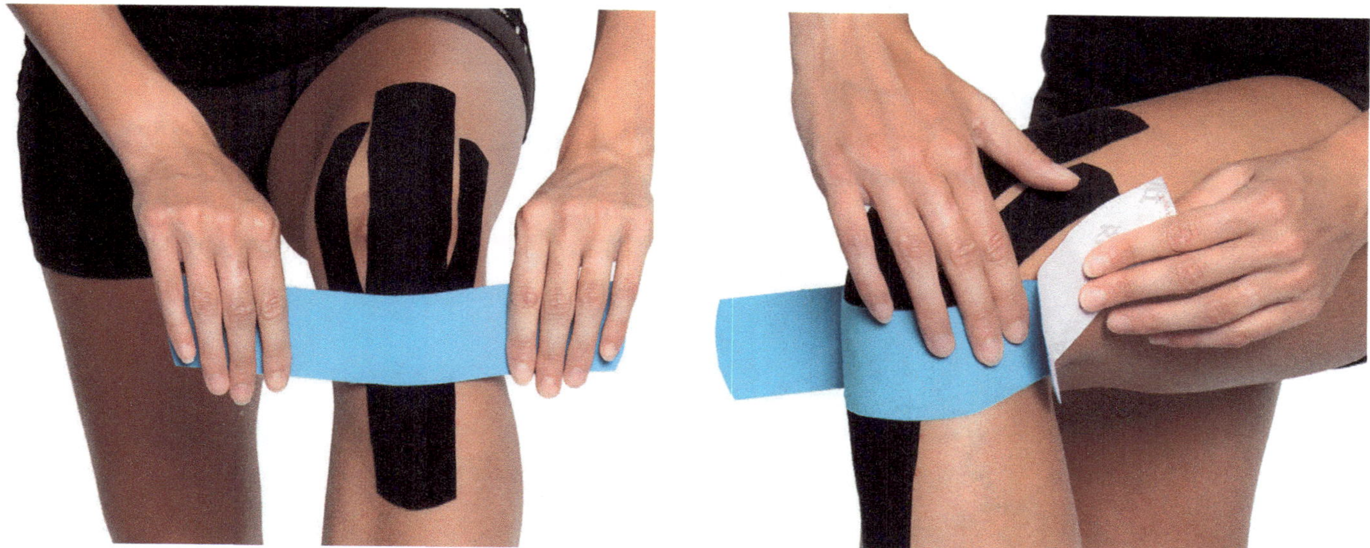

4. Take the blue tape strip and, if required, use the guide on the tape backing to cut the tape strip to the correct length. Using the tear line, remove the paper backing halfway down each side of the tape strip to expose the middle of the adhesive. Using minimal stretch, apply the middle portion just below the knee cap. Apply the remaining sides without stretch. *Rub the tape to activate the adhesive.*

PRECUT BACK INSTRUCTIONS

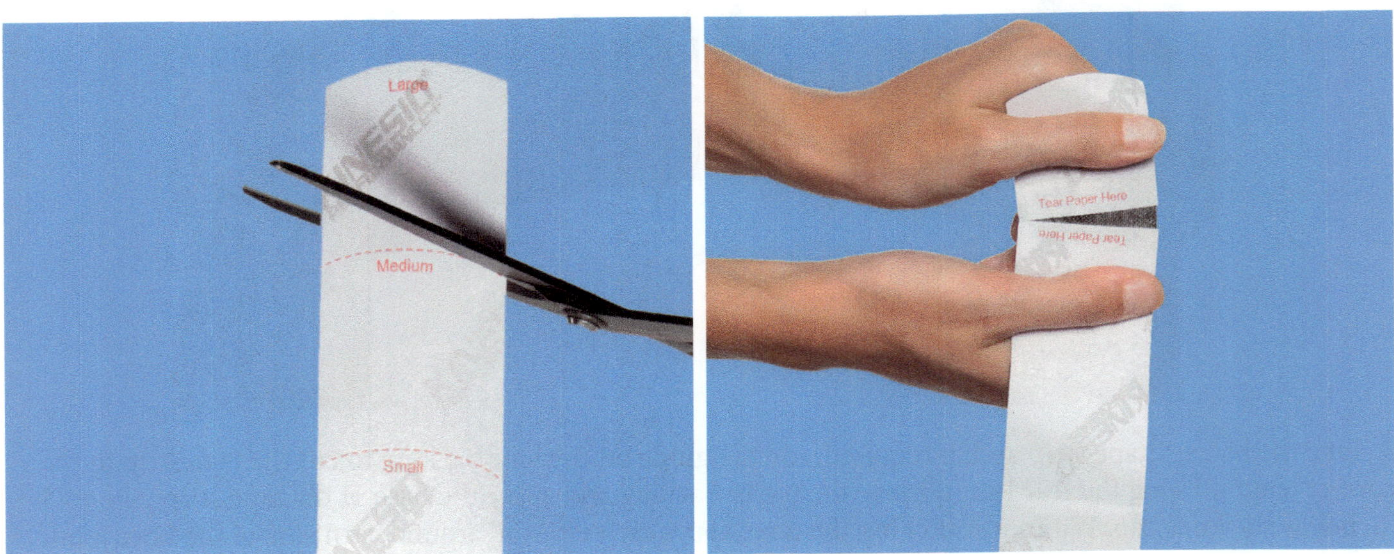

1. Take one black tape strip and, if required, use the guide on the tape backing to cut the strip to the correct length. Using the tear line, remove the small section of the backing paper from the strip.

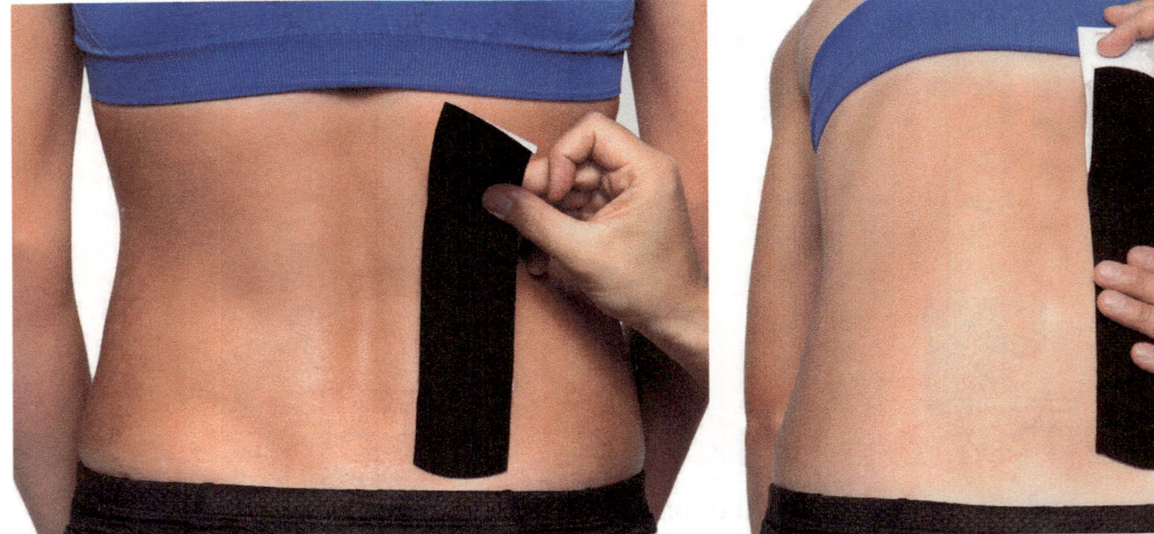

2. Place the base of the black strip above the lowest part of the back on one side of the spine. Bend forward to stretch the back muscles and begin removing tape backing. Without stretching the tape, extend the strip up and alongside the spine. *Once applied in the correct place, rub the tape to activate the adhesive.*

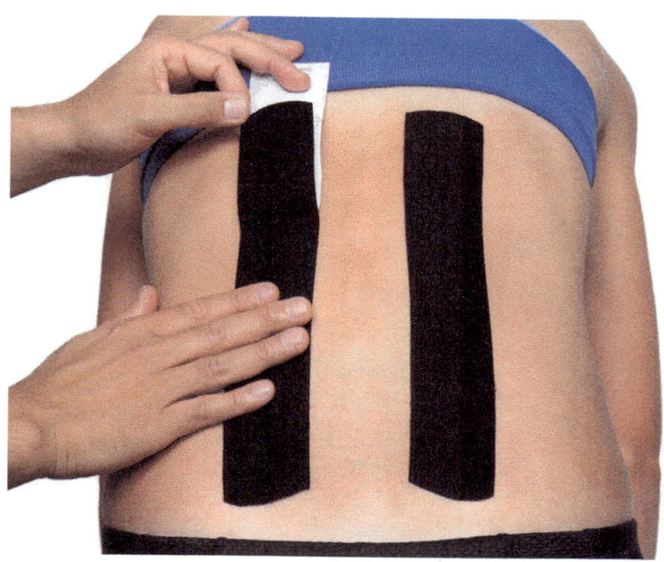

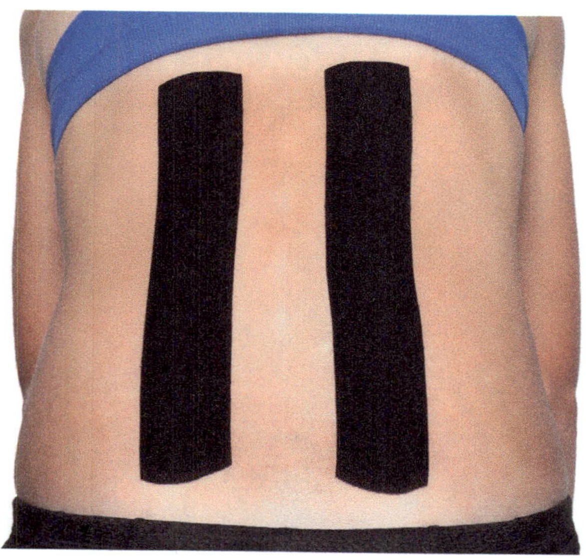

3. Take the other black strip and repeat the previous step for the opposite side of the spine. *Rub the tape to activate the adhesive.*

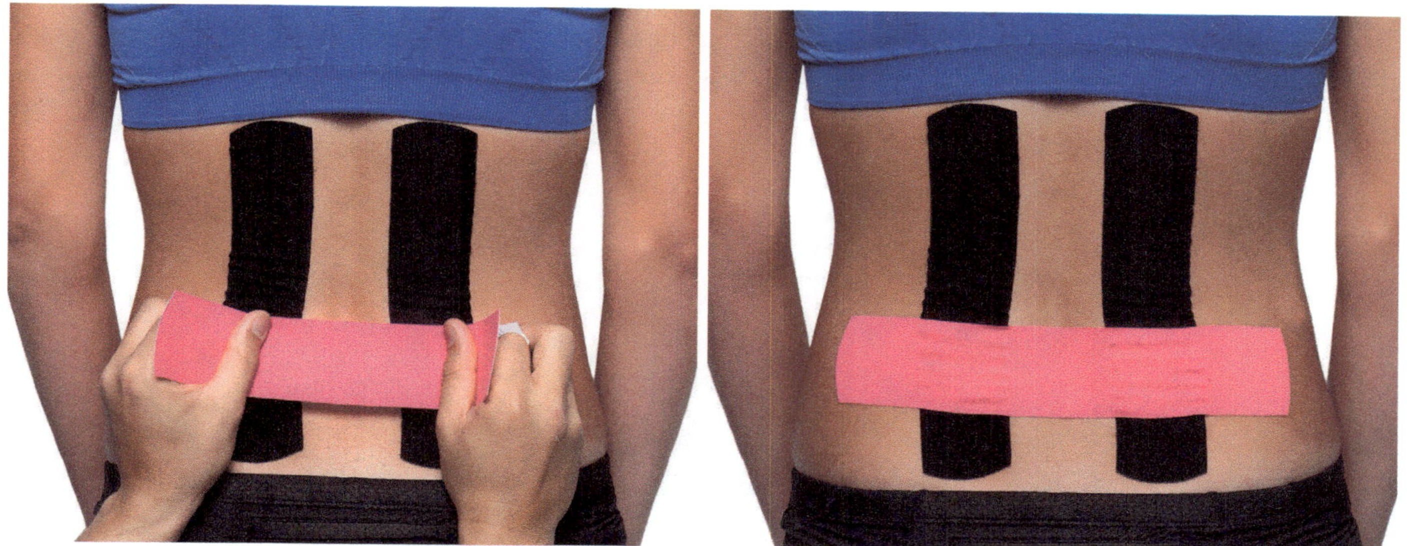

4. Take the pink strip and, if required, use the guide on the tape backing to cut the tape strip to the correct length. Using the tear line, remove the paper backing halfway down each side of the strip to expose the middle portion of the adhesive. Using minimal tension, apply the tape strip horizontally over the strained area on the lower back. *Rub the tape to activate the adhesive.*

PRECUT NECK INSTRUCTIONS

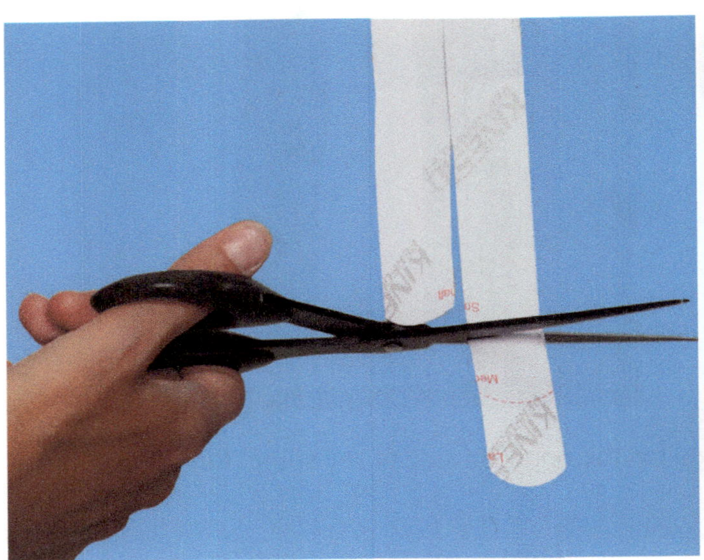

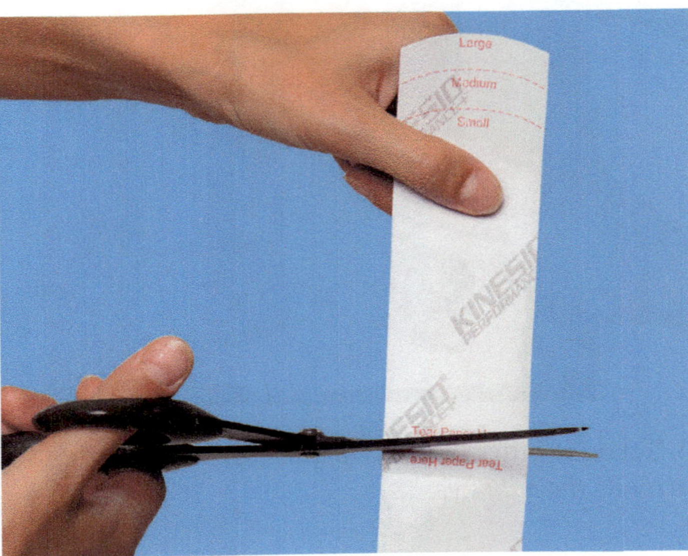

1. Take the beige tape strip and cut it to the small size using the guide on the tape backing. Take the black tape strip and cut it in half where the tape backing indicates "tear paper here."

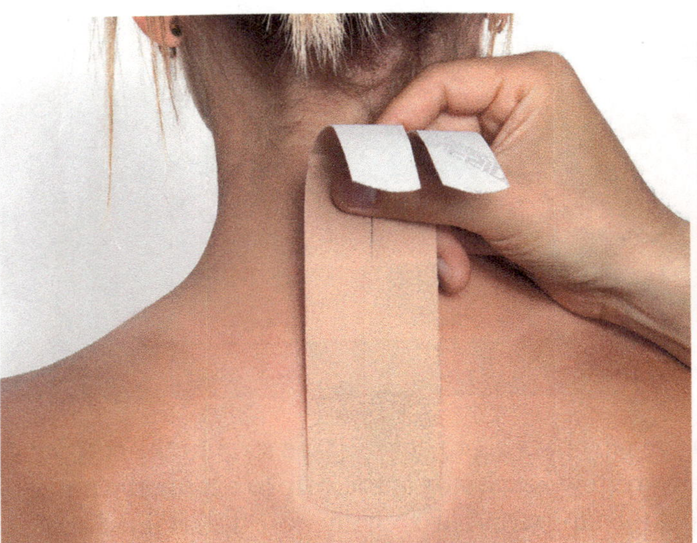

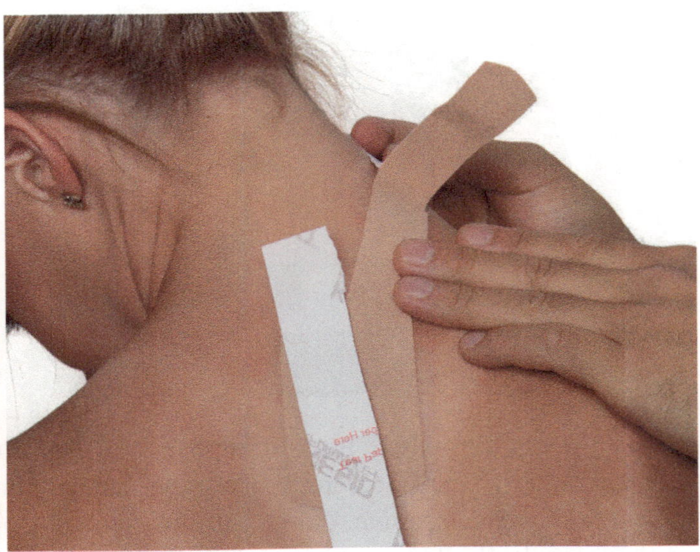

2. Using the tear line, remove the small section of the tape backing. Place the base of the tape strip in the center of the spine about 2 in. to 3 in. below the base of the neck. Tilt your head forward and to the left. Begin applying the right tape tail up the right side of the neck. Be careful not to apply the tape tail over loose hair. Once applied in the correct place, rub the tape to activate the adhesive.

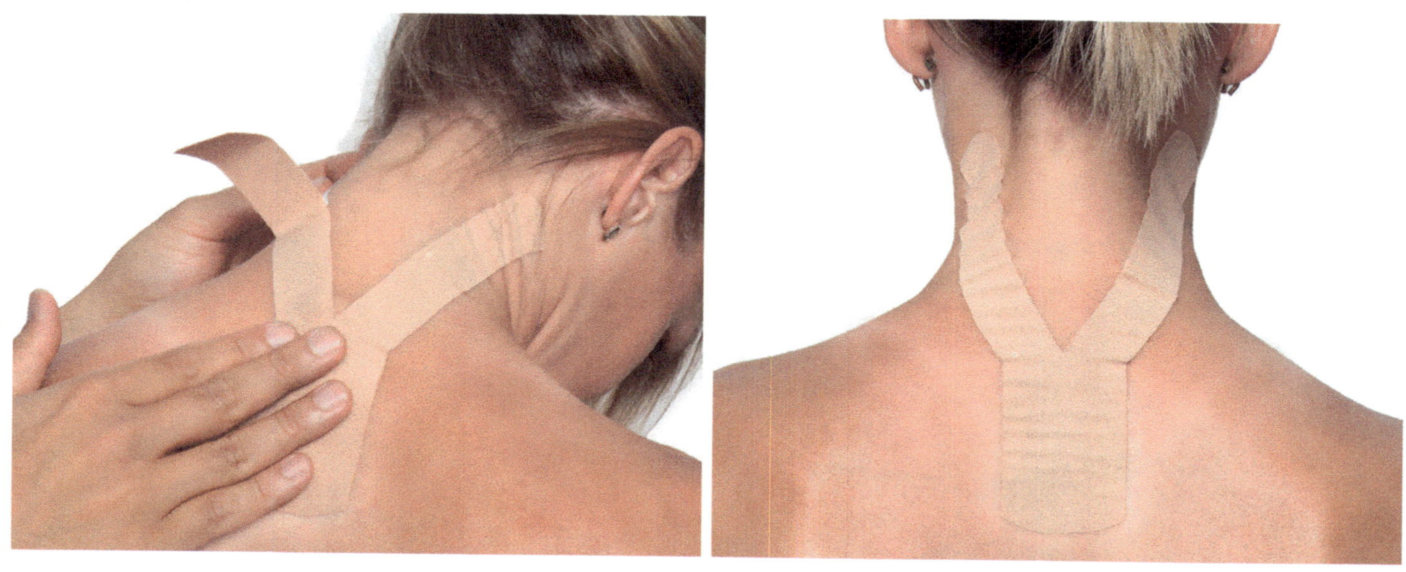

3. Using the left tape tail, repeat the previous step for the opposite side of the neck. *Rub the tape to activate the adhesive.*

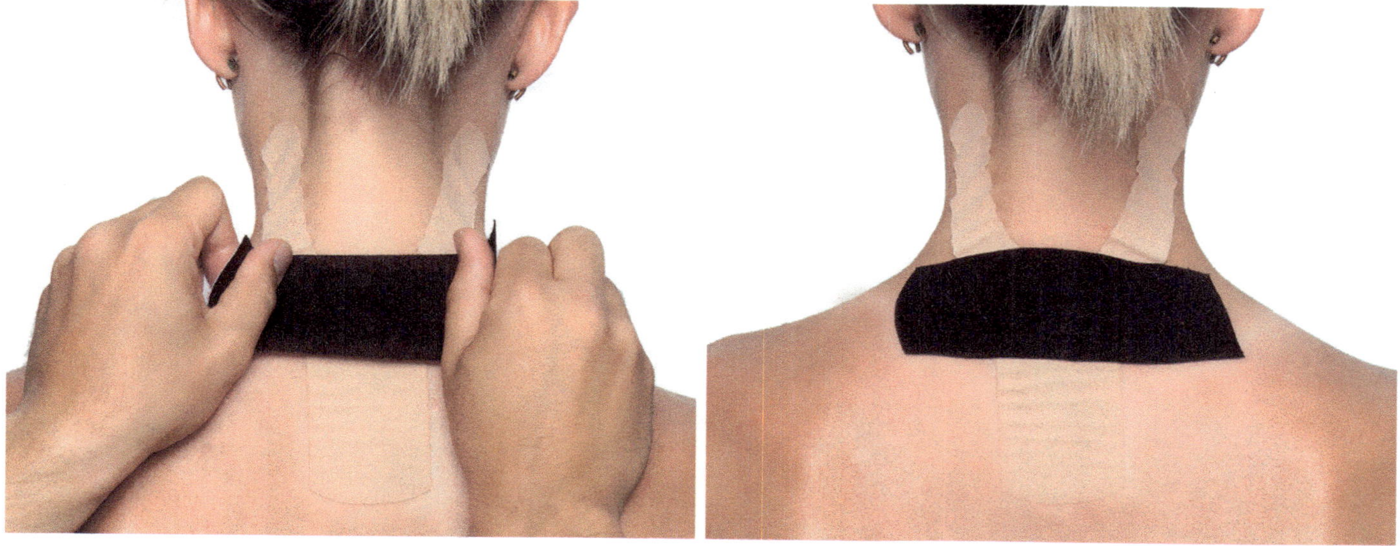

4. Take one of the black tape strips and fold it in half. After folding in half, tear the tape backing in the center of the tape strip. Remove the tape backing halfway down each side of the tape strip to expose the center portion of the adhesive. Using minimal tension, apply the tape strip over the strained portion of the neck. Apply ends without stretch. *Rub the tape to activate the adhesive.*

PRECUT SHOULDER INSTRUCTIONS

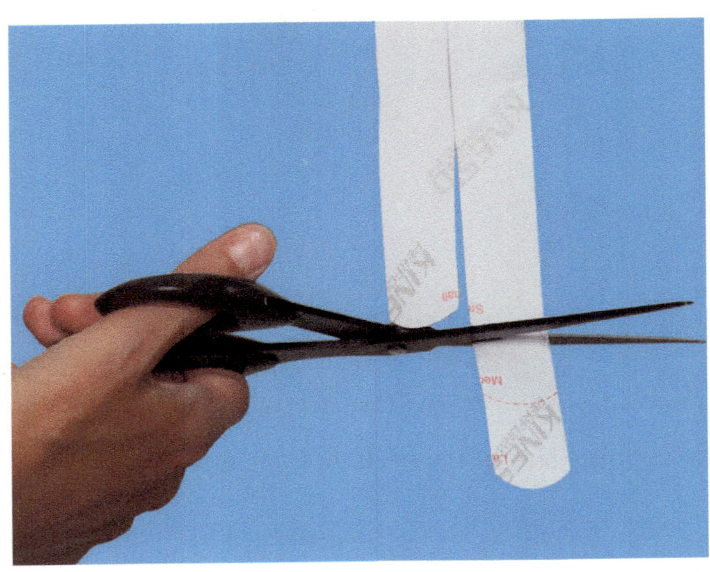

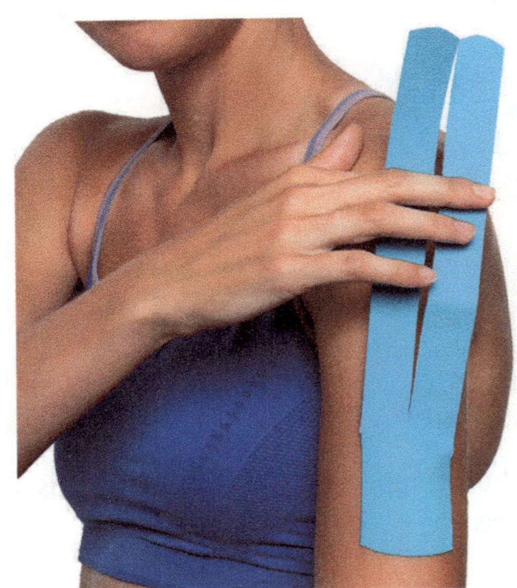

1. Take one blue Y tape strip and, if required, use the guide on the tape backing to cut the strip to the correct length. Using the tear line, remove the small section of the paper backing from the tape strip and apply the base of the tape strip at the midpoint of the arm.

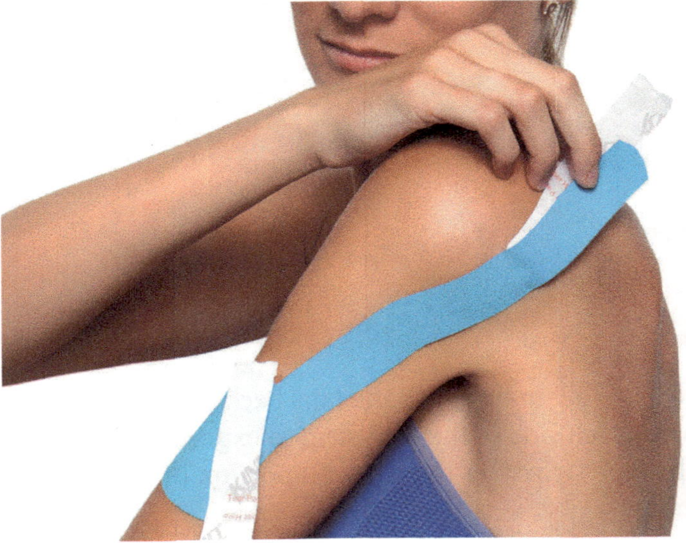

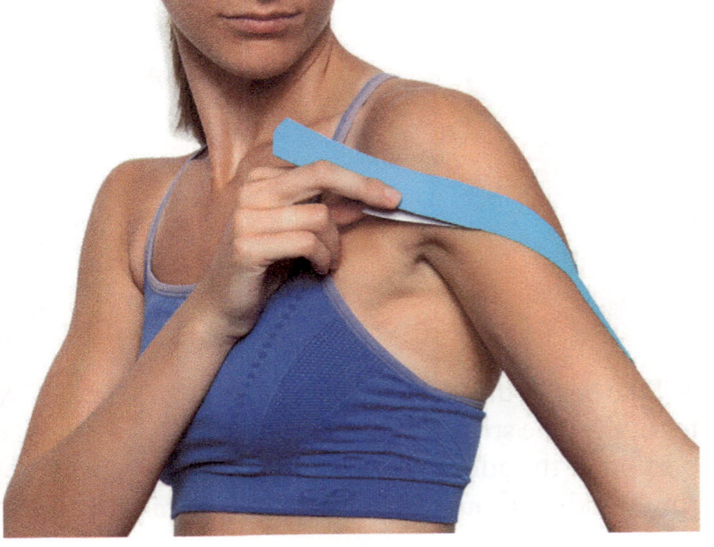

2. Move your arm in front of you, and without stretching the tape, apply the back tape tail along the back of your shoulder. Once applied in the correct place, both tape tails should be rubbed to activate the adhesive. Move your arm back at a 45-degree angle, and without stretching the tape, apply the front tape tail along the front of your shoulder. *Rub the tape to activate the adhesive.*

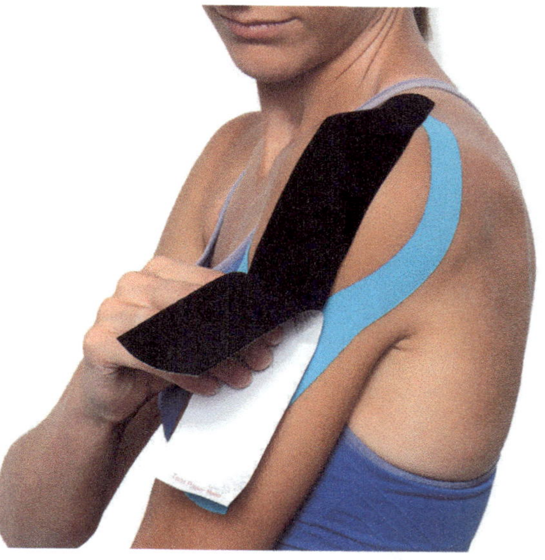
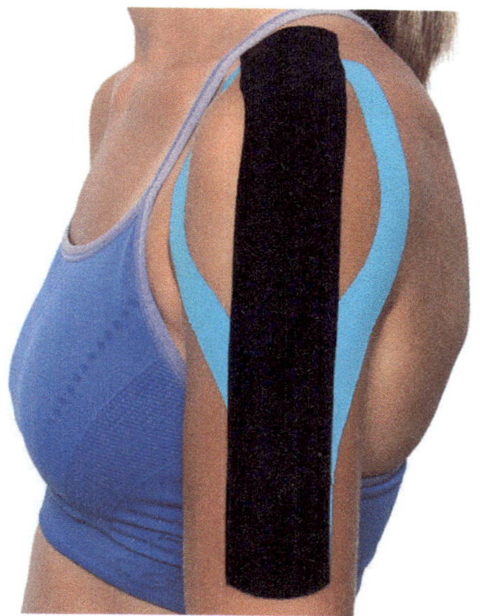

3. Take the black tape strip and, if required, use the guide on the tape backing to cut the tape strip to the correct length. Using the tear line, remove the paper backing and apply the base of the tape strip approximately 3 in. to 4 in. above the shoulder joint. Without stretching the tape, apply the tape strip over the shoulder joint and down the arm, ending over the base of the blue Y tape strip. *Rub the tape to activate the adhesive.*

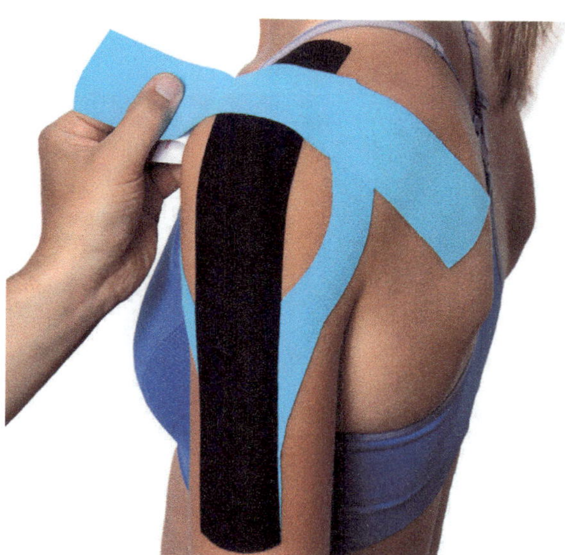
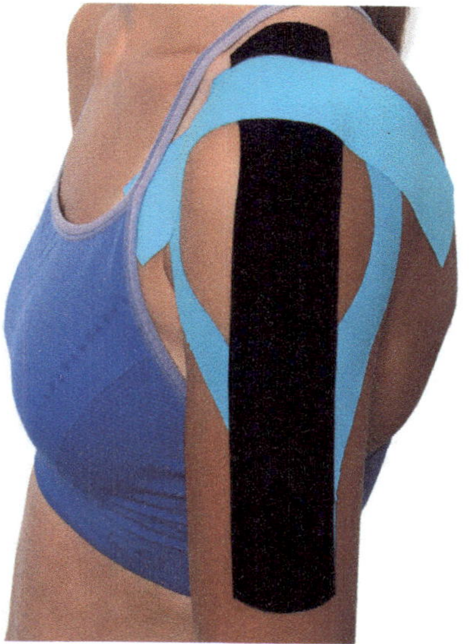

4. OPTIONAL (for more support): Take the remaining blue tape strip and, if required, use the guide on the tape backing to cut the tape strip to the correct length. With assistance, using the tear line, remove the paper backing and apply the base to the shoulder blade. Begin removing the remaining paper backing and apply the tape strip over the shoulder joint without stretching the tape. *Rub the tape to activate the adhesive.*

PRECUT WRIST INSTRUCTIONS

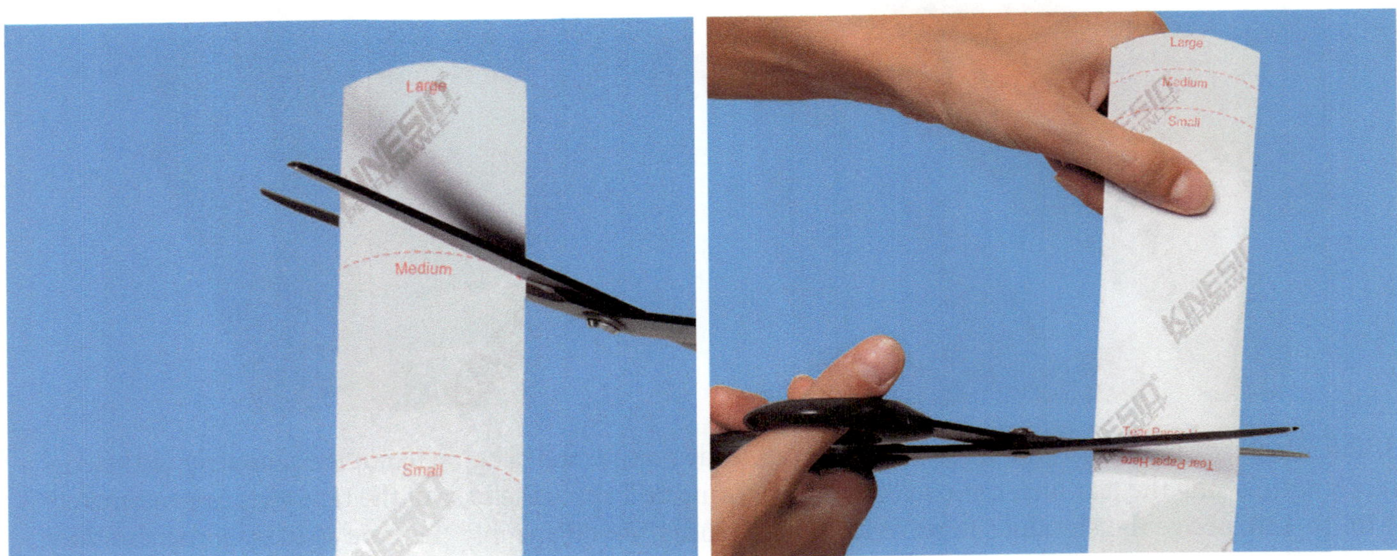

1. Take one blue tape strip and, if required, use the guide on the tape backing to cut the strip to the correct length. Take the black tape strip and cut it in half where the tape backing indicates "tear paper here."

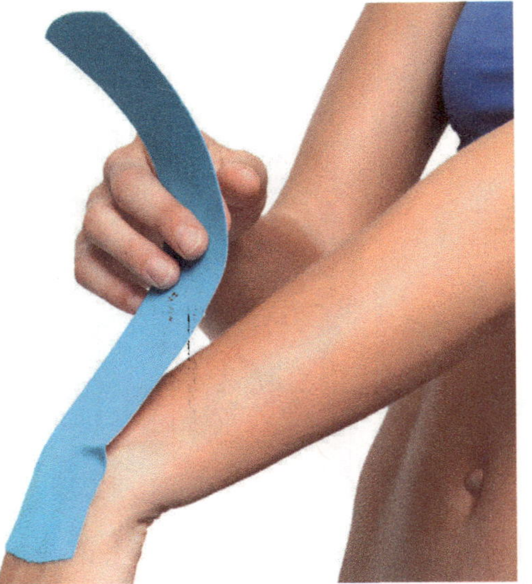

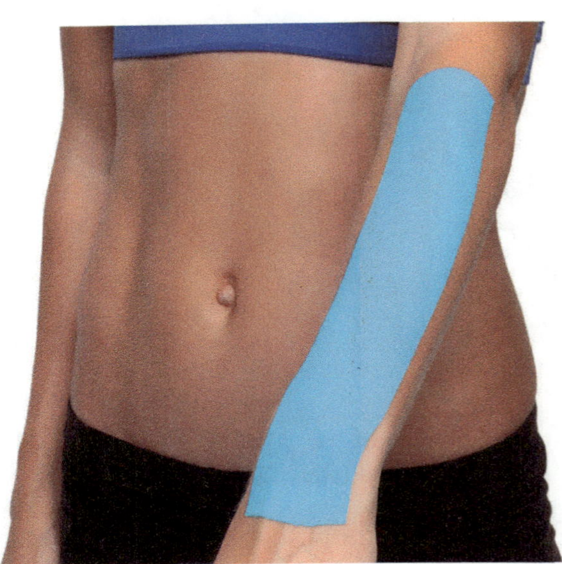

2. Using the blue tape strip, tear the paper backing where indicated on the tape backing. Remove the small section of the tape backing. Bend the wrist/hand downward and place the base of the blue tape strip above the knuckles. Without stretching the tape, begin removing the remaining paper backing as you apply the tape strip over the wrist joint and up the arm. *Once applied in the correct place, rub the tape to activate the adhesive.*

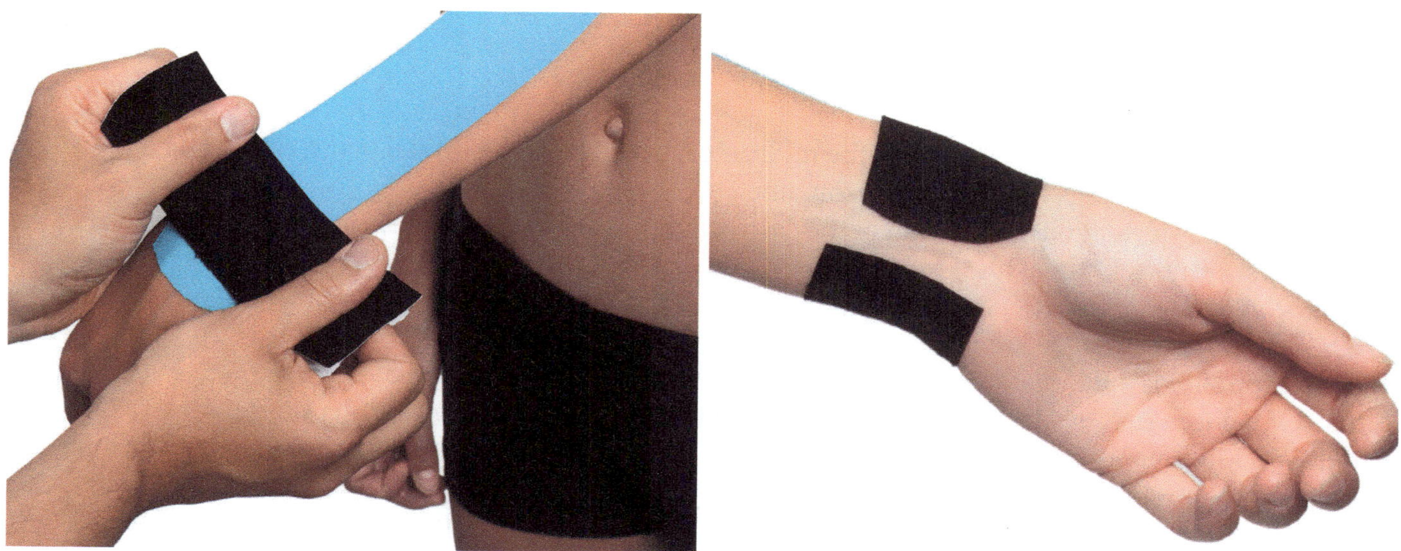

3. Take one black tape strip and fold it in half. After folding it in half, tear the tape backing in the center of the tape strip. Remove the tape backing halfway down each side of the tape strip to expose the middle portion of the adhesive. With assistance, apply the tape strip over the top of the wrist joint using minimal stretch. Apply ends with no stretch around wrist joint so that they do not overlap. *Rub the tape to activate the adhesive.*

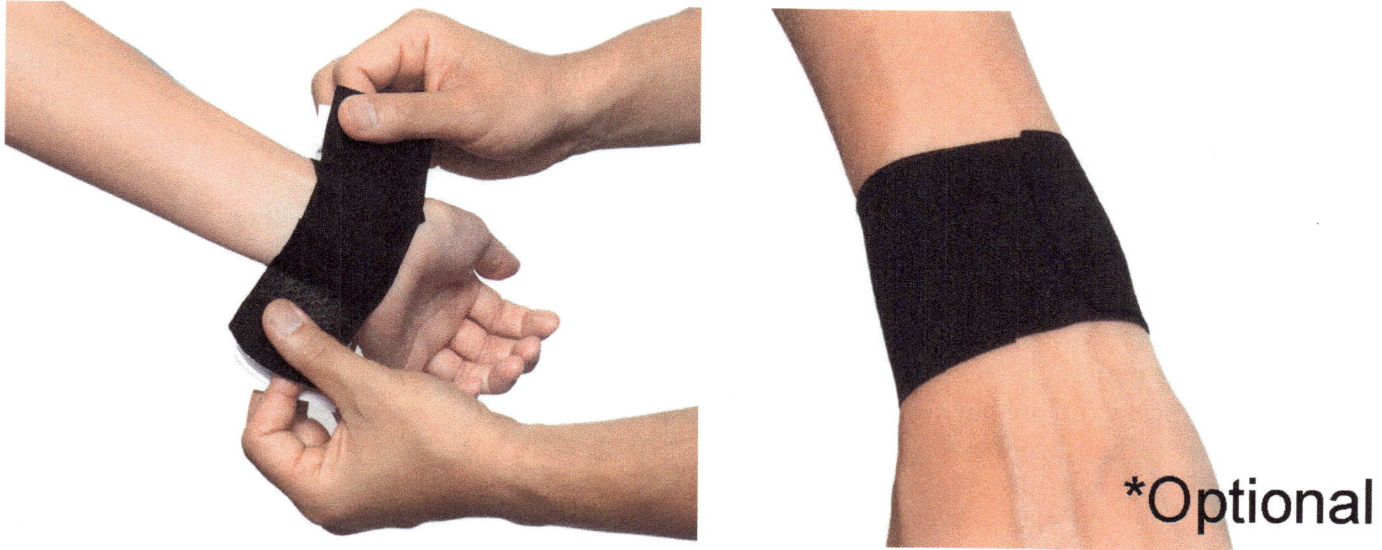

4. OPTION 1 (for more support): Using a second black tape strip, repeat the previous step but apply the tape strip to the bottom of the wrist joint. *Rub the tape to activate the adhesive.* OPTION 2: Using two black tape strips, repeat Step 3 and Option 1. Option 2 is only used to achieve support for the wrist joint if applied without the blue I tape. *Rub the tape to activate the adhesive.*

Appendix A: Glossary

A

Abduction. Lateral movement away from the midline of the trunk in the frontal plane. An example is raising the arms or legs to the side horizontally.

Achilles tendon. The tendon of insertion of the gastrocnemius and soleus muscles on the calcaneus; one of the strongest tendons in the body.

Acromioclavicular joint (AC). A gliding or plane joint between the acromion and the acromial end of the clavicle; sprain to joint is known as separate shoulder.

Action. In physiology, the motions or functions of a part or organ of the body.

Acute. Of pain, sharp, severe; of disease, having rapid onset, severe symptoms, and a short course.

Adduction. Movement medially toward the midline of the trunk in the frontal plane. An example is lowering the arm to the side or the thigh back to the anatomical position.

Adhesive felt (moleskin). Material contains an adhesive mass on one side, thus combining a cushioning effect with the ability to be held in a specific spot by the adhesive mass.

Adhesive (tape) mass. Adhesive applied to the cloth comprised of natural synthetic, zinc oxide, and so forth.

Anatomical position. The position assumed when a person is standing erect with arms at the sides, palms forward; the neutral stance of the individual.

Anatomical snuffbox. A depression in the skin formed at the posterior base of the thumb when the thumb is extended from the hand; the space at the base of the thumb created by the extensor pollicis longus and brevis tendons.

Anchor. Anything that makes something stable or secure, anything that is depended upon for support or security.

Antalgic gait. A gait in which the patient experiences pain during the stance phase and thus remains on the painful leg for as short a time as possible.

Anterior. Before; in front of; in anatomical nomenclature, it refers to the ventral or abdominal side of the body; the front of the body or body part.

Anterior cruciate ligament (ACL). A ligament crossing through the knee joint that attaches from the anterior tibia to the posterior femur. It limits anterior movement of the tibia from the femur, as well as rotation of the tibia.

Appendicular skeleton. The bones that make up the shoulder girdle, upper extremities, pelvis, and lower extremities; these bones form the appendages and attach to the axial skeleton.

Arch. An anatomical structure having a curved or bowlike outline.

Articular surfaces. The ends of bones which move on each other; these surfaces are covered with a thin layer of cartilage (hyaline cartilage) to ensure smooth movement.

Articulation. A joint; the site of close approximation of two or more bones; the manner of connecting by a joint.

Avascular. Lacking in blood vessels or having a poor blood supply, said of tissues such as cartilage.

Avulsion. A tearing away forcibly of a part or structure.

Axial skeleton. Composed of the bones of the skull, the thorax, and the vertebral column. These bones form the axis of the body.

Axilla. Armpit.

B

Base strip. Supportive strips to taping procedure.

Biceps. The muscle of the upper arm that flexes the elbow and supinates the forearm; muscle on front of upper arm.

Bloodborne pathogens. Bloodborne pathogens are infectious microorganisms in human blood that can cause disease in humans. These pathogens include, but are not limited to, hepatitis B (HBV), hepatitis C (HCV) and human immunodeficiency virus (HIV). Needlesticks and other sharps-related injuries may expose workers to bloodborne pathogens. Workers in many occupations, including first aid team members, housekeeping personnel in some industries, nurses and other health care personnel may be at risk of exposure to bloodborne pathogens.

Bone. A supportive rigid connective tissue consisting of an abundant calcified matrix enclosing many branched cells.

Brace. Any one of a great variety of devices used in orthopedics for increasing stability of joints or extremities.

Buckle. A fastening device for two loose ends that is attached to one and holds the other by a catch.

Bunion. Inflammation and thickening of the first metatarsal joint of the great toe, usually associated with marked enlargement of the joint and lateral displacement of the toe.

Bursa. A fluid-filled sac or saclike cavity that allows a muscle or tendon to slide over bone (thereby eliminating friction). Bursae means plural.

Bursitis. Inflammation of a bursa, especially between bony prominences and muscle or tendon, as in the shoulder and knee. It is typically caused by repeated stresses placed on a joint during work or play, but sometimes results from sudden trauma, from inflammatory joint disease, or bacteria. Common forms include rotator cuff, miner's or tennis elbow, and prepatellar bursitis.

Butterfly. Strips of tape that overlap in an X pattern; an adhesive bandage used in place of sutures to hold wound edges together.

C

Calcaneus. The heel bone; it articulates with the cuboid bone and with the talus.

Cantilever. Shapes and supports the arch; spreads force to front and rear of shell on flat or noncantilever pads.

Cap or Cup. Shoulder pad padding that covers deltoid/humerus.

Cartilage. A connective tissue characterized by its nonvascularity and firm consistency.

Cast. To produce a specific form by pouring material (metal, plaster, etc.) into a prepared mold; used to immobilize an anatomical body part.

Cervical. Pertaining to or in the region of the neck; seven vertebrae in the neck.

Check rein. Reinforced tape to prevent movement; restricts range of motion.

Chondral. Pertaining to cartilage.

Chrondromalacia patella. Chondromalacia at the front of the knee, accompanied by pain and crepitus, and often affecting younger athletes.

Chronic. Of long duration; long lasting; persistent.

Circumduction. Movement around an axis such that the proximal end of a limb is fixed and the distal end traces a circle.

Clavicle channel. Shoulder pad padding that is structured in such a way to provide a gap between the pad and the AC joint.

Closed cell foam. Material that is firm and is one layer, retains its shape quickly.

Close out strips. Final strips of adhesive or elastic tape that are applied to finalize taping procedure; usually applied distal to proximal.

Coccyx. A small bone at the base of the spinal column in humans, formed by four fused rudimentary vertebrae; it is usually ankylosed and articulated with the sacrum above.

Cohesive bandage (wrap and/or tape). A bandage made of material that sticks to itself but not to other substances, used to bandage fingers and extremities or to build up pads.

Collateral. Accompanying; side-by-side (i.e., medial and lateral).

Collateral ligament. A ligament that provides medial and lateral stability to joints, including the medial (ulnar) and lateral (radial) collateral ligaments at the elbow, the medial (tibial) and lateral (fibular) collateral ligaments at the knee, the medial (deltoid) and lateral collateral ligaments at the ankle, and the collateral ligaments of the fingers.

Compression. The act of applying pressure to a body part (i.e., applying an elastic wrap: begin the elastic wrap distally, farthest from the heart; cover the injury; and spiral the wrap toward the heart on the involved anatomical structure).

Condyle. A rounded protuberance at the end of a bone forming an articulation.

Contract. To draw together, reduce in size, or shorten.

Contusion. Compression to anatomical structure; injury caused by direct contact.

Costochondral. Pertaining to the rib and its cartilage.

Cotton. A soft, white, fibrous material obtained from the fibers enclosing the seeds of various plants of the Malvaceae, especially those of the genus Gossypium; the ability to absorb, to hold emollients, and to offer a mild padding effect.

Cover strip or bandage. A piece of soft, usually absorbent gauze or other material applied to a limb or other part of the body as a dressing.

Cranial. Pertaining to the cranium.

Cruciate. Cross-shaped, as in the cruciate ligaments of the knee.

Cubital Fossa. Triangular area on the anterior aspect of the forearm directly opposite the elbow joint (the bend of the elbow).

Custom brace. Made to individual specifications and fitted by a qualified health care professional and medical equipment specialist; used to protect specific anatomical structures.

Cutaneous. Pertains to the skin.

D

Depression (down). Just the opposite, as in lowering the shoulder.

Dermal. Pertaining to the dermis; cutaneous.

Dermatome. A band or region of skin supplied by a single sensory nerve.

Diagonally. A slanted or oblique direction.

Diamond shape. An object that is in the shape of two equilateral triangles placed base to base.

Diarthrodial joint. A joint characterized by the presence of a cavity within the capsule separating the bones, permitting considerable freedom of movement; ball and socket joint.

Digit. A finger or toe.

Disinfectant. A substance that prevents infection by killing bacteria.

Dislocation. The displacement of any part, especially the temporary displacement of a bone from its normal position in a joint.

Distal. Farthest from the center, from a medial line, or from the trunk; opposed to proximal.

Distal to proximal. A term commonly used in a taping or wrapping procedure that describes applying material distal (farther away) to proximal (closest); closure strips.

Dorsal. Upper surface (e.g., top of foot).

Dorsiflexion. Flexion movement of the ankle that results in the top of the foot moving toward the anterior tibia in the sagittal plane.

Dorsum. Pertains to the dorsum (back); lying on the back with the face upward; supine; toward the back of an organism.

Dual density foam. Material that has a hard side to disperse the blow and a soft side to absorb impact.

E

Elevation. A raised area that protrudes above the surrounding area; up, as in lifting the shoulder up.

Epaulet. The plastic flap on the shoulder region of shoulder pads, held in place by snubbers; allows movement but returns in place.

Epicondylitis. Inflammation of the epicondyle of the humerus and surrounding tissues.

Epiphysis. A center for ossification at each extremity of long bones; growth plate.

Eversion. Turning the sole of the foot outward or laterally in the frontal plane; abduction. An example is standing with the weight on the inner edge of the foot.

Exostosis. A bony growth that arises from the surface of a bone, often involving the ossification of muscular attachments.

Extension. Straightening movement that results in an increase of the angle in a joint by moving bones apart, usually in the sagittal plane. Using the elbow, an example is when the hand moves away from the shoulder.

External rotation. Rotary movement around the longitudinal axis of a bone away from the midline of the body. Occurs in the transverse plane and is also known as outward or lateral rotation.

F

Fascia. A fibrous membrane covering, supporting, and separating tissue; two kinds of fascia: deep fasciae for muscles and superficial fasciae for connecting the skin to the muscles.

Felt. A material composed of matted wool fibers pressed into varying thickness that range from 1/16 in. to 1 in.

Figure of eight. The bandaging of a joint where the initial turn circles the one part of the joint and the second turn circles the adjoining part of the joint to form a figure of eight (number 8).

Flexion. Bending movement that results in a decrease of the angle in a joint by bringing bones together, usually in the sagittal plane. An example is the elbow joint when the hand is drawn to the shoulder.

Foam. Material that is made in different thickness and densities that is usually resilient, nonabsorbent, and able to protect the body against compressive forces.

Friction. Rubbing; any force that resists motion that is generated when two surfaces move with respect to each other.

Frontal plane. A flat surface formed by making a cut, imaginary or real, through the body or a part of it. Planes are used as points of reference by which positions of parts of the body are indicated. In the human subject, all planes are based on the body being in an upright anatomical position.

G

Gamekeeper's thumb. An injury to the ulnar collateral ligament of the metacarpophalangeal joint of the thumb.

Gauze. Thin, loosely woven muslin or similar material used for bandages and surgical sponges; assembled in varying thickness and can be used as an absorbent or protective pad.

Glenohumeral joint (GH). Pertaining to the humerus and the glenoid cavity.

H

Hamstrings. Muscle group in the posterior thigh consisting of the semitendinosus, semimembranosus, and biceps femoris.

Heat plastic foam. Plastic that has difference in densities as a result of the addition of liquids, gas, or crystals.

Heel lock. Commonly used in ankle taping, this supportive technique aids in stabilizing the calcaneus.

Hematoma. A swelling comprising a mass of extravasated blood (usually clotted) confined to an organ, tissue, or space and caused by a break in a blood vessel.

Hip pointer. Bruise (contusion) to iliac crest and tissue.

Horizontal plane. A transverse plane at right angles to the vertical axis of the body.

Horizontal strip. A strip of tape or felt tape that is placed horizontal, as opposed to vertical.

Horseshoe. Padding made to resemble a U shape.

Hot spot. Early redness of the skin from friction that could result in a blister formation if preventive measures are not taken.

Hyper. Over, above, excessive.

Hyperextension. Extreme or abnormal extension of a joint, usually the result of trauma, increased muscle tone.

Hyperflexion. Increased flexion of a joint, usually the result of trauma, decreased muscle tone, or joint laxity.

Hypoallergenic. Having diminished potential for causing an allergic reaction.

I

Iliac crest. The anatomical landmark for the superior margin of the pelvis, located between the anterosuperior and posterosuperior iliac spines; a contusion to this area is called a "hip pointer."

Immobilizer. A device to protect and limit the mobility of a specific anatomical body part.

Impingement. Degenerative alteration in a joint in which there is excessive friction between joint tissues; this typically causes limitations in range of motion and the perception of joint pain.

Inferior. Beneath; lower; used medically in reference to the undersurface of an organ or to indicate a structure below another structure.

Insertion. The movable attachment of the distal end of a muscle, which produces shape changes or skeletal movement when the muscle contracts.

Internal. Within the body; within or on the inside; enclosed; inward; the opposite of external.

Internal rotation. Rotary movement around the longitudinal axis of a bone toward the midline of the body. Occurs in the transverse plane and is also known as inward or medial rotation.

Interphalangeal joint (IP). In a joint between two phalanges; in hand and feet, the distal interphalangeal joint (DIP) and proximal interphalangeal joint (PIP).

Inversion. Turning the sole of the foot inward or medially in the frontal plane; adduction. An example is standing with the weight on the outer edge of the foot.

J

Joint capsule. A sheath or continuous enclosure around an organ or structure; a capsula; articular capsule and/or synovial capsule—a saclike, fibrous membrane that surrounds a joint; often including or interwoven with ligaments.

Joint range of motion. The possible excursion of motion at a joint, accomplished by an examiner, without any muscle contraction by the patient. The excursion can be measured by a goniometer and is normally slightly greater than active range of motion. The examiner assesses the maximum excursion at both its beginning and its end; the maximum range of movement of a joint measured in degrees of a circle.

K

Kinesiology. The study of muscles and body movement.

L

Lace. A cord or string used for drawing together two edges such as a garment or shoe.

Lambs wool. A material commonly used on and around the athlete's toes when circular protection is required.

Lateral. Pertains to the side; farther from the midline plane; away from the midline plane.

Lateral epicondylitis (tennis elbow). Tendinitis occurring at the lateral epicondyle; this injury is commonly seen as a result of overuse of the elbow or repetitive wrist extension.

Ligament. A band or sheet of strong fibrous connective tissue connecting the articular ends of bones, binding them together to limit.

Longitudinal arch. The anteroposterior arch of the foot; the medial portion is formed by the calcaneus, talus, navicular, the three cuneiform bones, and the first three metatarsals; the lateral portion is formed by the calcaneus, cuboid, and the fourth and fifth metatarsals.

Lumbar. Pertains to the loins (the part of the back between the thorax and pelvis); vertebral column extending from the 20th through the 24th vertebrae; low back.

M

Major. Means greater or larger.

Malleable. Having the property of being shaped by press.

Malleolus. The protuberance on both sides of the ankle joint; the lower extremity of the fibula is the lateral malleolus and lower end of the tibia is the medial malleolus.

Mechanism of injury. The manner in which a physical injury occurred; the mechanism of injury is used to estimate the forces involved in trauma and thus the potential severity for wounding, fractures, and internal organ damage that a patient may suffer as a result of the injury.

Medial. Pertains to the middle; nearer to the midline plane; toward the midline plane.

Medial epicondylitis (baseball and/or golfers elbow). Tendinitis occurring at the medial epicondyle. This injury is commonly seen as a result of overuse of the elbow or repetitive wrist flexion.
Mallet finger. A flexion deformity of the distal joint of a finger, caused by avulsion of the extensor tendon.
Metacarpophalangeal joint (MCP). Joint between the metacarpus and the phalanges.
Metatarsal arch. The metarsal arch of the foot formed by the metatarsal and proximal bones of the foot.
Memory foam. Material that has varying thickness and slow recovery to impact.
Meniscus. Interarticular fibrocartilage of crescent shape, found in certain joints, especially the lateral and medial menisci (semilunar cartilages) of the knee joint.
Metal grommets. The material that protects/strengthens opening for eyelets.
Midsagittal plane. A vertical plane through the trunk and head dividing the body into right and left halves.
Minor. Of lesser or inferior importance, size, scope, or effect.
Morton's neuroma. Painful condition and swelling of interdigital nerves between the third and fourth metatarsal heads.
Muscle. A type of tissue composed of contractile cells; a contractile organ composed of muscle tissue, affecting the movements of the organs and parts of the body.
Muscle contracted. Active contraction of the muscle by the involved individual.
Myositis ossification. Bone formation occurring at an abnormal anatomical site, usually in soft tissue (e.g., ossification of the intramuscular fascia after an injury.

N

Nerve. Parallel axons running together inside a thick connective tissue sheath (an epineurium); a bundle of nerve fibers, usually outside the brain or spinal cord.

O

Off-the-shelf braces. Brace made in standard sizes and available from merchandise in stock.
Olecrannon. A large process of the ulna projecting behind the elbow joint and forming the bony prominence of the elbow.
Open cell foam. Material that is soft and layered.
Origin. The source of anything; a starting point.
Orthotic. Relating to orthosis; supportive device used for injuries to the foot and ankle.
Overuse syndrome. An injury that results from repetitive use or overuse of a part of the body or from external pressure or environmental conditions that can affect bones, joints bursae, muscles, tendons, nerves, or other anatomical structures.

P

Pad support. A pad placed in a certain area to sustain, hold up, or maintain a desired position.
Palmar. Ventral aspect of the hand; palm of the hand.
Patella. A lens-shaped sesamoid bone situated in front of the knee in the tendon of the quadriceps femoris muscle.
Peroneal tendinitis. Inflammation of the peroneal tendons.
Pes cavus. High arch; deformities of the foot.
Pes planus. Flat feet.
Phalanges. Bones of the fingers (hand) or toes (foot).
Plantar. Pertains to the sole of the foot; ventral aspect.
Plantar fascia. The fascia investing the muscles of the sole of the foot.
Plantar fasciitis. Painful inflammation of the heel and bottom surface of the foot caused by excessive stretching of the fibrous tissue (fascia) that attaches the heel to the forefoot.
Plantar flexion. Extension movement of the ankle that results in the foot and/or toes moving away from the body in the sagittal plane.

Plantar (Joplin) neuroma. A compression neuropathy affecting the nerve that supplies sensation to the medial side of the great toe. The condition often occurs in runners or in people whose shoes are too tight at the metatarsophalangeal joint, where the medial plantar proper digital nerve is found.

Popliteal space (fossa). The space behind the knee joint, containing the popliteal artery and vein and small sciatic and popliteal nerves.

Position. The place or arrangement in which something is put; the manner in which a body is arranged for examination.

Posterior. In human anatomy, pertains to or located at or toward the back; dorsal; in human anatomy, caudal, dorsal, and posterior mean the same thing: situated behind.

Posterior cruciate ligament (PCL). A ligament crossing through the knee joint that attaches posteriorly on the tibia and crosses to the inside of the knee on the anterior portion of the medial condyle of the femur.

PRICES. Acronym for protection, rest, ice, compression, elevation, and support.

Pronation. The act of lying prone or facing downward; the act of turning the hand so that the palm faces downward or backward.

Prone. Horizontal with the face downward.

Prophylactic. Any agent or regimen that contributes to the prevention of infection and disease; denoting something that is preventative or protective.

Proprioception. The awareness of posture, movement, and changes in equilibrium and the knowledge of position, weight, and resistance of objects in relation to the body.

Protraction. The extension forward or drawing forward of a part of the body such as the mandible.

Proximal. Nearest the point of attachment, center of the body, or point of reference; the opposite of distal.

Proximal to distal. A term commonly used in taping or wrapping procedure that describes applying material from proximal (closes) to distal (farther away).

Q

Q angle. The acute angle formed by a line from the anterior superior iliac spine of the pelvis through the center of the patella and a line from the tibial tubercle through the patella. The angle describes the tracking of the patella in the trochlear groove of the femur.

Quadriceps. The muscle group in the anterior thigh consisting of the rectus femoris, vastus medialis, vastus intermedius, and vastus lateralis.

R

Range of motion (ROM). The extent to which a body part can move through all of its planes of movement; types of range of motion include active, assistive, passive, and resistive.

Rehabilitation. The processes of treatment and education that help disabled individuals to attain maximum function.

Resilient material. The ability to regain shape after impact; commonly used in areas subject to repeated impact.

Retinaculum. A band or membrane holding any organ or part in its place.

Retraction. The act of drawing backward or the condition of being drawn back; shortening.

Rotary forces. A force generated by active or passive motion that rotates about an axis.

Rotation. Process of turning on an axis; movement around a longitudinal axis which passes through a joint as in turning the palm of the hand up or down with the arm abducted.

Rotator cuff. A musculotendinous structure consisting of supraspinatus, infraspinatus, teres minor, and subscapularis tendons blending with the shoulder joint capsule. The muscles, which surround the glenohumeral joint below the superficial musculature, stabilize and control the head of the humerus in all arm motions, function with the deltoid to abduct the arm, and rotate the humerus.

S

Sagittal plane. A vertical plane through the longitudinal axis of the body or part of the body, dividing it into right and left parts. If it is through the anteroposterior midaxis and divides the body into right and left halves, it is called a median or midsagittal plane.

Sesamoid bone. A type of short bone occurring in the hands and feet and embedded in tendons or joint capsules.

Sesamoiditis. Inflammation of a sesamoid bone.

Shin splints (medial tibial stress syndrome or medial tibial syndrome). Pain in the anterior, posterior, or posterolateral compartment of the tibia. It usually follows strenuous or repetitive exercise and is often related to faulty foot mechanics such as pes planus or pes cavus. The cause may be ischemia of the muscles in the compartment, minute tears in the tissues, or partial avulsion from the periosteum of the tibial or peroneal muscles. Proper shoes and foot orthotics may help to prevent onset of the condition.

Shoelace. A lace used for fastening shoes or orthopedic devices.

Shorten the angle of pull. Decreasing the range of motion of a joint.

Spica. A figure eight (8) bandage/wrap that generally overlaps the previous to form V-like designs; used to give support, to apply pressure, or to hold a dressing; figure of eight wraps are placed over ankle, knee, elbow, wrist, and hand joints.

Spiral. Applying a bandage around a limb that ascends the body part overlapping the previous bandage.

Sprain. Trauma to ligaments that causes pain and disability depending on the degree of injury to the ligaments.

Stirrup. Any U-shaped loop or piece.

Strain. Trauma to muscles and tendons from violent contraction or excessive or forcible stretch; it may be associated with failure of the synergistic action of muscles.

Strap. To support an injured joint with overlapping strips of adhesive or elastic plaster or tape.

Subluxation. Partial or incomplete dislocation.

Subtalar joint. Any of the three articular surfaces on the inferior surface of the talus.

Superficial. Pertains to or situated near the surface.

Superior. Toward the top of the body or body part.

Supination. The turning of the palm or the hand anteriorly or the foot inward and upward; the act of lying flat upon the back; the condition of being on the back or having the palm of the hand facing upward or the foot turned inward and upward.

Supine. Lying on the back with the face upward; dorsal; a position of the hand or foot with the palm or foot facing upward; the opposite of prone.

Support. To sustain, hold up, or maintain a desired position.

Surface anatomy. The study of the form and markings of the surface of the body, especially as they relate to underlying structures.

Swelling. An abnormal transient enlargement, especially one appearing on the surface of the body. Ice applied to the area helps to limit swelling.

Syndesmosis ankle sprain. Damage to the ligamentous structures of the distal tibiofibular syndesmotic joint, resulting from dorsiflexion or external rotation of the talus within the ankle mortise, or both, which in turn causes spreading of the joint. The distal tibiofibular syndesmosis is formed by the anterior tibiofibular ligament, the interosseous membrane, and the posterior tibiofibular ligament.

T

Tendinitis. Inflammation of a tendon.

Tendon. Fibrous connective tissue serving for the attachment of muscles to bones and other parts.

Tendinosis. Noninflammitory degeneration of tendon from repetitive stress.

Tenosynovitis. inflammation of a tendon sheath.

Thenar eminence. A prominence formed by muscles on the palm below the thumb; known as thenar web space

Thoracic. Pertains to the chest or thorax (chest).

Transverse arch. The transverse arch of the foot formed by the navicular, cuboid, cuneiform, and metatarsal bones.

Transverse plane. A horizontal plane at right angles to the vertical axis of the body. A plane that divides the body into a top and bottom portion.

U

Ulnar (medial) collateral ligament (elbow). Ligament that provides medial stability to the elbow joint.

Ulnar collateral ligament (thumb). Ligament that provides medial stability to the thumb joint.

V

Valgus. Bent or turned outward, used especially of deformities in which the most distal anatomical part is angled outward and away from the midline of the body.

Varus. Bent or turned inward, used especially of deformities in which the most distal anatomical part is turned inward and toward the midline of the body.

Ventral. Bottom surface; opposite of dorsal.

Vertical strip. A strip that is placed perpendicular to the line of the horizon, opposed to horizontal strip.

Viscoelastic material. Substance having both viscous and elastic properties.

Volar. Ventral aspect of the hand.

X

X pattern. The crossing of three or more pieces of tape in the shape of a fan.

Appendix B: Bibliography

American Academy of Orthopaedic Surgeons. (2005). *Athletic training and sports medicine.* Chicago, IL: Author.

Anderson, M., & Hall, S. (2012). *Foundations of athletic training.* Baltimore, MD: Lippincott Williams & Wilkins.

Abian-Vicen, J., Alegre, J., Fernadez-Rodriquez, J. M., & Auguando, X. (2009). Prophylactic ankle taping: Elastic versus in-elastic taping. *Foot Ankle International,* (30), 218–225.

Bachmann, L., Kolb, E., Koller, M., Steurer, J., & Ter Riet, G. (2003). Accuracy of Ottawa ankle rules to exclude fractures of the ankle and mid-foot: A systematic review. *British Medical Journal, 326*(7), 417–419.

Barker, S., Wright, K., & Wright, V. (2001). *Sports injuries 3D* (3rd ed.). Gardner, KS: Cramer Products.

Beam, J. (2012). *Orthopedic taping, wrapping, bracing and padding* (2nd ed.). Philadelphia, PA: F. A. Davis.

Bleakley, C. M., Glasgow, P. D., Phillips, N., Hanna, L., Callaghan, M. J., Davison, G. W., Hopkins, T. J., & Delahunt, E. (2010). Management of acute soft tissue injury using protection rest ice compression and elevation from the Association of Chartered Physiotherapists in Sports and Exercise Medicine. *SKIPP, Good Practice Panel.*

Booher, J., & Thibodeau, G. (2000). *Athletic injury assessment.* St. Louis, MO: McGraw-Hill Higher Education.

Cordova, M., Ingersoll, C., & Palieri, R. (2002) Efficacy of prophylactic ankle support: An experimental perspective. *Journal of Athletic Training, 37*(4), 446.

Deere, R., Wright, K., & Gibson, F. (2003). Open basket taping for acute ankle sprain. *KAHPERD Journal, 39*(1), 26–27.

Deivert, R. (1994). Functional thumb taping procedure. *Journal of Athletic Training, 29*(4), 357.

Des Rochers, D. M., & Cox, D. E. (2002). Proprioceptive benefits derived from ankle support. *Athletic Therapy Today, 7*(6), 44.

Draper, C. E., Besier, T. F., Santos, J. M., Jennings, F., Fredericson, M., Gold, G. E., Beaupre, G. S., & Delp, S. L. (2009). Using real-time MRI to quantify altered joint kinematics in subjecs with patellofemoral pain and to evaluate the effects of a patellar brace or sleeve on joint motion. *Journal of Orthopedic Research,* (27), 571–577.

Fleet, K., Galen, S., & Moore, C. (2009). Duration of strength retention of ankle taping during activities of daily living. *Injury,* (40), 333–336.

Fletcher, S., Whitehill, W., & Wright, K. (1993). Medicated compress for blister treatment. *Journal of Athletic Training, 28*(1), 81–82.

Floyd, R. T. (2012). *Manual of structural kinesiology* (18th ed.). New York, NY: McGraw-Hill Higher Education.

France, R. (2011). *Introduction to sports medicine and athletic training* (2nd ed.). New York, NY: Thomson Delmar Learning.

Fratesi, G. R. (1992) Thigh and knee protective device. Retrieved from www.google.com/patents/US5107823?dq=protective+devices+in+athletics

Gallaspy, J., & May, D. (1996). *Signs and symptoms of athletic injuries.* St. Louis, MO: McGraw-Hill Higher Education.

Gehlsen, G. M., Pearson, D., & Bahamonde, R. (1991) Ankle joint strength, total work, and ROM: Comparison between prophylactic devices. *Athletic Training Journal, 26*(2), 62–65.

Green, T. A., & Hillman, S. K. (1990). Comparison of support provided by a semiridgid orthosis and adhesive ankle taping before, during, and after exercise. *American Journal of Sports Medicine, 18*(5), 498–506.

Hardy, L., Huxel, K., Brucker, J., & Nesser, T. (2008). Prophylactic ankle braces and star excursion balance measures in healthy volunteers. *Journal of Athletic Training,* (43). 347–351.

Harrison, L. (2014). Should police replace rice as the ankle therapy of choice. Retrieved from http://www.medscape.com/viewarticle/823217_2.

Hawke, F., Burns, J., Radford, J. A., & Toit, V. (2008). *Custom-made foot orthoses for the treatment of foot pain.* Cocharane Database Syst RE (3) CD006801.

Herrinton, L., Simmonds, C., & Hatcher, J. (2005). The effect of a neoprene sleeve on knee joint position sense. *Research in Sports Medicine*, (13) 37–46.

Hewston, T. J., Austin, K., Gwynn-Brett, K., & Marshall, S. (2009). An illustrated guide to taping techniques. (2nd ed.). St Louis, MO: Mosby Elsevier.

Holmes, C., Wilcox, D., & Fletcher, J. (2002). Effect of a modified, low-dye medial longitudinal taping procedure on the subtalar joint neutral position before and after light exercise. *Orthpo Sports Physical Therapy, 32*(4), 305–309.

Hoppenfeld, S. (1995). *Physical examination of the spine and extremities*. New York, NY: Appleton-Lang.

Johnson & Johnson Consumer Products. (1986). *Athletic uses of adhesive tape*. Skillman, NJ: Author.

Johnson & Johnson Consumer Products. (1993). *Athletic uses of adhesive tape*. Skillman, NJ: Author.

Kaneko, S., & Takasaki, H. (2011). Forearm pain, diagnosed as intersection syndrome, managed by taping: A case series. *Journal of Orthopaedic & Sports Physical Therapy, 41*(7), 514–519.

Kase, K., Wallis, J., & Tsuyoshi, K. (2003). *Clinical therapeutic applications of the kinesio taping method* (2nd ed.). Kinesio Taping Association: Albuquerque, NM.

Knight, K., & Brumels, K. (2009). *Assessing clinical proficiencies in athletic training*. Champaign, IL: Human Kinetics.

Lacroix, V. J. (2000). A complete approach to groin pain. *Physician and Sports Medicine, 28*(1), 66.

Lun, V. M., Wiley, J. P., Meeuwisse, W. H., & Yanagawa, T. L. M. (2005). Effectiveness of patellar bracing for treatment of patellofemoral pain sysndrome. *Clinical Journal of Sports Medicine*, (15), 235–240.

Lynch, S., & Renstrom, P. (1999). Groin injuries in sport: Treatment strategies. *Sports Medicine, 28*(2), 137–144.

Magee, D. (2007). *Orthopedic physical assessment* (5th ed.). Philadelphia, PA: W. B. Sanders.

Martin, N. M., & Harter, R. A. (1993). Comparison of inversion retraint provided by ankle prophylactic devices before and after exercise. *Journal of Athletic Training, 28*(4), 3245–329.

McDonald, R. (2004). *Taping techniques: Principles and practice* (2nd ed.). Oxford, UK: Butterworth- Heinemann.

McDonald, R. (2010). *Pocketbook of taping techniques: Principles and practice*. London, UK: Churchill Livingstone Elsevier.

Mellion, M., Walsh, W., Madden, C., Putukian, M., & Shelton, G. (2001). *The team physician's handbook* (3rd ed.). Philadelphia, PA: Hanley and Belfus.

Mitchell, A., Dyson, R., Hale, T., & Abraham, C. (2008). Biomechanics of ankle instability. *Medicine and Sports Exercise*, (40), 1522–1528

Myer, G., Ford, K., & Hewett, T. (2004). Rationale and clinical techniques for anterior cruciate ligament injury prevention among female athletes. *Journal of Athletic Training, 39*(4), 352–364.

National Athletic Trainers' Association. (2005, March). Official statement from the National Athletic Trainers' Association on community-acquired MRSA infection. Retrieved from http://www.nata.org/official-statements

National Center for Safety in Sport. (2012, June). PREPARE sports safety courses. Retrieved from http://www.sportssafety.org

Neumann, D. A. (2013). *Kinesiology of the musculoskeletal system: foundations for rehabilitation*. St. Louis, MO: Elsevier Health Sciences.

Ng, G. Y. (2005). Patellar taping does not affect the onset of activities of vastus medialis obliquus and vastus lateralis before and after muscle fatigue. *American Journal of Physical Medicine and Rehabilitation*, (84), 106–111.

Olmsted, L., Vela, L., & Denegar, C. (2004) Prophylactic ankle taping and bracing: A numbers-needed-to-treat and cost-benefit analysis. *Journal of Athletic Training, 39*(1), 95.

Olmsted-Kramer, L., & Hertel, J. (2004). Preventing recurrent lateral ankle sprains: An evidence-based approach. *Athletic Therapy Today, 9*(6), 19.

Occupational Safety and Health Administration. (2011a). Bloodborne pathogen exposure incidents. Retrieved from https://www.osha.gov/OshDoc/data_BloodborneFacts/bbfact04.pdf

Occupational Safety and Health Administration. (2011b). OSHA's Bloodborne pathogen standard. Retrieved from www.osha.gov/OshDoc/data_BloodborneFacts/bbfact01.pdf

Paris, D. L. (1992). The effects of the swede-o, new cross, and mcdavid ankle braces and adhesive ankle taping on speed, balance, agility, and vertical jump. *Journal of Athletic Training, 27*(3), 253–256.

Perrin, D. (2012). *Athletic taping and bracing* (3rd ed.). Champaign, IL: Human Kinetics.

Pfieffer, R., & Mangus, B. (2011). *Concepts of athletic training* (6th ed.). Boston, MA: Jones and Bartlett.

Pietrosimone, B. G., Grindstaff, T. L., Linens, S. W., Uczekaj, E., & Hertell, J. (2008). A systematic review of prophylactic braces in the prevention of knee ligament injuries in collegiate football players. *Journal of Athletic Training*, (43), 409–415.

Prentice, W. (2011). *Principles of athletic training* (14th ed.). New York, NY: McGraw-Hill Higher Education.

Reeves, D. A., & Emel, T. J. (2009). Ankle taping and bracing. Retrieved from http://emedicine.medscape./article 86495-overview.

Rome, K., Handoll, H. H. G., & Ashford, R. L. (2005). Interventions for preventing and treating stress fractures and stress reactions of bone of the lower limbs in young adults. *Cochran Database Syst Rev*, (2) CD000450.

Rosenbaum, D., Kamps, K., Bosch, B., Thorwesten, L., Bolker, K., & Eils., E. (2005). The influence of external ankle braces on subjective and objective parameeters of performance in a sports–related agility course. *Knee Surgery Sports Traumatology Arthroscopy*, (13), 419–425.

Royal College of Nursing, Society of Orthopaedic and Trauma Nursing. (2012). *A practical guide to casting* (3rd ed.). London, UK: BSN Medical.

Ruhi Soylu, A., Irmak, R., & Baltaci, G. (2011). Acute effects of Kinesio Taping on muscular endurance and fatigue by using surface electromyography signals of masseter muscle. *Medicina Sportiva, 15*(1), 13–16.

Smith, T. O., & Davis, L. (2008). A systematic review of bracing following reconstruction of the anterior cruciate ligament. *Physiotherapy*, (94), 1–10.

Starkey, C., Brown, S., & Ryan, J. (2010). *Examination of orthopedic and athletic injuries* (3rd ed.). Philadelphia, PA: F. A. Davis.

Stedman's medical dictionary for the health professions and nursing (7th ed.). (2011). Baltimore, MD: Williams & Wilkins.

Street, S., & Runkle, D. (2000). *Athletic protective equipment: Care, selection, and fitting.* St. Louis, MO: McGraw-Hill Higher Education.

Taber's medical dictionary (22nd ed.). (2012). Philadelphia, PA: F. A. Davis.

Thelen, D., & Stoneman, P. D. (2008). Clinical efficacy of Kinesio® Tape for shoulder pain. *Journal of Orthopaedic & Sports Physical Therapy, 38*(7), 389–395.

Tiggelen, D. V., Coorevitis, P., & Witvrouw, E. (2008). The effects of a neoprene sleeve on subjects with a poor versus good joint position sense subjected to an isokinetic fatigue protocol. *Clinical Journal of Sports Medicine.* (18), 259–265.

Tsai, H.-J., Hung, H.-C., Yang, J.-L., Huang, C.-S., & Tsauo, J.-Y. (2009). Could Kinesio® Tape replace the bandage in decongestive lymphatic therapy. *Supportive Care in Cancer, 17*(11), 1353–1360.

Tulley, M. A., Bleakley, C. M., O'Connor, S. R., & McDonough, S. M. (2015). Functional management of ankle sprains: What volume and intensity of walking is undertaken in the first week postinjury. Retrieved from http://bjsm.bmj.com.

van den Bekerom, M. P. J., Struijs, P. A. A, Blankevoort, L., Welling, L., van Dijk, C. N., & Kerkhoffs, G. M. M. J. (2012). What is the evidence for rest, ice, compression, and elevation therapy in the treatment of ankle sprains in adults? *Journal of Athletic Training, 47*(4), 435–443.

Warden, S. J., Hinman, R. S., Watson, M. A., Avin, K. G., Bialocerkowski, A. E., & Crorssley, K. M. (2008). *Arthritis and Rheumatology*, (59), 73–83.

Wilkerson, G. (2002). Biomechanical and neuromuscular effects of ankle taping and bracing. *Journal of Athletic Training, 37*(4), 436.

Wilkerson, G., Kovaleski, JE., Meyer, M., & Stawiz, C. (2005). Effects of subtalar sling ankle taping technique on combined talocrural-subtalar joint motions. *Foot Ankle Internation*, (26), 239–246.

Williams, S., Whatman, C., Hume, P. A., & Sheerin, K. (2012). Kinesio taping in treatment and prevention of sports injuries: A meta-analysis of the evidence for its effectiveness. *Sports Medicine, 42*(2), 153–164.

Wright, K., Barker, S., & Whitehill, W. (2007). *Basic athletic training* (5th ed.). Gardner, KS: Cramer Products.

Wright, K., & Deere, R. (1990). Comparison of results concerning the use of ankle taping/strapping and ankle braces. *Applied Research in Coaching and Athletics*, 93–104.

Wright, K., & Hendrix, S. (1989). Perceptions of ankle strapping techniques versus bracing in collegiate basketball. *Sports Medicine Update, 4*(3), 19–20.

Wright, K., Lewis, M., Barker, S., & Deere, R. (2014). *Comprehesive manual of taping, wrapping, protective devices* (4th ed). Urbana, IL: Sagamore.

Wright, K., & Whitehill, W. (1991). Preparation of the athlete for protective taping/wrapping techniques. *Sports Medicine Update, 6*(1), 26–29.

Wright, K., & Whitehill, W. (1993). How to tape & wrap ankles. *Topics in Sports Medicine, 1*(4), 4–6.

Wright, K., & Whitehill, W. (1996a). *The comprehensive manual of taping and wrapping techniques* (2nd ed.). Gardner, KS: Cramer Products.

Wright, K., & Whitehill, W. (1996b). *Sports medicine taping series* [Video series]. St. Louis, MO: McGraw-Hill Higher Education.

Wright, K., Whitehill, W., & Lewis, M. (2005). *Preventive techniques: Taping/wrapping techniques and protective devices* (3rd ed.). Gardner, KS: Cramer Products.

Zinder, S. M., Granata, K. P., Shultz, S. J., & Gransneder, B. M. (2009). Ankle bracing and the neuromuscular factors influencing joint stiffness. *Journal of Athletic Training*, (44), 363–369.

Appendix C:
Websites for Health Care and Sport Industry Professionals

American Academy of Dermatology *www.aad.org*
American Academy of Family Physicians *www.aafp.org*
American Academy of Neurology *www.aan.com*
American Academy of Ophthalmology *www.aao.org*
American Academy of Orthopaedic Surgeons *www.aaos.org*
American Academy of Otolaryngology *www.entnet.org*
American Academy of Pain Management *www.aapainmanage.org*
American Academy of Pediatrics (AAP) *www.aap.org*
American Academy of Podiatric Sports Medicine (AAPSM) *www.aapsm.org*
American Academy of Physical Medicine and Rehabilitation (AAPMR) *www.aapmr.org*
American Chiropractic Association *www.acasc.org*
American College of Foot and Ankle Surgeons *www.acfas.org*
American College of Sports Medicine *www.acsm.org*
American Dental Association *www.ada.org*
American Dietetic Association *www.eatright.org*
American Heart Association *www.americanheart.org*
American Kinesiotherapy Association *www.akta.org*
American Massage Therapy Association *www.amtamassage.org*
American Medical Association *www.ama-assn.org*
American Medical Society for Sport Medicine *www.amssm.org*
American Occupational Therapy Association *www.aota.org*
American Optometric Association *www.aoa.org*
American Orthopaedic Foot and Ankle Society *www.aofas.org*
American Orthopaedic Society for Sports Medicine *www.sportsmed.org*
American Osteopathic Academy of Sport Medicine *www.aoasm.org*
American Osteopathic Association *www.osteopathic.org*
American Physical Therapy Association (APTA) *www.apta.org*
American Physical Therapy Association Sports Physical Therapy Section *www.spts.org*
American Alliance for Health, Physical Education, Recreation, and Dance *www.aahperd.org*
American Association for Physical Activity and Recreation (AAPAR) *www.aapar.org*
America's Health Insurance Plan *www.hiaa.org*
American Red Cross *www.redcross.org*
American Red Cross – Athletic Training Education Competencies *www.redcross.org/athletictrainers*
American Sports Medicine Institute *www.asmi.org*
Athlete Performance Institute *www.athletesperformance.com*
Andrews Institute *www.theandrewsinstitute.com*
Academy for Sports Dentistry (ASD) *www.academyforsportsdentistry.org*
Association for Applied Sport Psychology *www.appliedsportpsych.org*
Association for Sports Medicine in Industry, Business, and Military *www.theindustrialathlete.com*
Association of Sport Performance Centres *http://forumelitesport.org*
Canadian Academy of Sport and Exercise Medicine *www.casem-acmse.org*
Canadian Athletic Therapists Association *www.athletictherapy.org*
Centers for Disease Control and Prevention *www.cdc.gov*
Collegiate Strength and Conditioning Coaches *www.cscca.org*
Collegiate and Professional Sport Dietitians Association (CPSDA) *www.sportrd.org*
International Olympic Committee *www.olympic.org*

International Society for Sports Psychiatry (ISSP) *www.sportspsychiatry.org*
Joint Commission on Sports Medicine and Science *www.jcsportsmedicine.org*
Kinesio Taping Association International *www.kinesiotaping.com/global/association*
Mayo Clinic *www.mayoclinic.org*
National Athletic Trainers' Association *www.nata.org*
National Athletic Trainers' Association Board of Certification *www.bocatc.org*
National Association for Sport and Physical Education *www.aahperd.org/naspe*
National Center for Drug Free Sports *www.drugfreesport.com*
National Center for Sports Safety *www.sportssafety.org*
National Collegiate Athletic Association *www.ncaa.org*
National Federation of State High School Athletic Associations (NFHS) *www.nfhs.org*
NFHS Coach Education *www.nfhslearn.com*
National Interscholastic Athletic Administrators Association *www.niaaa.org*
National Institutes of Health *www.nih.gov*
National Operating Committee on Standards for Athletic Equipment (NOCSEA) *www.nocsae.org*
National Strength and Conditioning Association (NSCA) *www.nsca.com*
National Safety Council *www.nsc.org*
North American Society for Pediatric Exercise Medicine (NASPEM) *www.naspem.org*
Occupational Safety and Health Administration (OSHA) *www.osha.gov*
Sports, Cardiovascular, and Wellness Nutrition (SCAN) *www.scandpg.org*
Sport Information Resource Centre (SIRC) *www.sirc.ca*
Stop Sports Injuries *www.stopsportsinjuries.org*
United States Olympic Committee (USOC) *www.usoc.org*
World Federation of Athletic Training and Therapy *www.wfatt.org*

Appendix D: Websites for Medical Health Care Companies

Cramer Products, Inc. *www.cramersportsmed.com*
Medco Sports Medicine *www.medco-athletics.com*
Johnson & Johnson *www.jnj.com*
PRO Orthopedic *www.proorthopedic.com*
FCX Global *http://www.fcxglobal.com*
Kinesio Taping *www.kinesiotaping.com*
Ambra LeRoy Medical *www.ambraleroy.com*
3M *www.3m.com*
DonJoy *www.djoglobal.com*
Amerx Health Care *www.amerigel.com*
Vasyli Medical *www.vasylimedical.com*
Breg *www.breg.com*

Appendix E: Informational Websites

http://ahealthyway.net/kinesio-taping/kinesio-tape-vs-others/

http://emedicine.medscape.com/article/86495-overview

http://physical-therapy.advanceweb.com/Article/Taping-or-Bracing.aspx

http://www.ncbi.nlm.nih.gov/pmc/articles/PMC164375/

http://fingerlakessportsmedicine.com/taping-vs-bracing/

http://usatoday30.usatoday.com/sports/2005-11-07-taping-work_x.htm

http://running.competitor.com/2014/03/injury-prevention/tape-it-up-does-kinesiology-tape-really-work_51973

http://vype.com/houston/2015/01/25/houston-methodist-sports-medicine-compares-braces-and-taping-in-youth-sports/

http://meredithatwood.tripod.com/

http://sportsmedicine.about.com/od/ankletaping/a/kinesio_tape.htm

http://www.physioadvisor.com.au/11855950/shoulder-taping-shoulder-strapping-physioadvis.htm

http://www.mccc.edu/~behrensb/documents/TherapeuticTapingTechniques-May2006.pdf

http://www.medicinenet.com/kinesio_tape/article.htm

Index

D

E

F

G

H

I

K

L

M

N

O

P

Q

R

S

T

U

W

Instructions for Online Companion Resource Access

Online companion resources include videos, images, and other resources that the authors have provided as supplemental information for the text. These resources are found online and accessible only by creating an account using the one-time pass code provided at the bottom of this page. For more information about the use of or policies regarding the code for online companion resources, please visit www.sagamorepub.com.

Steps to redeem access code if you DO NOT currently have a Sagamore account

1. Go to **http://www.sagamorepub.com**
2. Click on the **Create Account** link and fill out the requested information
3. Enter the code provided at the bottom of this page in the **online access code field.**
4. Click on **Create New Account.**
5. Click on **My Materials** tab to access all additional materials provided with your book purchase.

Steps to redeem code if you currently DO HAVE a Sagamore account

1. Go to **http://www.sagamorepub.com**
2. Click on the **Login** link and proceed to login
3. Click on the **Access Codes** tab for your account, enter the code provided at the bottom of this page and click **Submit**.
4. Click on the **My Materials** tab to access all additional materials provided with your book purchase.

If this book was purchased as a used book and the activation code is no longer valid, please call (800) 327-5557 to purchase a new activation code

Online Materials Access Code

CompTap5-fW1aYbsFwppo

Related Books

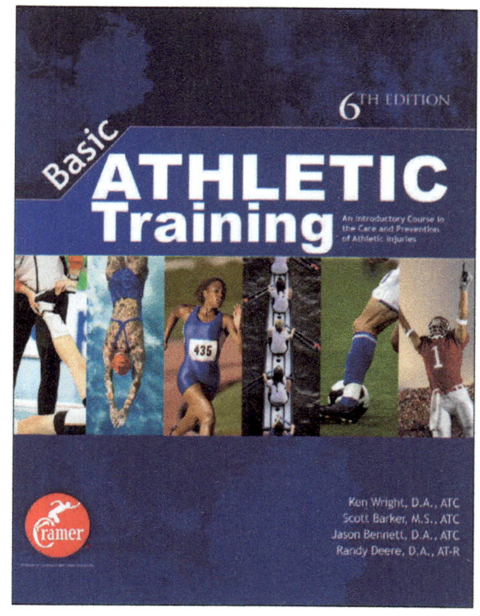

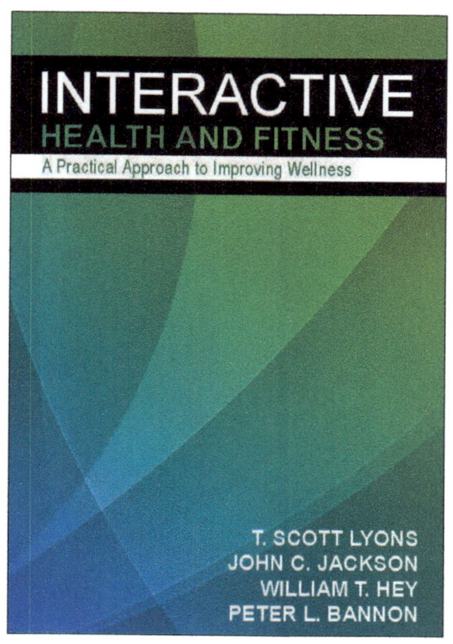

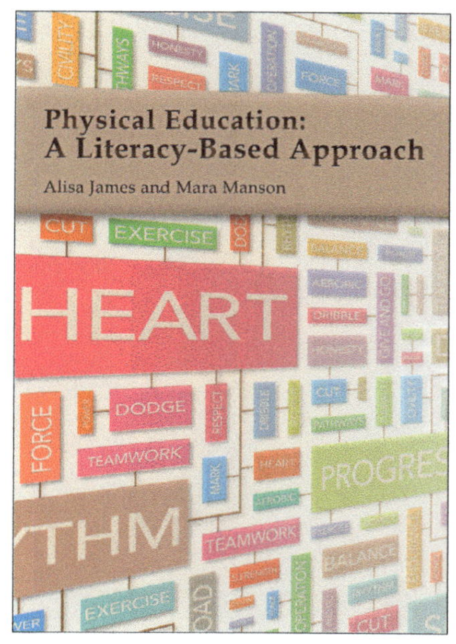

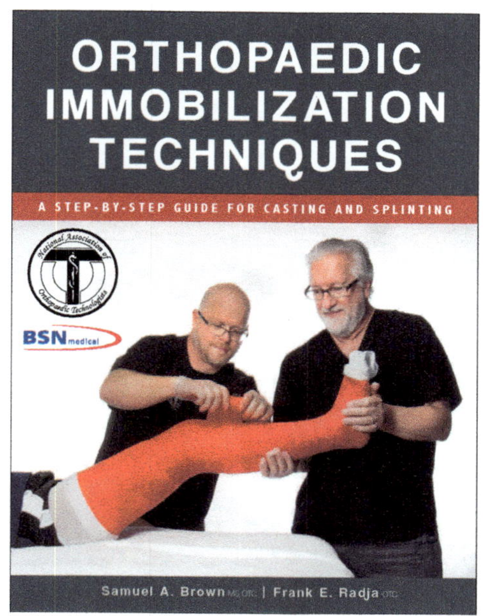